2nd Edition—Completely Revised and Updated

Don't Go To The Cosmetics Counter Without Me

An Eye Opening Guide To Brand Name Cosmetics

by

Paula Begoun

Editor: Miriam Bulmer
Typography: Rescue Control
Cover Design: Patrick Howe
Printing: RR Donnelley & Sons Company
Research Assistance: Elizabeth Janda, Ona Kircher, and Stephanie Bell

©Copyright 1993, by Paula Begoun
Publisher: Beginning Press
        5418 South Brandon
        Seattle, WA 98118

ISBN 1-877988-09-X

7 8 9 10

This book is distributed to the United States book trade by:
        Publishers Group West
        4065 Hollis Street
        Emeryville, CA 94608
        (800) 788-3123

and to the Canadian book trade by:
        Raincoast Book Distribution Limited
        8680 Cambie Street
        Vancouver, BC
        Canada V6P 6M9
        (604) 323-7100

Table of Contents

TABLE OF CONTENTS

TABLE OF CONTENTS

CHAPTER EIGHT—EVALUATION OF SKIN CARE PRODUCTS

TABLE OF CONTENTS

CHAPTER NINE—THE PRODUCTS YOU AND I LIKED THE MOST

CHAPTER TEN—BEAUTY THAT RESPECTS NATURE

Publisher's Note

The intent of this book, as it was with the first edition, is to present the author's ideas and perceptions about the marketing, selling, and use of cosmetics. The author's sole purpose is to present consumer information and advice regarding the purchase of makeup. Nowhere herein does the publisher endorse the use of one product over another. The information and recommendations presented strictly reflect the author's opinions, perceptions, and knowledge about the subject and products mentioned. Some women may have found success with a particular product that is not recommended or even mentioned herein, or they may be partial to a $250 skin care routine. It is everyone's inalienable right to judge products by their own criteria and standards and to disagree with the author.

More important, because everyone's skin can, and probably will, react to an external stimulus at some time, any product may cause a negative reaction on your skin at one time or another. If you develop a skin sensitivity to a cosmetic, stop using it immediately and consult your physician. If you need medical advice about your skin, it is best to consult a dermatologist.

*"Other moisturizers make you look
10 years younger; this one makes you look
20 years younger."*

Lancome Saleswoman to a 30 Year Old Woman

Don't Go To The Cosmetics Counter Without Me

MAKING A DIFFERENCE

Some things never change: there still isn't one cosmetics line that I like best. There are many good and bad products in every line. I can help you sort through the confusion and make the best, most economical decisions.

From the first moment I decided to set out and write the original *Don't Go To The Cosmetics Counter Without Me* two years ago, the task at hand seemed insurmountable. I gritted my teeth, took my charge card in hand, and began the process of evaluating cosmetics. Two years later the job was no less daunting. As I once again tackled the cosmetics counters, drugstores, infomercials, direct (in-home) sales lines, and mail-order makeup and skin care products, I found myself being overwhelmed by the number of products available in the world of cosmetics.

More than 300 cosmetics lines are presently being sold in Canada and the United States. That number includes everything from the products sold at your local hairdresser's to the latest celebrity-endorsed miracles, health food store products, major drugstore chain lines, and the long-established brands we all know by name. Amazing. And somehow, in this maze of products, a consumer has to figure out which cosmetics are the best—which ones will deliver and which will disappoint. For example, if you want a red lipstick you have to select from hundreds of possibilities. Not only are there varying shades of red but do you want a creamy or matte texture? What about a tint or gloss? Should it contain a sunscreen? And what about shine? Whether it be lipsticks or moisturizers, there are literally thousands to pick from. Making a selection is not easy.

Given that the cosmetics companies won't provide a critical forum for their products, we—you and I—will just have to do it on our own. For the past ten years I have been in a unique position as a consumer advocate who specializes in the arena of cosmetics, and I am constantly impressed by the need for what I do. The letters of thanks I receive from hundreds of women a month are absolutely wonderful. I can't express my gratitude and appreciation for this feedback. I also want to stress how much I value the criticism and challenges I receive from readers. It helps to keep me on my toes and gives me new insights I might have overlooked. Balanced input is the best way I can think of to make an educated decision about what products are worth considering.

My goal has always been to provide open-minded, impartial information and professional opinions about the cosmetics women purchase. Leaving this job to the cosmetics companies has given women a parade of pubescent models selling wrinkle creams, salespeople dressed in smocks to make them look like clinicians, and an arsenal of sales rhetoric that is indecipherable and, for the most part, unbelievable, at least if you have enough information to analyze what is really being said in the ads, on product labels, and in brochures, and what the salespeople tell you.

In spite of my genuine resentment toward the deluge of exaggerated claims and promises made by the cosmetics industry, including products that simply don't work or are just not very good, I have to admit I am rather impressed by the many improvements that have taken place in many of the lines reviewed for this book. (Of course, my ego would like to believe that I had an impact on these changes. After selling more than 500,000 books and beginning the second year of publishing my bimonthly newsletter, *Cosmetics Counter Update*, perhaps that is a justified notion.) What I found is a tremendous number of matte eyeshadows, a wide variety of water-soluble cleansers that don't irritate the skin or burn the eyes, an ample assortment of toners that really are irritant-free, an outstanding group of nonchemical sunscreens that can block almost all of the sun's ultraviolet radiation, great mascaras that don't smear or clump, an improved selection of foundation colors (particularly for women of color), and a large array of silky blush colors. There are still problems out there, but it is a pleasure to see these changes for the better.

What you still have to watch out for are the chronic array of wrinkle creams that have a mindboggling spectrum of names: Anti-aging Microemulsion, Restorative Fluid, Emergency Tonic, Nighttime Revitalizer, Defense Cream, Anti-Stress Restorative Cream, Moisture

Intensifier, Moisture Regulating Emulsion, Nourishing Hydrating Emulsion, Moisture Active Emulsion, Urgent Moisture, UV Defense, Environmental Defense, Fortifying Complex, Daily Vitalizer, and Advanced Night Repair. I could list hundreds, perhaps thousands, more, but the emphasis is always the same: women's skin is being attacked and in desperate need of help requiring crucial and immediate moisture and nourishment.

What they don't tell you is that the ingredients in the thousands of moisturizers being sold are surprisingly similar. Even when there are differences, the differences are minor in comparison to the similarities. Furthermore, what you are supposed to believe about these products is almost embarassing. Spleen extracts? Liver extracts? Herbal extracts? Do these really affect the skin in any significant way? All the dead livers and spleens or thyme and chamomile thrown into a cosmetic aren't going to change your skin one little bit. Even something that can make a difference (suich as alpha hydroxy acids or liposomes) won't be the huge wondrous skin care sensation you were led to believe it would be. Just because a product works or is good for the skin doesn't mean it will get rid of one wrinkle. It may temporarily make your skin look smoother, but that doesn't warrant a $25 price tag.

The latest hype promotes environmental, anti-aging ingredients, which are mostly either antioxidants or sunscreens. Antioxidants (mineral oil and vitamin E) keep air off the face; sunscreens offer ultraviolet protection (depending on their SPF rating). These standard additions to any cosmetic can bring a glut of sensational, dramatic claims pledging freedom from a woman's worst enemies—wrinkles and dryness.

Wrinkle creams and moisturizers are the most expensive and the most emotional purchases most women make when it comes to their cosmetics purchases. If the cosmetics industry can logically persuade you that something in the environment (such as pollution) or something inside of you (such as stress) causes wrinkles or any other skin problem, they can further convince you that they have creams and lotions to combat it. It doesn't matter whether they work or not, it doesn't even matter whether or not pollution or stress can even affect your skin; convincing you that it can, even in the smallest, almost imperceptible, way, is all it takes to get your money. Propagating myths about skin care is one of the things the cosmetics industry does best. There is no evidence that pollution causes wrinkles, and the same is true for stress. Yet the number of creams being sold to combat these made-up skin maladies is remarkable.

Before I go much farther it is important to mention that I don't have the last word when it comes to makeup and skin care. The last word inevitably is yours. This book is not about my being right, it is about disseminating independent ideas and opinions so that the cosmetics industry is not your only source of information about cosmetics. My fantasy is that you will take this book with you to cosmetics counters, drugstores, and in-home sales demonstrations, and keep it nearby when you are watching television and an infomercial comes on. Then, when the salesperson carries on about how superb this or that product is, you can say, "Excuse me, I would like to see what Paula has to say about this product." You may not agree with me, but you will have more input than just advertising and marketing language.

SELLING COSMETICS—THE AGONY AND THE ECSTASY

Over the past eight years I've written a lot of information about the world of makeup and skin care. I've complained, taught, instructed, researched, and spent a great deal of time immersed in the cosmetics industry. Regrettably, through all of this, I've had little straightforward interaction with cosmetics salespeople. Most of the time I don't announce who I am. I usually act like any other consumer, which helps me get a better feel for what everyone else is hearing and experiencing when shopping for cosmetics. (I also don't say who I am because I often get thrown out of department stores when I do tell them why I'm really there.) Because of this necessary charade I have only limited personal dialogues with the people who sell makeup. I regret the distance imposed by what I do for a living and what they do for a living. I regret that I am perceived as the enemy. Although most of the people who sell cosmetics might find this hard to believe, I understand the struggles of their occupation and it has never been my intention to make their lives harder. On the other hand, I would be a fool if I didn't realize that, to a great extent, I get in their way.

I know that many cosmetics salespeople would rather I shrivel up and go away like the Wicked Witch of the West. I understand their animosity. I am only trying to make the consumer's life easier, which has to get in the way of anyone selling a wrinkle cream or an over-priced mascara. Although my efforts are more directed at the cosmetics executives and their advertising departments, it has to affect the bottom line of the people selling makeup and skin care products. I sincerely apologize for putting them in an awkward position in the middle of all this, but it is essential that consumers get information from someone who doesn't have a vested interest in what they purchase. Over and above objectivity, the consumer also needs to talk to people who know what they are doing.

Insufficient education is a recurring protest from the cosmetics sales-people I've interviewed. They receive minimal makeup application lessons and the skin care information is almost entirely sales jargon, leaving little room for questions or skepticism. If a salesperson has any doubts or concerns about what she is selling she assuredly cannot tell management—that would be like asking to be fired. The lack of training leaves the uninformed consumer at the mercy of the cosmetics sales-person she encounters, or, turned around, the cosmetics salesperson is at the mercy of the informed consumer. There isn't much a cosmetics salesperson can do about this until the cosmetics companies change their direction. As long as the cosmetics companies believe they can continue fooling the consumer, they have no incentive to provide their staff with more expertise than the little they currently receive.

IF YOU SELL MAKEUP THIS IS FOR YOU

Although there were numerous cosmetics salespeople I did not reveal my identity to (I feel like a spy sometimes), there were many to whom I did, and a number of them have read my books. On the chance that they might read this one too, I'd like to take the time to speak to them directly.

First, I want to say thank you to all of the cosmetics salespeople who helped me (and even those who didn't help me) while I was working on this update. You have a difficult job and I understand your frustration and defensiveness. You are underpaid, and the consumer, most of the time, doesn't appreciate or trust you. (I know many of you think that I'm accountable for a lot of that and I willingly accept some of the responsibility, but that side effect has never been my intent.) Many of you told me how consumers come to your counters or in-home sales presentations with my book in hand. It isn't that I want to make your job harder, I just want the consumer to get a fair shake. Having spent part of my life in your position, I understand your sore feet and bruised egos when you apply makeup to a woman and she winces at her appearance in the mirror with disdain. She won't even buy the lipstick and another half hour goes by without any commission. Also, many cosmetics counters are economically slower than ever and department stores in general are having a rough time. Women are cutting back and aren't easily convinced that a $50 product is that much better, or even a little bit better, than the $25 product at the counter across the aisle. Plus, many of the lines you work for have recently been bought and sold many times over, and the resulting inventory problems and poor management are a strain.

There isn't much glory in all of this and yet you play an integral role in the life of the woman who comes to you for information about what she should be doing to and using on her face. Every woman just wants someone who can show her how to be beautiful without wasting money or time, and she wants the salesperson to be sensitive to her frustration with the world of cosmetics. After all, if a woman is over the age of 35, she has used a few products in her life. How do you, as a salesperson, handle all that? It is a large responsibility and your companies rarely provide enough training to help you with your job. That puts you in a no-win situation. Without the knowledge you need to respond to a consumer's needs, all the advertising in the world won't save a sale or bring the customers back. Personal ability aside, the vast majority of people selling makeup, I am told over and over again, simply do not know what they are doing.

However, I want more than just a better-educated sales force out there behind the counters and at in-home sales presentations, although this would be a great advantage for the consumer, at least when it comes to makeup purchases (skin care is another entire discussion, but one thing at a time). Take it easy on shiny eyeshadows, don't say something looks good when it doesn't, and don't be a snob or aloof; even though you think I can't afford a $40 or $50 foundation you don't have to be rude, and, besides, you could be wrong, which means you lose a sale.

THERE IS STILL A LOT TO DO

I've written quite a bit about the cosmetics industry over the years. My books *Blue Eyeshadow Should Be Illegal* (1985), *Blue Eyeshadow Should Still Be Illegal* (1988), and *Blue Eyeshadow Should Absolutely Be Illegal* (1992) gave detailed explanations of the cosmetics industry's advertising and promotion techniques. I also explained at length why many astringents are a waste of money, why wrinkle creams can't do what they claim, and why most advertising rhetoric is empty and meaningless. I also described how to tell the differences between blushes, eyeshadows, mascaras, and highlighters, and how to apply makeup quickly with fewer products than the salespeople encourage you to buy. In essence, almost every page divulged what the cosmetics companies would never reveal to you.

The thrust of those books was to teach you how to take care of your skin without any of the product-driven information you receive from the cosmetics companies. Conceptually, it was about doing the best for your skin and still being able to spend the least amount of money. I described at length in each of the *Blue Eyeshadow Should Be Illegal* books how to use a $15 to $20 skin care routine that works (it used to cost $10 back in 1985, when I wrote the first book), how to apply makeup, and what to look for in a particular blush or foundation. That still didn't clear up the confusion of how to choose one product over another. What was true when I first wrote this book will probably always be true: women want to know exactly which cosmetics to use. They want to know which foundations go on the lightest or cover the best; which mascaras don't smudge but make lashes thick and long; which blushes blend on smooth and soft; which eyeshadows blend evenly and don't crease; which cosmetics lines are the most reliable and which ones are overpriced. The answers to these questions and more required a radically different kind of research than I used for *Blue Eyeshadow.*

For most women, the social need for makeup and skin care products does not wane. Women need information about looking their best and buying the right products if they are going to achieve a confident appearance. For many women the major, if not only, source of advice on what to buy when it comes to their face is fashion magazines. It is no secret that I have repeatedly criticized the inadequate and misleading information the fashion magazines continue to print when it comes to the cosmetics industry. As I am told over and over again by beauty editors who call me for information they can't get anywhere else, their hands are bound by lucrative advertising accounts. I have none of that headache. Without any constraints from advertisers I can tell you what I learn without fear of loosing a $600,000 advertising account from Estee Lauder or Borghese. I don't have to worry if La Prairie wants to take their advertising someplace else because I think their products are ridiculously overpriced. Every fashion magazine you read pays homage to the cosmetics industry with every article and overstated editorial regarding cosmetics; you will find none of that in these pages.

Beauty Note: I shouldn't put the onus entirely on fashion magazines. Exercise or health magazines such as *Longevity* and *Self* are notorious for writing articles that sound more like ads than anything else. If you read an article that only elaborates on how wonderful and superior a product is, whether it be for your thighs or face, and no critical information is provided, you most likely have been reading an ad disguised as an article. These deceptive stories often quote studies or research that sound very impressive, but the research is almost always produced by the cosmetics line or a company hired by that line and the results are rarely impartial. I can't tell you the number of times I've read article endorsements that involved a study that looked at 15 people, eight or nine of whom showed positive results, without specifying what those positive results were. General rule of thumb: if it sounds too good to be true, it is.

I should add that one change over the past few years is an attempt by many fashion magazines to introduce or portray themselves as an objective source for cosmetics information. Fashion magazines rarely used to want to interview me, but now I get several calls a month. At first this seemed to be an exciting breakthrough, but what quickly became apparent was the limitation of what would eventually be printed. Carefully they would reword everything I said to make it sound harmless, almost deferential to the cosmetics industry. I was repeatedly told that they could not "insult the advertisers." I wanted to know how they justified insulting the reader.

Practically every fashion magazine writer who interviewed me apologized for the constraints placed on her. Some were considerably chagrined, but there was nothing they could do about it. Whenever I am asked what rip-offs are taking place at the cosmetics counters, I am asked to never name names—it all has to be vague generalizations because they can never mention specific products or they might insult their advertisers or potential advertisers. I usually can't praise directly either; that seems to be saved for the cosmetics companies who spent the most on advertising in that issue.

In my book you don't have to worry about any of that. You may not like what I have to say, but I am giving you what my research and experience have uncovered, nothing more and nothing less. I have no constraints except the truth as I see it, and that is what I will present as best I can.

COSMETICS COUNTER UPDATE

More than a year ago, after receiving thousands of letters from women who had read my books and wanted ongoing information, I decided to start a newsletter. In July 1992 the first issue of *Cosmetics Counter Update* was published. Every issue continues the effort to bring sanity to the insane world of beauty and fashion. Continuing product reviews, editorials about skin care news, and honest information about cosmetics lines appear in each issue. I've written about how products get named; reviewed lines that were not included in the original *Don't Go* book such as Nu Skin, Clarins, Clarion, Beauty Without Cruelty, and Rachel Perry; discussed at length what you need to know about alpha hydroxy acids (AHAs); reported what makeup companies are being bought and sold by other makeup companies; told which exercise videos won't hurt your body; found out which waterproof mascaras are the best; and much more.

This effort has been really exciting. It keeps me on top of what is happening in the world of cosmetics and gives the consumer an alternative source of information besides fashion magazines. If you want to know more about this bimonthly newsletter, you can receive a one-time free introductory copy and see for yourself if the stories and reviews are what you want to read on a regular basis. Please use the form at the front of the book or call *Cosmetics Counter Update* at (206) 722-7200 and get your introductory copy today.

WHAT YOU'LL FIND INSIDE THIS BOOK

Don't Go To The Cosmetics Counter Without Me presents a product-by-product review of cosmetics for sale from more than 60 of the most popular lines. That is 30 more cosmetic lines and 5,000 more products than the first edition of the book. I have to admit that maintaining my adopted job description as the "Ralph Nader of Rouge" is not always thrilling: I find the cosmetics counters as frustrating, intimidating, and annoying as you do. I did not relish the prospect of spending money on $40 foundations that I knew weren't any better than $6 to $12 foundations, nor did I savor the thought of dealing with the salespeople. I knew that most of the information they would give me would be nothing more than sales pitches, hype, anecdotes, and scientific cosme-babble. Who wants to put up with that? Not exactly a great way to spend a hundred afternoons. But there was no other way to go about gathering the information for this book. I also increased my budget, spending more than $5,000 on cosmetics.

If you've ever felt uncertain or didn't have the time or energy to figure out for yourself which foundations are too pink or too orange, which eyeshadows are too shiny or too difficult to use, which powders go on too chalky, which cleansers are too greasy, or which toners are too harsh, read the product-by-product and line-by-line reviews in the following chapters, covering 60-plus cosmetics lines. There is a summary chapter of best finds, but don't jump to that one first. It is important to read the individual product reviews so you understand exactly what you are buying. There may be 20 good mascaras available, but each one might be good for a different reason.

Each product is described in terms of its reliability, value, texture, application, and effect. Within every category of product I established specific criteria and went about finding which products lived up to that list. If a foundation is supposed to be light, sheer, and match your skin exactly, it can't be oily or thick, blend poorly, or be orange or rose. There are no orange- or rose-colored people. The same determinations were made for mascaras, blushes, eyeshadows, concealers, pressed powders, lipsticks, and pencils. Skin care products were reviewed almost entirely by ingredient list versus claim. If a toner asserts that it is designed for sensitive skin it shouldn't contain ingredients that irritate the skin. If a moisturizer claims it can hydrate the skin it should contain ingredients that can do that. I have also challenged the inflated claims made about such ingredients as yeast, herbal extracts, botanicals, alpha hydroxy acids, vitamins, and liposomes.

I have also included the results of a survey I mailed to more than 1,500 women, 600 of whom responded about the cosmetics products they use. Although their information does not always agree with mine, it is wonderful additional feedback about what you can expect from the cosmetics you might want to purchase. With this information, you no longer have to rely on your own random search-and-test method, accept the sales clerk's pitch, or be seduced by cosmetics ads. I have done a lot of the work for you.

WHAT ELSE SHOULD BE ILLEGAL BESIDES BLUE EYESHADOW?

Unfortunately, even though I am impressed with many improvements on the cosmetics front, there are still many disappointments. Some of the more irksome things you may encounter when shopping for cosmetics are: shiny eyeshadows; wrinkle creams; rejuvenating creams; astringents; toners that contain irritating ingredients; special eyelid foundations; bright green, lavender, or pink eyeshadows; bright blue eye pencils; nonsurgical eye-lift creams; eyeshadow sets; sponge-tip eyeshadow applicators; compact-size brushes; models under the age of 30 posing for wrinkle cream ads; models with perfect skin posing for skin care ads in general; models with tans posing for sunscreen ads; ingredient names no one understands; "all day" lipstick claims; brown lipsticks; brown lip liners; mascaras that clump and flake; water-soluble mascaras that don't rinse off completely; overly aggressive cosmetics salespeople; poorly lit makeup counters; miracle ingredients; "dermatologist tested" claims; "hypoallergenic" claims; "noncomedogenic" and "nonacnegenic" claims; "all natural" claims; pink- and orange-colored foundations; and tanning powders, bronzers, and tinted moisturizers.

WHY YOU STILL SHOULDN'T GO TO THE COSMETICS COUNTERS ALONE

Whenever you shop for makeup the choices are dazzling, provocative, and extensive, and the sales methods fetching and slick. Enticing names and colors suggest the very essence of beauty. Wondrous claims sound too good to pass up. The thought flickers, If I buy that I will look really great, or, If I use that my skin may really look younger. Elegance, glamour, and sensuality, all for the asking. What difference does price make when all that matters is looking and feeling beautiful? A bevy of options, from gleaming wet lipsticks to perfectly pressed eyeshadows to skin-enhancing foundations, are lures hard to ignore.

Then you notice the skin care items and listen to the encouragement and scientific-sounding information the salesperson chants. A little of this here and there and those lines or that blemish will vanish before your very eyes. Your hand is in your wallet before you know it.

That is when the deja vu begins. An unsettling voice in your ear says, "Didn't this happen a few months or a year ago? Did the last wrinkle cream I bought really make a difference? Why should this one work? How did the last lipstick color I bought that looked so luscious on the counter turn out so wrong at home?" Even if you like the products you bought, the next eye-catching ad can make you doubt what you are using. Perhaps there is something better out there you might be missing. Another $50 or $75 later you have new products at home, and nothing changes until the next incentive or media suggestion takes place. This cycle gets you nowhere and that's why you need me.

There are several major obstacles to overcome when tackling the cosmetics buying process: (1) the vast number of choices; (2) the number of products that are nothing more than a waste of time and money; (3) the salespeople who are trained primarily on how to sell products and not how to apply them; and (4) the dilemma of knowing what looks good on you and what doesn't.

The purpose of this book is to help you narrow down the choices. Yes, it's hard to know what looks the best and what skin care products work, but it gets easier once you learn what to avoid. In all honesty, shopping the cosmetics counters may never be an easy experience, but it can be a fun, challenging adventure, and with usable information you can make it just that. This means that you can't go to the cosmetics counters alone—at least not yet, especially when the fashion magazines and the media make rational decisions so incredibly difficult.

FOR WOMEN OF COLOR

Many cosmetics lines are trying to make up for their past inequities by adding makeup products appropriate for women of color. Previously, the foundations offered in this area were too orange and greasy, the eyeshadows were strictly shiny, and the skin care products fairly drying. It seems unbelievable that it's taken so long for the major cosmetics companies to finally acknowledge and try to meet the needs of such a diverse group of women. Maybelline, Revlon, Prescriptives, and M.A.C. are the leaders in this area, and they are to be commended. Not only are their color products appropriate, but they offer a large number of choices. Although some lines were designed specifically for women of color, such as Flori Roberts and Fashion Fair (both are reviewed in Chapter Seven), the options from these lines had limitations. Now the options are endless and the selections are beautiful.

Beauty Note: A handful of cosmetics lines coming on the scene claim they are designed for Asian women. I have read their brochures and seen the claims about how Asian skin is supposedly so different from Caucasian, Spanish, and African-American skin that it requires a separate product line. Nothing could be further from the truth, and the products from these lines aren't any different in formulation than products from all the other lines on the market. Creating a special marketing niche where none exists might be good business, but it isn't necessarily good for the consumer. As it turns out, most Asian women do not want a line directed specifically at them; they would rather buy mainstream cosmetics, just as they have always done.

SEX AND THE CONSUMER

Admittedly, I am a conservative dresser of sorts, and my body type doesn't lend itself to being draped in tight, revealing clothing. But aside from my restrained nature and possible jealousy, there is still a critical problem with the cover of *Cosmopolitan* and with most of the fashion images in women's magazines all over the world. From *Elle* to *Glamour* to *Allure* to *Harper's Bazaar,* the recurring monthly theme is how much breast you can show without fully displaying the nipple and how much leg you can reveal without exposing the vagina. Every issue extols the desirability of a sultry come-hither look, the value of full lips semi-parted in breathless expectation, and the prestige of wearing clinging outfits.

And what message does this recurring theme convey? That a woman's only interest and full-time job is to be sexually irresistible—not what I call a lofty message. How confusing for the majority of women who are struggling with their identities as working women, home-makers, or mothers. How useful is the perpetual suggestion that a woman's sole purpose is to attract a man? When are we supposed to get down to taking care of our professional and personal lives?

How often does a women need to be reminded that her focus in life is to oblige a man's fantasy? And what a boring, redundant reminder that is. Don't we have this one down solid by now? Besides, if the issue is sexuality why is it only the responsibility of the woman? There is no male counterpart for this one. Men don't dress in a sexually revealing manner for women, at least not in public. In fact, men who do unbutton their shirts to bare their chests are considered somewhat tacky, not the least bit sexy.

None of these magazines use images that are suitable for the workplace. Even the outfits that are suggested for the office are oftentimes too revealing for a woman who is trying to be taken seriously. Attempting unconsciously to appear tantalizing to your male coworkers or boss, even in the name of fashion, won't get you a raise or promotion, but it can cause you problems and, as many studies indicate, a lateral career cycle.

I am not suggesting that the way women dress is the cause or even the main reason for women lagging behind men in the workplace, but it is a factor just as it is for men. Imagine Donald Trump or any other male executive you can think of wearing skintight pants or a sheer see-through shirt. If part of what we need to achieve independence and career advantages is to maintain a bearing of power and ability, then none of these magazines are helping. They are eroding our power.

If it sounds like I am a proponent of a conservative public wardrobe and makeup as the best mode of dress for a woman, particularly during the day, for the most part you'd be right. I am aware that for some women the way they achieve their power is by being sexual and voluptuous, and conservative clothing would get them nowhere. But for most of us, exposed cleavage, naked thighs, and parted red lips net us very little. If there is one arena we are still novices at, it is establishing our power as women and not as sex objects. Many fashion magazines take this cause back to the dark ages.

The obvious, nagging question that comes to mind is why. Why does the bait of young hard bodies cause consumers to spend their money? Why are women all over the country willing to be seduced by images of subtle to hard-core sensuality? (Calvin Klein's Obsession ads have sold a lot of cologne.) We know that buying Elizabeth Taylor's perfumes (White Diamonds and Passion) isn't really going to improve our sex lives and we will not gain one iota of Ms. Taylor's popularity. And no matter how well our lipstick stays on or how smooth our skin looks, it isn't going to change anything in our bedrooms. We can rub all the cellulite cream we want into our legs, but Richard Gere (or even someone who looks like him) isn't showing up tonight (whether it works or not).

Some of us throw logic out the door when confronted with the hope of increased desirability. Common sense doesn't come into play when we are titillated by enticing ads and promises. A more comely exterior is our sole reason to buy, buy, buy. We want to be more sexually appealing than we were before we bought that new cream or lipstick. And not only more desirable but younger too, because younger is better.

For many the attraction of the ads has nothing to do with the prospect of increased sexuality. The hook isn't in what we get in terms of actual sex, but rather if a product becomes a sexual experience in and of itself. What manufacturer doesn't want the consumer to feel turned on by their product? Forget a real attraction to or lust for the opposite sex. If a product makes you feel sexy, haven't you gotten your money's worth? And that is exactly the goal of most advertising—a sexual experience for less money and trouble than it takes to find a significant other or to convince your significant other to be sexy with you. Advertising executives understand the concept of promise her anything, but give her sex.

Unfortunately, this "sell by seduction" technique is the absolute worst way to make decisions involving cosmetics. Perfume ads are the most flagrant. They offer only images, not even bothering to mislead you with deceptive sales rhetoric. Designed strictly to tantalize and excite, these ads are incredibly powerful. Do not for one second believe that any of us are above the pull of sensational images telling us how we can look and feel like them, even if only a little bit.

The more aware we are of this influence in our lives, the more we will remember that these are only glossy fantasies dancing before our eyes and nothing more. There are no facts or information in these illusions and flashing pictures. Consumer decisions should be based on facts and information. Let's be more careful where we spend our money. We can't look like them even a little bit. We can look like ourselves, with a fashionable flair and style, and that is more than good enough to make life interesting and intriguing. With this attitude we can save hundreds of dollars in a year or two.

STAYING OBJECTIVE

One of the interesting side notes to having sold quite a few "beauty" books is that the cosmetics companies have noticed me. I think they prefer to ignore me, but once in a while they can hardly help themselves. After *Don't Go To The Cosmetics Counter Without Me* was published, several cosmetics companies' representatives, including The

Body Shop, Borghese, and Elizabeth Arden, wanted to let me know that I had made some dreadful mistakes in my assessment of their products. One very passionate phone call had no follow-up letter, but the two others were accompanied by a letter. The outrage, of course, was directed only toward the products I had criticized; I was obviously very accurate about the products I had praised. My response was and always is the same. I list the reasons why I said what I said, I offer all my research and documentation, and in return I ask that they send me documentation of their research and evidence. Once I receive enough information to suggest I have made an error, I say, I would be willing to retract or change my statement. That is always where the conversation stops. I never hear from them again.

It is practically impossible for me to get an interview, assistance, information, press kit, ingredient lists, or even prices from any of the public relations people at the major cosmetics companies. I've asked many times to be treated like any other beauty editor. Having sold more than 500,000 books and a steady circulation from my newsletter, I didn't think my request was so out of the ordinary, and I thought I deserved similar consideration. At least prices and ingredients, there on the containers, are not a big secret or anything. However, it was more often than not very difficult for me to get the sort of information and sample products other beauty editors receive. There are a few exceptions that I'd like to point out: Cheeseborough Ponds, Maybelline, Noevir, Nailbirth, Alpha Hydrox, Arbonne, Artistry by Amway, Aveda, Avon, Clinique, Murad, M.D. Formulations, NeoStrata, and Almay. Thank you for being willing to take the risk that your products would receive an honest evaluation. Although I didn't like all of your products, I did like many of them, and consumers should be aware of your willingness to be helpful on their behalf.

Another intriguing facet is that on occasion I have received requests from a few cosmetics lines to represent their products. I think these proposals come before they've read my book, because once I explain what I've written about their company they apologize for wasting my time. I'm flattered by the attention and don't mind getting these calls, but I couldn't possibly represent their companies. Once you are a paid spokesperson to represent a product line you must love all the products in that line. You can't have an honest opinion. To sign away my freedom to say what I believe would be antithetical to what I am trying to do with my work and books.

OVERCOMING MAKEUP ADDICTION

If any of the following quotes sound the least bit familiar, you may be one of the thousands (if not millions) of women addicted to buying cosmetics. As with any other addiction, there is often a fine line between responsible behavior and the endless routine of acting on impulse or reflex without logic or reason. And just like any other addiction, the first way to cure the problem is to recognize that it exists. You have to admit you're addicted to buying cosmetics before you can stop the behavior. See if any of these attitudes regarding cosmetics fits you or someone you know.

"It's fun to buy makeup and skin care products. I love the cosmetics counters. A new lipstick or eyeshadow just makes my day. I love all the glamour and beauty stuff. It's not a waste of money, it's fun."

"I'll try anything to stop my face from aging."

"I think I'm different from all those women who buy expensive products, because I only buy the cheap stuff. I know these products are all the same, so I'm saving money and I look better than my friends who buy the expensive lines. If it's under $10 I buy it. The problem is I buy all of the inexpensive stuff, everything and anything. I've spent hundreds of dollars on hundreds of products. For what? I still look the same no matter what I use."

"I'm an executive for a major real estate company. I was considered one of the top salespeople several years in a row, yet I'm a sucker for every cosmetics sales pitch I've ever heard. Can you imagine how many cosmetics lines I've bought? And I mean every product they tell me to use."

"I never believe what they tell me at the cosmetics counter, and I know all those cosmetics ads are of tall, disgustingly thin, naturally flawless 20-year-olds who wouldn't recognize a pimple or a wrinkle if it hit them over the head and yelled 'I'm here.' Yet none of that stops me. Once they get my attention and start describing how this product protects my skin from the environment and stress or this other product prevents wrinkles and all kinds of other nonsense, my charge card is out on the counter and the products are in a bag on their way home with me."

"I never buy the cheap lines. I would never put that stuff on my face. I take very good care of myself. I use only the best lines regardless of the price; that way I know I'm getting the best. I take care of each part of my body with just the right product. I feel very elegant and pampered. The money is incidental when it comes to how I look."

"I thought I was doing better but now the television cosmetics ads make it too easy to try something new. I just pick up the phone and order and new toys come in the mail. I spent over $1,200 last year on skin care and makeup without even leaving my house."

Admitting that you are addicted to buying cosmetics is much harder than it seems on the surface, because cosmetics buying is not considered socially unacceptable. In fact, just the opposite is true. Much as drinking is considered an essential part of any social event, buying makeup is considered an essential detail for the contemporary woman. Women shopping for cosmetics are just taking good care of themselves, aren't they? For some women that is exactly what is happening; others are wasting hundreds, if not thousands, of dollars unnecessarily.

One problem with recognizing cosmetics addiction is that for the most part there is nothing really harmful about it. Seven cleansers, 4 toners, 10 moisturizers, 6 foundations, 15 lipsticks, 18 eyeshadows, 9 blushes, and a dozen or so highlighters, concealers, and wrinkle creams are not going to hurt you, at least not as far as your face is concerned. Your pocketbook and self-esteem are an entirely different story and the heart of the problem.

The issue of being addicted to buying makeup is primarily a financial dilemma for most women. A typical cosmetics drawer can have between $500 and $700 of half-, never-, or rarely used products. That's not loose change, yet a cosmetics addict can have more than twice that amount of unused products. Even more insidious than the waste of money is what this preoccupation with buying makeup represents.

The true makeup addict unconsciously or consciously believes that somewhere the perfect skin care product or makeup color will bring her the beauty and self-esteem she longs to possess. Surely cosmetics that will deliver perfect skin and a cover-girl image hide behind a counter somewhere waiting to be discovered, purchased, taken home, and applied. Then, *voila*, instant self-acceptance. But it never happens. The search never ends. There are only so many shades of lipstick or types of toner to try before the issue is no longer a quest for products but a deeper understanding that an emotional need is not being met, one that has nothing to do with applying makeup or taking care of the skin. But the cosmetics addict never gets to that awareness.

The women I've talked to over the years who were caught in that cycle of accumulating a never-ending reservoir of skin care and makeup products all fell into many of the same emotional traps. Here are my suggestions to help you start the process of letting go of cosmetics as your self-esteem crutch. It doesn't mean never wearing makeup. This isn't about cold turkey. This is about balance and reason. This is about saving money and not being gullible or susceptible to every cosmetics sales pitch you hear. This is ultimately about enjoying makeup without being preoccupied with it, about liking the way you look and using cosmetics as an accessory or tool and not a cure or disguise.

All of these suggestions can help save you a lot of money, not to mention a great deal of time and emotional energy.

1. All the makeup and skin care products in the world can't cover up an unhealthy life-style of no exercise, smoking, and/or a high-fat diet. Although this sounds corny and boringly redundant, this first point is essential.

2. There is no such thing as the perfect cosmetic or cosmetics line. There are a lot of good products available. Once you find a product that is good, your search is over until it is gone and then you can start again or you can even buy the same product again.

3. No one needs more than a daytime moisturizer with an SPF of 15 or greater and a nighttime moisturizer without a sunscreen. Your face cream does not need to be different from your body moisturizer. Specialty creams for various parts of your body are a waste of money.

4. Spending more money does not mean you will look more beautiful. Knowing how to apply makeup is the key to looking put together. Expensive mascara that smears is not glamorous. Buying expensive cosmetics may make you feel like you're doing something good for yourself, but don't be fooled. Expensive shiny eyeshadows or toners with alcohol don't look good on anyone.

5. There are no anti-aging products available besides sunscreens. Searching for and buying these on a regular basis are a sure sign of a tendency toward cosmetics addiction.

6. Find ways to feel good about yourself that don't come from your appearance: pursuing a hobby, volunteering at your favorite charity, reading, singing, or visiting with good supportive friends. Then, on days when you are feeling less than attractive (and it happens to all of us no matter who we are), you have other qualities to concentrate on to boost your self-esteem.

7. The information you get at the cosmetics counters is rarely accurate, particularly when it comes to skin care. Do not fall into listening to a sales pitch. If you can't say "no" or "I'm not interested," don't go near them ever again.

8. Do not get sucked into the elite craze of spa treatments for the skin. There are no quick repairs for the skin. The idea is to simply take good care of your skin daily.

9. It is a waste of money to buy more than one or two shades of any color. No one needs eight shades of pink lipstick or coral blush.

10. And last, but not least, there is nothing wrong with shopping for makeup. But keep in mind how much energy you spend trying to look glamorous instead of getting out and being beautiful by living life.

"A woman's intense desire to be beautiful makes her desire anything the cosmetics industry wants to sell her."

A La Prairie salesperson when asked why their products were so expensive

CHAPTER

T · W · O

The Language of Cosmetics

SELLING DREAMS

What's in a name? That which we call a rose by any other name would smell as sweet.

Let's get one thing straight from the beginning: Juliet's assertion that Romeo's last name didn't matter was wrong. She was too young to recognize that part of his allure *and* the cause of their downfall was the forbidden genealogy represented by his last name. You and Juliet should be very aware that in fact names do matter. Subconsciously they can be very powerful and seductive, particularly cosmetics names.

Perhaps no single part of the process of inventing and marketing a product is as important to the selling process as giving a product its name. Skilled wording can serve several functions: (1) it can tell you what the product is; (2) it can define (more or less accurately) what the product promises to do; and, (3) *most important*, at least for the cosmetics companies, the name can make you want to buy the product. Knowing how all this works can make you less likely to be lured by enticing but essentially unsubstantiated promises.

When it comes to skin care most of us want prettier, softer, smoother, clearer, or younger-looking skin. In a nutshell, cosmetics companies are trying to convince us they can make that dream come true if we buy their products. The most important factor in naming a product (even more important than the ingredients, which are all fairly similar) is to create a short name that immediately identifies what promise you are buying. The industry calls this promise the product's *benefit*. A good name (one that makes you want to buy the product) will encapsulate the implied benefit in the name unobtrusively, persuasively, and *naturally*—in as few words as possible.

Take Elizabeth Arden's *Visible Difference* skin care line. You know from the name exactly what the products promise: a noticeable change in your skin. Or consider Prescriptives' *Comfort Cream*; it sounds simple and cozy. What woman wouldn't want that for her skin? These are clear and concise names; they convince with their matter-of-fact, easily understood language. One of Prescriptives' recent successes is their *All You Need* moisturizer. What a perfect name. It absolutely says it all. It doesn't matter that it isn't all you need (it doesn't contain a sunscreen and isn't very good for someone with dry skin)—the name is too enticing to ignore.

But there are many styles of names, and if you pay attention you'll notice that companies adopt a kind of "signature" approach in the wording they choose for their products. Clinique, for example, revolutionized the industry in the early 1970s by being the first company to center its whole identity on the suggestion that medical authorities had participated in the development of the products. The motto "dermatologist tested" was, and is, their claim to fame. The implication, of course, is that you are practically under a doctor's care when you use Clinique. (No dermatologists were quoted nor were any research studies available, but cosmetics companies don't have to prove any of their claims to consumers.) *Dramatically Different Moisturizing Lotion* (which, in reality, is far from different or dramatic), *Clarifying Toner,* and *7-Day Scrub Cream* all sound like something a doctor might prescribe. Physicians Formula does the same thing with the very nature of their name. It doesn't matter that there is only one dermatologist on the medical committee that reviews their products and ingredient lists. Just because the company name sounds authentic, it doesn't mean its products are medically reliable.

Other companies seek to distinguish themselves with foreign names and images. Consider L'Oreal's *Plenitude* line; the name, easily understood in both French and English, suggests an abundant capacity to take care of the skin. L'Oreal is a moderately priced drugstore line owned by the same company that owns Lancome. L'Oreal offers *Eye Defense Gel-Cream with Liposomes* and *Plenitude Action Liposomes* "created by the Skincare Laboratories of L'Oreal." Very European, with the aura of "active" science thrown in. Chic but clinical at the same time. In effect, Lancome offers the same image but in an even more abbreviated style; *Progres Eye Creme* and *Niosome* and *Noctosome* creams "from Lancome, Paris" sound very French and very scientific. The same is true for Borghese with an Italian twist and La Prairie with a Swiss emphasis. Both companies are using the same two psychological enticements: (1) they are trading on the American woman's belief that European women are beautiful and know how to take good care of their skin; and (2) they are suggesting, with pseudoscientific names, that an elite medical team designed these products. (Every cosmetics company wants you to believe this one. Of course, cosmetic chemists *are* involved in developing products, but that is true for the entire industry. Many cosmetic chemists "free-lance" for several companies at the same time and share information at conventions. There are no cosmetics secrets that will change one wrinkle or cure a blemish on your face.)

Another prime example of this amalgamation of European-sounding elegance and high-tech science is embodied in the Princess Marcella Borghese line. Here's the insider information: the company was previously owned by Revlon and recently sold to a group of Saudi Arabian businessmen; the actual princess lives in Europe and is an informal *advisor* to the company. But *La Dolce Cura Anti-Stress Restorative Creme* and *Effetto Immediato Spa Lift for Eyes* are named very carefully to seem very Italian, very specialized, and very clinically efficient.

Once in a while a cosmetics company comes up with a product name that is so effective the whole industry sits up and takes notice. Such a name is Estee Lauder's *Night Repair* and *Fruition*. In one or two words these products promise everything. *Night Repair* implies an instant overnight fix, fast and direct, and the product's packaging supports the name; *Night Repair* looks like medicine. *Fruition* suggests that your dream of perfect skin can be attained.

A straightforward name, one you can easily understand that also suggests medical and pharmaceutical authority, helps stimulate sales regardless of what the product contains or really does. Other Estee Lauder products follow this clever naming psychology: *Skin Defender*, *Skin Perfecting Lotion*, and *Future Perfect* all sound like simple yet hard-working "miracle" products.

Another Estee Lauder company, Origins, has had great success borrowing ideas from natural cosmetics lines. Perhaps the most innovative thing that Origins has done is to name its products with emotional names that address our 1990s life-style concerns: *Stress Buffer On-the-Spot Gel, Constant Comforter*, and their smash best-seller, *Peace of Mind*. If that's not a temptation for almost all of us, I don't know what is. Skin care, Zen meditation, and efficiency in a two- to four-ounce jar.

As you've probably noticed, there's a new skin care product or new skin care line born every minute. The cosmetics companies are under extreme economic pressure to convince you to try something new. What's next? For now, probably more of the same: science mixed with European flair and ecology integrated with emotional, New Age relief. One thing is certain: the companies are carefully researching what you want, what you worry about, what you're dreaming of, and what name they can assign to a product that will convince you to buy it. Every time you feel yourself falling for a product name that articulates your fantasies and concerns, remember that you now know better. With a little self-discipline, you can rise above manipulative, psychological seduction.

> *To think that a moisturizer with herbs, vitamins, botanicals, or some other skin care ingredient can feed the skin, is like thinking that you can put a bologna sandwich on your face and have lunch.*

HOW THEY CONVINCE YOU TO SPEND MONEY

Over the past several years little has changed in the advertising, marketing, and selling techniques used by the cosmetics industry to get consumers to purchase makeup and skin care items. The copious brochures, product labels, informational inserts, packaging, and advertisements contain the most exaggerated and extreme claims of any business you'll encounter. Take the package insert for Christian Dior's *Mascara Parfait with Cashmere*. It states, "A perfect formula that helps protect and envelop each lash with colour ensuring its supple feel . . . Using a totally original and perfect brush. . . ." Sounds very impressive, particularly the cashmere, but the mascara is not perfect or all that different from a number of other mascaras. Here's one of my favorites, from Yves St. Laurent's *Hydro-Light Day Creme*, "The skin's surface is immediately smoothed as siliaqueous micro-pearls deliver effective moisturizers and humectants." Wow! I wonder where they found the word "siliaqueous," and "micro-pearls" is so much more enchanting than "mircronized," but the sentence still says only that the product will moisturize your skin, something all moisturizers can do.

The essence of this art of compelling cosmetics language is found in an ad for Clarins' *Multi Eclat Foundation*: "One complex, composed of two synergistic molecules, provides filmogenic, yet non-occlusive properties to effectively promote more youthful-looking, more radiant skin." *Filmogenic?* Where did they get that word? And synergistic molecules are nothing unique; that's how molecules work, by staying connected. I think the idea is to assure you that this product will keep the air off the face. Mineral oil does that very well without all this fancy language. But then the cosmetics industry needs all the merchandising ammunition it can get. What else really sets apart one product from another when they often have more similarities than differences? Besides, if you can confuse a consumer enough and keep her attention away from the ingredient list, the consumer will end up making an emotional decision instead of an educated one. What a great way for a cosmetics company to make a bigger sale.

Another aspect of marketing cosmetics that you should be aware of is the vague and empty promises. Unlike any other commodity, cosmetics can't live up to their claims. When you buy a clothes dryer, the chances are fairly good that it will dry your clothes. If you buy a car, no matter what assertions the salesperson has made about the vehicle, it will probably take you from here to there when you turn it on. (It may break down more than you'd like, but when it works it will take you where you want to go.) The same cannot be said for cosmetics. A moisturizer label that says or implies the product will revitalize, regenerate, and rebuild the skin, or prevent wrinkles, or lift and firm, cannot fulfill the promise. Astringents and masks that claim to close pores, or give you perfect skin, or perfect anything, will never come through. These products are simply not what they seem, at least not to the extent the manufacturers and salespeople would lead you to believe. That doesn't mean cleaning and moisturizing the skin won't make a positive, wonderful difference to your face—it will. And sunscreens with a sun protection factor (SPF) of 15 or greater will indeed prevent some amount of sun damage when used religiously. But all the other language you hear and read is vastly more fanciful than realistic.

CELEBRITY LANGUAGE

It has finally happened. We are drowning in a sea of skin care products. A tidal wave of makeup colors has engulfed us, and we are knee-deep in moisturizers and cleansers, swamped with concealers, saturated with shadows and lipsticks. None of this would be so bad if we weren't beleaguered by all the chicanery that is part and parcel of the glamour flood. Unwittingly, in the midst of all this hoopla, we consumers safeguard the cosmetics industry, protecting it from accountability by remaining loyal to the media's full frontal assault, ever hopeful that our next purchase will put an end to wrinkles, breakouts, oozing oil, and dry skin.

Every time I begin to think that consumers just can't take any more (think about it: How many more cosmetics lines can one society use? How many more products can we buy as we wait for our skin to become "good enough"?), I receive a deluge of requests for information about every new (and old) product from such and such a celebrity or such and such a "natural, pure" line. Cher, Victoria Principal, Tova Borgnine, Connie Stevens, Elizabeth Taylor, and even George Hamilton are just a few who have put their names to products. Joan Rivers, Kathie Lee Gifford, and a slew of famous models have all endorsed different lines of cosmetics. And what about the amazing number of impressively titled personalities such as "doctors," "cosmetic chemists," and "pharmacists" who want you to put your trust in their supposed high-tech formulations?

Bottom line: Celebrities don't know any more about skin care than you do; they get lucrative endorsement contracts because there is money to be made. And cosmetic chemists, dermatologists, and pharmacists do not have secret miracles available to you for the low price of $39.95 if you order now. The idea that pharmacists would know anything about cosmetic formulations is unrelated to what they do for a living. Dermatologists might know something about skin care ingredients, but they are not cosmetic chemists or makeup artists and you would not want them to (nor do they want to) design cosmetics. But it all sounds so reliable and scientific.

Celebrities are running to the television with new product lines because there is so much profit in selling cosmetics. The financial bottom line is enough to make any businessperson drool with expectation. If a "wrinkle" cream costs $2 to manufacture and package and you can sell it for $15, that is a remarkable return on your investment. Of course, it is even better if you can make it for $1.25 and sell it for $25 or $50 or $100, which, as you know, most companies do.

If you hear or read about a celebrity or some other authority praising the miraculous effect of a product and you feel motivated to get out your checkbook or charge card, stop a moment and think about the celebrity's contract before you buy a thing. You would get hot and bothered over a cosmetic too if you were making that kind of money.

LISTENING OBJECTIVELY

Examining the claims of packaged youth or flawless skin is the most fascinating part of dissecting the cosmetics business. I must point out that there is a stark difference between the things said at the counters and the things said on TV and in magazine ads. Unlike claims made by cosmetics salespeople, which vary wildly from person to person and, as a result, are hard to pin down and refute, cosmetics advertising and promotional literature are bold, direct, and in full color. The one- and two-page ads or 30-minute television infomercials assert clearly what you are supposed to believe about an individual product or product line. Most of these ads are beautiful and beguiling; they have all the trappings of authenticity and veracity. But more often than not, the claims couldn't be further from the truth, or at best they're misleading. What isn't smothered in scientific jargon is shrouded in confusing rhetoric. Anyone who has heard phrases like "a two-week treatment synchronized to your skin's natural rhythm" or "cellular balancing complex" knows that it all sounds good, but no one is quite sure what it means. Are your cells imbalanced? Exactly what cells are we talking about? Does skin have a rhythm? And if it does, how does the product play everybody's tune?

More so than ever before, environmental language sells cosmetics. Keeping the environment off the face is essential for good skin care, at least that's what the cosmetics industry wants you to believe. And it is so believable. If pollution is killing the world, just imagine what it must be doing to the skin. Or if stress causes heart attacks, it must be really doing a number on the face. This is all very logical, and perhaps the cosmetics companies have found a way to prevent that damage from taking place. You'll see terms like "mobilizes your skin's defenses," "protects against pollution," "soothes environmental stress," "defends against environmental hazards," "rebalances the skin's natural defense systems," and "keeps pollutants off the face." A little sunscreen and oil are all it takes to make these claims accurate. Oil keeps the air off the face (and no oil does that better than mineral oil—vitamin E does a good job but can cause allergic reactions). "Rebalances the skin" is always a good one. The skin's only real natural defense is oil, so if the product contains oil you're back in business. It's not fancy, it's not costing the manufacturer a lot of money, but it does sound good.

Does stress age the skin? Given how intense stress can get in our daily lives it seems logical that the answer would be yes. But that's not the case. Stress does not age the skin. There is no evidence that someone who is stressed out has better or worse skin than someone who is perfectly calm. But even if this premise were true, how would a cream reduce stress? Stress is an internal process, and there is no cream that when applied to the outside of the face can affect your emotions. You may enjoy rubbing the cream on your skin, but that won't change the problems you're having at work or the pressure from your family. Nice idea, but it's impossible.

On the other hand, if you're talking about *environmental stress,* a term only cosmetics companies use, that does have an impact. The sun, not pollution, causes most of the aging we see on the face, which is what sunscreens are for. Air dehydrates the skin, but that's what moisturizers are for. You can't repair, defend, revive, or change any of this without those two basics—sunscreen and moisturizer. There are no distinctive formulas that can combat these problems in any mysterious, exotic way.

Why then does it sound like all these products can do such glorious things for your skin? How do you get so misled? Why do all the claims sound so convincing? It's all in the words that are used to describe what a product can do. These catchy phrases say everything you want to hear and yet say nothing at all. The terms you need to be most aware of are the ones that show up in connection with a vast number of skin care products. In order to comply with the Food and Drug Administration's (FDA) ruling in regard to cosmetics advertising, the claim on any given product can only *suggest* that your skin will be better; it can't say that it actually will. A cosmetic cannot say it will change or alter the skin's structure (if it could, it would be a drug and therefore subject to radically different federal regulations). But if a cosmetics company can lead you to believe their products can change your skin without actually stating this, no FDA rules will have been broken. In other words, misleading consumers is perfectly legal. And because the number of products is vastly greater than the number of inspectors at the FDA, bending the rules too far is all part of the cosmetics game.

See how many of the most typically used catchy, albeit meaning-less, phrases you recognize: "appears to" (doesn't say it will, just that it can *seem* that way); "leaves the skin looking smoother" (looks that way doesn't mean it *is* that way); "changes the appearance of" (doesn't say it changes the skin structure, only the way it looks, which any moistur-izer can do); "lessens the signs of" ("signs" refers to dryness, and almost any moisturizer can do this too); "reduces the chances of" (chances can mean 100 to 1 odds against reducing, but it's still a chance); "reduces the temporary signs of aging" ("temporary" means dryness), "anti-aging" (as opposed to pro-aging? This term has no meaning); "affects the visible signs of aging" ("visible" means superfi-cial, as in dry skin, not anything deeper); "reverses the visual damage of aging" ("visual" also means what you can see on the surface and refers only to dry skin); and "accelerates cell renewal" (if something helps peel the skin it can affect cell turnover, but so can a washcloth). The number of products that make these claims and a dozen more is staggering. Just remember that nothing specific, long-lasting, or permanent can be guaranteed because nothing specific, long-lasting, or permanent can be proved.

Beauty Note: The main difference between a drug and a cosmetic as far as the FDA is concerned is that a cosmetic claim does not have to be proved and a drug claim does. A cosmetic product can come to market without any testing or proof of efficacy. A drug has to follow strict guidelines as to how well it works and whether or not it will cause any problems. Any claim for a cosmetic, no matter how vague or seemingly genuine, does not have to be substantiated.

READING BETWEEN THE LINES

Many cosmetics companies produce elaborate four-color brochures touting the special effects of their skin care products. These "scientifically generated" promotions are often accompanied by very official-looking test charts and diagrams. The layouts are most impressive in their technical dramatization and clinical appearance, but they are produced by graphic artists and marketing departments rather than by bona fide scientists in a neutral laboratory. They amount to little more then pretty pictures with enigmatic headings and descriptions. Even when illustrations do represent a scientific study of some type, there are still important questions to ask regarding the test results. Take, for example, a brochure that depicts a microscopic section of skin before and after a product was applied. The manufacturer is trying to demonstrate that when water is retained in the skin over a period of time, the skin is measurably more elastic. But a microscopic picture of skin that shows improvement after a cream is applied, or a graph depicting a similar change, in and of itself is meaningless.

You are given no information about the condition of the skin before the cream was applied, how old the test subject or subjects were, how many people (or animals) were tested, and whether the results were uniform among all the subjects. You don't know who performed the test, whether double-blind scientific procedures were used, who analyzed the results, how long the effects lasted, and whether the results were the same for a placebo cream placed on another part of the skin. There is no way those pictures or graphs have any legitimate scientific significance whatsoever.

The words that sound scientific are often the most presumptuous and carry the least information. I've yet to find a salesperson who, when pressed, can define "micro-refining," "micro-targeted," "micro-bubbles," "isotonic energy," "bio-synergetic," "bio-performance," and "micro-lipid-concentrate." Often these terms have been created by the company to sound impressive, but that's about all they stand for.

Then there are the untranslatable foreign words: "multi-regener-ante," "hydro-serum," "lipo-serum," "multi-reparateur restructurant," "resultante creme," "hydra-systeme" (water system?), "synchro serum," and "hydrafilm." Who knows for sure what they mean?

The terminology applied to products that supposedly ward off acne is less varied, but the general ad approach is the same. It attempts to convince the consumer that certain formulations can correct oily or combination skin because they are some, if not all, of the following: "dermatologist tested," "allergy tested," "laboratory tested," "noncome-dogenic," "oil-free," "natural," and "designed for sensitive skin." All of that sounds great, but the words can't guarantee that your skin won't react adversely to the product or that the product will keep you from developing acne or even help the acne you already have. I've stated before that although there are no absolutes about what elements cause acne or blackheads, some ingredients are considered to be higher risks than others. As surprising as this sounds, despite what the label says, some "noncomedogenic" products contain ingredients that may exacer-bate blackheads and acne.

KEEPING YOUR EMOTIONS AT HOME

All of these advertising terms make an appeal to our emotions—the part of us that wants to believe that we can win the battle against the clock or against acne. Even if the product provides only a temporary victory, most people feel that it is better than no victory at all. This sliver of hope, and the sensational allure of skin care ads, keeps many people, especially women, hooked on spending a lot of money on skin care and makeup products in general. But the satisfaction they obtain is usually emotional rather than physical.

The major problem with this advertising and marketing verbiage is that we want to believe it all. What woman over the age of 35 doesn't want to have her skin firmed and restructured? Who doesn't want to believe that there are scientists in the Swiss Alps or in some fancy labo-ratory designing products that can rid us of wrinkles? After all, if I can fax a letter to Australia in less than a minute and satellites can bring me live, up-to-the-minute coverage of world events, surely the technology exists to make skin look younger. Sigh. If I thought for one second that there was a moisturizer or astringent or specialty cream that could truly change the wrinkles on my skin or close a pore, I'd buy it for myself, recommend it to you, and buy stock in the company that makes it. To a large extent, it is our *willingness to believe* that drives the marketing hype behind each of these products. Only our commitment to reality and a raised consumer awareness will prevent us from buying products that can't possibly do what they say. The first step is to stop being deluded by slick packaging and advertisements.

PUTTING TO REST THE NATURAL AND PURE CRAZE

Many, if not all, cosmetics companies utilize the concept of all natural and pure ingredients as one of the primary inducements to buy their products. Over the years this has been an exceedingly effective sales gimmick in the world of cosmetics, and when combined with scientific jargon the combination is too much for most consumers to ignore. Pure and natural fused with anything that sounds like modern technology can make products jump off the shelf into a woman's bathroom or makeup bag.

I'm not saying that pure and natural ingredients aren't good, but they aren't essential or even necessary for good skin care. It is important to note that many cosmetics ingredients are naturally derived. You might not realize it from their names, but ingredients such as cetyl alcohol, stearic acid, stearyl alcohol, acetic acid, sodium cocoyl isethionate, oleoresin, cocamidopropyl, and caprylic glycerides are all derived from natural sources. On the other hand, you probably are familiar with ingredients such as chamomile, lavender oil, and vegetable oil, which appear to be quite natural, but the label doesn't tell you what processing that plant went through to get into the cosmetic. What started out as natural doesn't resemble anything natural in a cosmetic. Over and above the chemical process of combining ingredients, simply because an ingredient is natural or derived from natural sources doesn't tell you anything about its value or irritation potential. Natural is just too vague a term; it gives you no consequential information. Many natural ingredients can even be bad for the skin.

In addition, many ingredients, such as mineral oil, get a bad rap because they are derived from coal tar, but coal tar is as natural as any plant. It isn't enough that something sounds good or appears to be good for your skin; whether it is genuinely good should be the question. Words like natural and pure may be a powerful sales tool, but what they truly are is superficial and ambiguous.

It is interesting to note that the terms "100 percent natural" and

"100 percent pure" are not regulated by the FDA. Every cosmetics manufacturer uses the term as they see fit. Natural can mean that the ingredient in question is part natural and part synthetic, that the product itself has some natural ingredients and some that are not, or that all the ingredients are natural but synthetically extracted. To hold the blind belief that natural means good and chemical (synthetic)—interpreted to mean artificial and unnatural—means bad is to ignore a wide range of substances that can be combined to make great skin care and makeup products. In fact, there is little evidence that natural ingredients are even worth all the effort or significantly improve a product. A bunch of herbal extracts and essential oils without standard cosmetics ingredients wouldn't be much of a product. You can do without the extracts and oils, but you can't make a cosmetic without the usual ingredients that sound, and usually are, anything but purely natural, and even natural ingredients are synthetically treated so they can be blended into a cosmetic.

Please, stop being misled by cosmetics lines that claim to be made from plant extracts, botanicals, essential oils, or any other pure or natural-sounding ingredients. Do not let the cosmetics industry entice you with meaningless emotional language. We should know better by now, right?

THE GREENING OF COSMETICS

Like never before, the value of a product today lies not only in how natural it appears to be but in how *sincerely* natural it is. Everything from volcanic minerals to mangos, Dead Sea salts to oatmeal, and sea kelp to peaches, when added to an ordinary effective moisturizer, can make it seem sensational. It's still ordinary, but perception is everything in cosmetics.

Now, if everyone is using food in their products, how do you get yours to stand out? How much more natural can you get? The Body Shop has taken the search for (and marketing of) "green" ingredients to the seemingly ultimate degree, obtaining oils through natives of foreign countries, including the Maasai people of Africa and the Kayapo Indians of the Amazon rain forest. Has this search produced better products? There is no evidence that the oils and herbs they've utilized provide any benefit for the skin or for the earth. In fact, the use of nonrenewable sources such as sandalwood is a problem. The exotic sounding babassus oil is very similar to palm oil and could therefore become quite popular. It is found in the rain forest and may be one more reason this precious area becomes overcultivated. It isn't happening as yet, but it could if the consumer does not see beyond the label and demands more and more exotic-sounding natural ingredients. The exotic ingredients serve nothing more than the emotional need of the consumer who wants to believe that natural will finally be the thing that keeps the skin young.

What you really need to know is whether or or not a natural ingredient (particularly anything labeled "botanical" or essential oils) interacts better with the skin than a synthetic ingredient. Even substances found in human skin that have been manufactured synthetically for cosmetics cannot become a permanent part of your skin, nor do they necessarily provide any better protection. All the collagen, hyaluronic acid, protein, vegetable oils, plant extracts, or amino acids in the world cannot perform wonders for your skin. They can keep water in the skin, add texture to a product, and perform a number of other functions, but they are not automatically better for the skin simply because they originated from the earth, a plant, a person, or an animal.

According to the June 1992 issue of *Household and Personal Products Industry* magazine, "the concentration of plant extracts used in cosmetics is rarely enough to make a difference in a product. . . . [Cosmetics companies] use a little [amount of botanicals] and then rely on consumer perceptions." Although cosmetics companies will vow they are using botanicals due to their effect and not as a sales tool, the jump-on-the-bandwagon evidence is hard to ignore.

My favorite quote of all is from the March 1992 issue of *Drug and Cosmetics Industry* magazine, which critically stated: "Aromatherapy . . . is a newly emerging science that isn't yet understood. But why lose time by waiting until scientists can prove that essential oils work." That is basic cosmetics industry logic—convince the public, whether or not there is any supporting evidence. As long as the consumer believes you, what else counts? It doesn't matter whether or not it works.

Think twice before falling for a new spa line of cosmetics with tiny amounts of creams and lotions in attractive containers for a large amount of money. Traces of plant extracts suspended in standard cosmetics ingredients are not worth $30 for one ounce when it is less than 1 percent of the product. When was the last time you bought an assortment of herbs for several thousand dollars a pound?

INGREDIENTS YOU NEED AND DON'T NEED FOR DRY SKIN

This list hasn't changed much since I first compiled it. That isn't so surprising; cosmetics ingredients haven't changed much either. Even alpha hydroxy acids are nothing new on the cosmetics scene and the same is true for titanium dioxide, the ingredient used in nonchemical sunscreens. Yet, despite the many cosmetics ingredients that continue to show up in product after product, nothing is more unintelligible than an ingredient list. What a shame, because it is the only part of the product that tells you the absolute truth. The ingredient list is the only area where the FDA rules with an iron fist. My primary concern is to help you better understand this fundamental element of all cosmetics products. I don't expect you to be a chemist, but the more knowledgeable you are, the less likely you will be fooled by fancy language when worthwhile ingredients aren't included. This is a necessity if you are going to be able to look past the claims and company effusions.

Most of us know that skin care is important to our health and essential to how we look, but most of us are also bewildered by meeting that need. Everyone has individual skin care needs (discussed in Chapter Seven), but it is important to know what beneficial ingredients to look for in skin care products. That way the ingredient list will be much less cryptic and ambiguous. All of the ingredients listed below are good ingredients, but they are not miracles, skin rejuvenators, or defenders against stress and pollution, and none prevent skin from aging—except for sunscreens—or cure acne and blackheading.

The most beneficial ingredients to look for in products designed for dry skin are: allantoin, alpha hydroxy acids (glycolic and lactic acid), amino acids, ascorbic acid (vitamin C), avocado oil, basil oil, butylene glycol, caprylic/capric/lauric triglycerides, carrot oil, castor oil (yes, castor oil), cholesterol, coconut oil, collagen, egg oil, elastin, fatty acids (stearic acid), fennel oil, glycerin, glycosaminoglycans, hyaluronic acid, hydrolyzed animal protein, jojoba oil, lanolin, lanolin oil, lecithin, liposomes, macadamia oil, mineral oil, mucopolysaccharides, NaPCA (a water binding ingredient), oils of any kind, palm oil, petrolatum, phospholipids, polyethylene glycol (PEG), propylene glycol, proteins, retinyl palmitate (vitamin A), rice bran oil, sandalwood oil, sodium PCA (similar to NaPCA; this is also a water binding ingredient), soybean oil, squalane, sunflower seed oil, sweet almond oil, tocopherol (vitamin E), water, and wheat germ oil.

These ingredients can help maintain soft, moist skin. There is no guarantee, however, that you won't be allergic to one or many of them. There is also no guarantee that any or all of them will make a difference on your skin. However, if your moisturizer contains one or more of these, and most moisturizers do, it likely can help make your skin look softer, smoother, and, yes, *younger* for as long as you use the product. But the effect lasts only as long as you use the product. Once it is washed off or absorbed into the skin, the effect is gone. If your skin is not dry there is little to no benefit gained from using a moisturizer that contains any of these ingredients.

The above ingredients are found in moisturizers in all price ranges. I recommend that you experiment with lower-priced products before venturing into the range above $15. If the less expensive ones work just as well—and they do—why bother with the high-end stuff? If your skin looks good, what difference does it make how little you spend on skin care or makeup?

Beauty Note: For some reason lanolin has undeservedly snared a bad name in the world of cosmetics. Although some skin care products boast that they are lanolin-free, this doesn't make them any better. In fact, lanolin is a superlative moisturizing ingredient. It is taken from sheep during the sheering process and the animal is not harmed in any way. There is some risk of breakouts, but no more or less than from any other emollient of this type. If you have dry skin, do not stay away from lanolin unless you know for sure you are allergic to it.

The ingredients to disregard or ignore in products designed for dry skin are: adenosine triphosphate, algae extract, amniotic fluid, animal thymus extract, animal tissue extract, epidermal lipid extract, neural lipid extract, serum albumin, serum protein, spleen extract, tissue matrix extract, herb extracts, infusions of anything, and placenta extracts (both animal and human).

WORDS OF EMPTY HYPE FOR OILY SKIN

Most of us have sought relief from the emotional pain and humiliation that often accompany acne, whether it be one blemish or many, by going to drugstores or cosmetics counters where acne products and skin care regimes line the shelves. Myriad products promise clear skin and several pledge to zap zits, dry up blemishes, and drink up oil. The commercials and ads sound fairly convincing, but a closer look reveals that these products can't zap zits or dry up oil, much less stop either from occurring, and the irritation they cause can create more problems than they clear up.

These products claim they are designed for skin that breaks out, offering choices for oily, dry, and sensitive skin. But when you read the label, where the real information is, you find an array of ingredients that can often make acne worse and cause problems for sensitive skin. Several main ingredients show up repeatedly: salicylic acid (a peeling agent); benzoyl peroxide (a disinfectant); sulfur (a mild antiseptic); boric acid (a toxic antiseptic); and camphor, menthol, eucalyptus, and clove oil. All of these are potential skin irritants. Some of these ingredients do make sense. Sulfur and benzoyl peroxide can help to disinfect skin that breaks out, and salicylic acid can peel the skin, which can keep pores from getting clogged. My concern is that almost all of these ingredients are too strong for the face and end up overly irritating the skin, making things even worse than before. There are gentler ways to do the same things. For example, alpha hydroxy acid products can do the same thing as salicylic acid with much less irritation.

But what are menthol, camphor, eucalyptus, clove oil, and boric acid used for in acne products? They have no positive effect on acne whatsoever. They only irritate the skin, which serves no purpose with any skin type, plus they make oily skin more oily. Alcohol is also used in many acne products. It is a very irritating and drying ingredient. It is not even a good disinfectant, because the concentration used isn't strong enough. Alcohol is something every skin type should avoid. Bottom line: If an acne product is working for you, stay with it. If your skin is red and irritated, still oily, and you still have blemishes (as most people do who use these products), reconsider what you are doing.

Above and beyond the standard promise of dried-up oil, cosmetics labels now flaunt a new promise for women who are prone to breakouts. Of course the promise is fatuous, but that's never stopped the cosmetics industry before. Buying a product that boldly claims it is "noncomedogenic" or "nonacnegenic," only to find it makes you break out, is aggravating. It is preposterous to assume that a combination of ingredients, particularly waxy ingredients (notorious for clogging pores), won't react on someone's skin. Those two terms have slowly but surely begun to replace "hypoallergenic" on cosmetics labels. Most consumers by now know that they have occasionally had an allergic reaction to cosmetics that said they were hypoallergenic. Hopefully, we can extrapolate from our previous experiences and recognize that these new cosmetics terms are just as meaningless.

INGREDIENTS YOU NEED AND DON'T NEED FOR OILY SKIN

The ingredients listed below are considered soothing, cleansing, or antiseptic for oily skin. They are also, for the most part, considered ingredients that won't cause blackheads. They may or may not work on your skin; there's no way to know in advance because each individual's skin reacts differently to the same ingredients.

The most beneficial ingredients to look for in products designed for oily skin are: allantoin, alpha hydroxy acid (glycolic or lactic acid), ammonium glycerhizinate, bentonite, butylene glycol, glycerin, hexylene glycol, kaolin, magnesium laureth sulfate, polyethylene glycol, propylene glycol, sodium laureth sulfate, sodium lauroyl sarcosinate, and triclosan.

It is harder to heal an oily, acned skin condition than we would like to believe, but that's the painful truth. There are steps you can take to calm down acne as well as steps you shouldn't take. But you can't completely eliminate the problem with products from the cosmetics counters or the drugstore—those of us who have acne and have tried everything have come to understand this.

Naming ingredients to avoid if you have oily skin is fairly controversial. Some of you are using products right now that contain several of these ingredients, and you may feel that your skin is doing just fine. So much for tests, and so much for my opinion. As I said, this is a complicated, tricky area of skin care. But if your skin is not doing well or you are experiencing skin irritation and you're wondering what to do about it, you may want to start by eliminating some products that contain the questionable ingredients in this list.

I can personally attest that skin care products containing irritating ingredients are usually more harmful than helpful. The list below contains ingredients that are recognized by most dermatologists and cosmetic chemists as causing breakouts—such as lanolin and isopropyl myristate—and those ingredients that I feel make oily skin worse—such as alcohol and camphor—because of the irritation they can cause.

The ingredients to avoid or disregard in products designed for oily skin if you are experiencing skin irritation are: acetone, acetylated lanolin, ammonium lauryl sulfate, benzalkonium chloride, benzoyl peroxide, camphor, isopropyl lanolate, isopropyl myristate, lanolin, lanolin acid, lanolin alcohol, magnesium lauryl sulfate, SD alcohol, shea butter, witch hazel, and zinc lauryl sulfate.

INGREDIENTS YOU NEED AND DON'T NEED FOR SENSITIVE SKIN

First of all, let me state plainly that to one extent or another we all have sensitive skin. Do not skip over this section because you think you have a tough exterior. At some time almost all of us will experience a skin reaction to something. You can prevent some skin reactions, however, if you are aware of what often causes them.

The best part of the cosmetics world is that many products just feel good on the skin. Silky smooth creams and lotions glide over the skin, leaving a dewy, moist gloss behind that can make skin look and feel beautiful and provide a blissful emotional lift as well. Same thing with makeup; as you artfully, or even not so artfully, apply an appealing shade of eyeshadow to your lid in a velvety soft tone that sets off the depth of your eyes perfectly, you may feel a surge of self-esteem as you admire the way you look. Now that's what makeup should be all about.

Unfortunately, for those of you with even slightly sensitive skin, finding products that enhance but don't irritate is indeed a challenge. I would love to list ingredients that I could guarantee won't cause your skin to flare up, but there is no single ingredient or combination of ingredients that can live up to that sweeping claim. Numerous combinations exist, in all sorts of mixtures and formulations, but what and how they will react on your skin is anyone's guess. Your only recourse, and this is not the best news, is to keep experimenting until you find what works for you. If you do get a reaction, stop using the product immediately, consult your physician if the reaction is serious or prolonged, return the products that are suspect, and keep track of the ingredients included in products to which you seem to be allergic. Also, just because you've used a cosmetic for a long time doesn't mean you won't develop an allergic reaction to it.

When you review the list of recommended ingredients and the list of ingredients to avoid in the dry and oily skin sections, it is vital to keep in mind that how much of a specific ingredient is contained in the product can determine how it will affect your skin. The less there is of an ingredient, the farther down in the ingredient list it is, the less likely you are to have a reaction to it. Just because the ingredient is suspect doesn't mean it will always cause problems. Listen to your skin and be cautious.

It is also important to understand that some potentially irritating ingredients, such as many preservatives present in cosmetics, are critical to the products' stability, but are not good for skin and are known to cause allergic reactions. But chemists have few options when it comes to preventing microbes from taking up residence in their products. Fragrances are another known source of skin irritations, and often they are used simply to mask the unpleasant odor of many cosmetic ingredients. But more often than not, particularly in cosmetics that have strong, noticeable scents, fragrances are used to increase sales. It appears that many cosmetics consumers want their lotions and creams to exude an obvious bouquet. That isn't the fault of the cosmetics companies, although it does reflect a need for consumer education. If you want perfume, use perfume, but choose skin care products that are fragrance-free!

It would be impossible to predict with any accuracy why, where, when, and how a single ingredient or a combination of ingredients in one of any number of products will affect your skin. When you consider the hundreds of chemicals a woman places on her face in such varied products as cleansers, toners, moisturizers, foundations, blushes, lipsticks, eyeshadows, and mascaras, it is surprising to realize how really safe and nonirritating cosmetics usually are.

Although I'm sure that many of you already are aware of this, it can never be said too often: if you have an allergic reaction of any kind to a cosmetic product, stop using it immediately and consult your physician if the problem persists. Do not hesitate to return the product to the place where you purchased it and get your money back. It is not your fault that the product caused you problems. Also, returning the product gives the cosmetics company essential information about how their formulas are working.

CANADIAN INGREDIENT LISTS: WHERE DO WE STAND?

In Canada, you can know what's in a $2 box of cereal, but you're left in the dark about a $60 moisturizer. Cosmetic products sold on the U.S. side of the border list ingredients, but when the boxes come up here the ingredient lists are nowhere to be found. It's one of the most frustrating things about shopping for cosmetics in Canada (and other parts of the world besides the United States). Manufacturers are not required to list ingredients, so they don't. If you're allergic to a certain chemical or want to avoid products with alcohol or are curious about what kind of preservatives are in a cosmetic, you're out of luck.

But take heart and take notice! The process of making ingredient lists mandatory is under way. In 1989, an informational letter sent to manufacturers outlining the government's intention to regulate labeling got the ball rolling. Or maybe I should say crawling. Like all government processes, this one is taking years, and finding out anything about its status is harder than pulling teeth. The informational letter was circulated so that manufacturers could peruse the information and comment. Their comments were always the same: the two-language requirement in Canada already takes up too much space; there's no more room. Of course, when you look at a box there is always plenty of room, but myopic vision can be a problem when the goal is to not give the consumer too much information.

The Health Protection Branch of Health and Welfare Canada, Pharmaceutical Assessment and Cosmetic Division, currently oversees cosmetics. They tell me that the manufacturers' responses are coming back and that the first draft of the government regulations is almost ready. There will then be a grace period of one to two years so that manufacturers can sell off their stock with the old labeling before bringing out the new.

On a more assertive note, the Canadian Cosmetic, Toiletry and Fragrance Association in Mississauga, Ontario, has suggested to its retailers that they keep orders to a minimum so they will have very little stock to sell off once regulations are in place. The process is in the works, the industry is committed to it, and we should see ingredients listed on all products within the next two years. It's possible that manufacturers may comply sooner, but don't hold your breath.

For now, if you have to know what's in a product, you are limited to the few lines that *do* list ingredients. I suggest that you concentrate your energies at those counters: Ultima II, Shiseido, Monteil, Clarins, Chanel, Borghese, Intelligent Skin Care, Prescriptives, La Prairie, Natural Sea Beauty, Fashion Fair, Juvena, Stendhal, and Beaute Benetton. Companies that are beginning to put ingredient lists on their products are: Lazlo, Marcelle, Max Factor, and Revlon. M.A.C. cosmetics and The Body Shop keep binders of ingredient lists at their counters, so be aware of this and ask to see them.

Though this process is under way, if you feel compelled to write, which you should do lest they drop the ball, you can write to: Dr. Norman Pound, Pharmaceutical Assessment and Cosmetic Division, Bureau of Non-Prescription Drugs, 355 River Road, Place Vanier, Ottawa, Ontario K1A 1B8, Canada.

Beauty Note: Canadians might not have ingredient lists on their products but the testers available in drugstores are very impressive. That makes shopping for inexpensive quality makeup much easier. Once Canada secures madatory ingredient listing on all cosmetics they will have the best of both worlds.

CHAPTER

T · H · R · E · E

Shopping Wisely

IT'S STILL A JUNGLE OUT THERE

There is only one way to get through the cosmetics jungle and that is to change the way you've shopped for cosmetics in the past. Even if you have read this list before, I encourage you to read it again. This is the only game plan that is going to keep your budget and sanity intact while maintaining the health and welfare of your skin. The main goal is to never leave the store with something you don't want, don't like, can't afford, or that doesn't work. There is no other way to be a better consumer when it comes to your cosmetic purchases. From my point of view, the worst thing consumers do is overbuy or buy something in vain hope. Following my recommendations in the review section of this book (see Chapter Nine) is a start, but even then you can search endlessly for the best product or get waylaid the next time you read a testimonial about the latest, newest, unequaled cosmetic creation.

1. You must be willing to change some of your beliefs about the world of skin care and makeup. A cosmetics company does not necessarily have your best interests at heart. As is true of most businesses, a cosmetics company's interest is the bottom line, and what you buy affects that bottom line. If you are willing to buy stuff that is overpriced, doesn't work, or isn't fashionable, they will keep selling it, because there is no reason for them to change. No one's pores have ever been closed by a toner, and no permanent wrinkle has gone away because of a wrinkle cream, but we continue to buy toners and wrinkle creams. So why should the cosmetics companies stop selling them?

2. Every cosmetics line has good and bad products. For the sake of emphasis, I repeat: Every cosmetics line has good and bad products. That includes skin care items as well as makeup. I have yet to find a cosmetics line anywhere in the world that is 100 percent or even 60 percent wonderful. All lines have their share of useless, overly perfumed, glaringly shiny, overpriced, and unreliable products. They also have products that work, but these products are often still overpriced. Also, just because a product works doesn't mean it is worth $50; there is certainly a $5 or $10 equivalent available elsewhere.

3. Give up line loyalty. It is great when you find a line that you are comfortable with. For example, you might like Prescriptives' lipsticks, foundations, and eyeshadows (only the nonshiny ones, right?) or you may prefer Clinique's blushers and foundations. That doesn't mean that every other product in those lines is also guaranteed to please you or be good for you. No matter how enthusiastic salespeople are about their terrific line, they are not unbiased bystanders; they have a vested interest in what you decide to buy.

4. Do not buy impulsively or quickly. You can take notes, wear a color for a while, take a sample of a skin care item, and then make a decision. In fact, buying a product you've just tried on and haven't worn for at least an hour or two is almost always a mistake. You have nothing to lose if you take your time and consider your purchase. How does it look in different light? How does it look and feel after it's been on your face for a while? I cannot tell you how many women I watched buy foundations, lipsticks, eyeshadows, or blushes after looking at them in store light that was little better than a dimly lit restaurant. The same was true for skin care products.

5. Cosmetics advertising may be alluring and interesting, but they are ads, not documentaries. Just because the ads are sensual doesn't mean the products featured in the ads are sensual, and it doesn't mean they'll make *you* more sensual. Accept seductive ads for what they are—seductive ads, not a reliable source of facts.

6. Trying to pretend you are above being affected by cosmetics advertising is to ignore a very, very powerful stimulus in all our lives. Cosmetics advertising, just like any advertising, is designed to make us buy that specific product or be attracted to that specific company. Whether we like it or not, advertising strongly affects the way we make decisions at the cosmetics counters. It is also unwise to ignore the fact that advertising sells products, and sells them very well, because the cosmetics companies wouldn't keep throwing money at something that produced no financial return. The next time you think you are not being affected by cosmetics advertising, think again.

7. Figure out your cosmetics budget and stick to it. There are excellent products available in all price ranges. A good cosmetics salesperson can sell you a line of skin care products for $200 before you know it. You'd like to think you're stronger than that and aren't capable of overspending to that extent, but we've all done it, and many of us have done it more than once. Admitting that you are weak in this regard and setting a solid, nonnegotiable limit on what you are willing to buy is your first step. The second step is sticking to it.

8. When it comes to cosmetics there are no miracle ingredients, trade secrets, exotic ingredients, or doctor-tested formulas that will permanently change the appearance of permanent wrinkles or keep the skin from wrinkling (this does not apply to sunscreens) or cure acne. I know I've said this before, but more than anything else it bears repeating. If there were a magic potion, it wouldn't stay under wraps. Every line would get their hands on it, just like they did with alpha hydroxy acids. Chemists are capable of analyzing a product's ingredients and duplicating whatever they want. Sophisticated technologies make reproducing a product's components as easy as assembling a jigsaw puzzle when all of the pieces are included. If one wrinkle cream really worked, it wouldn't take long for a million copies to show up on the market right behind it (and I would be one of the first people to tell you to buy it and give it a try).

9. Truly superior mascaras, foundations, lipsticks, blushes, and eyeshadows can be found in inexpensive lines. Formulations might vary and some products are better than others, but on the whole that is not reflected in the price. I found just as many great products at the drugstore as I did at the department store. Marketing creates the mystique of makeup. If spending $50 on foundation makes you look $50 better, then I guess it's worth it. But if spending $50 makes you look the same as if you had bought the $5 product, then I recommend that you reconsider your decision process.

SHOPPING FOR COSMETICS IN A DEPARTMENT STORE

There is something very intimidating yet elegant about shopping for cosmetics in a department store. The sales pressure is evident from the moment you approach the glass-and-chrome cases outlining the cosmetics area. The elegance lies in the pampered feeling you get from the earnest, helpful information and advice the salespeople provide. How can you have your cake and eat it too? How can you enjoy the luxury of the service without taking a bath in purchases? The following directives are essential to surviving makeup shopping.

1. Don't browse at the cosmetics counters; they are designed for spontaneous impulse shopping. Know ahead of time what you need or want. If you're looking for a lipstick, you should not leave with a mascara, eye cream, and lip liner. The worst question I hear women ask when shopping for makeup is: "What else do I need?" Also, don't get sucked into a standard sales technique where the cosmetics salesperson says, "Would you like to try our new_____? Everyone just loves it, it can change the metabolism of your skin to that of a teenager."

2. Have a mirror with you so that you can leave the store and look at yourself in the daylight. Never trust the interior lighting in the store. At almost every cosmetics counter the lighting is a bad joke. No matter how you stretch your face toward the light or adjust the mirror, it just isn't going to reflect what you need to see.

3. It is rarely necessary to change eyeshadows if you are wearing a good neutral eye design. Lipstick and blush can change to complement new colors of clothing, but the eye design can remain the same. If you are trying to match colors to a particular outfit, bring part of the outfit with you. Yes, it's a pain to bring it along, but the benefits of getting the right color outweigh the inconvenience of getting the wrong color.

4. Expect the product to live up to its claim and ask if you can return the product if it doesn't do whatever it is supposed to do. It is the best way to guarantee your satisfaction. Do not hesitate to return a product that doesn't live up to its claim—regardless of what the claim is. If the "signs of aging" don't go away, if the all-day lipstick barely makes it through the first coffee break, if the creaseless eyeshadow creases and the shineproof foundation shines, if the toner doesn't "refine" your pores and the promise of flawless skin is flawed, take it all back for a refund!

5. Remember that the salesperson does not necessarily know anything about makeup artistry or skin care. While researching cosmetics counters, I encountered many salespeople who chose the wrong foundation for me or selected skin care products that were inappropriate for my skin type. Quite often different products from the same cosmetics line would be recommended by different salespeople. What happens at the cosmetics counters often has nothing to do with expertise and everything to do with ringing up sales. To rely on what the cosmetics salesperson tells you about skin care or skin care products would be like getting a nutritional evaluation from a waitress or waiter.

6. If you are shopping for a foundation, do not wear a foundation to the store, or be prepared to take it off. Never, absolutely never, test a makeup product over the makeup you are wearing. If you can't persuade yourself to enter a store without wearing makeup, then use the moisturizer demos that are displayed on the counter to help rub it off when you get there.

7. Testing cosmetics is, in my opinion, one of the most important ways to discover what works best for you and what doesn't. But this is still a controversial issue. Concern over bacteria and germs is valid. A few companies offer small, individually packaged demo brushes; these neat giveaways, however, are not always available, so you can't count on being able to use them. Cotton balls and cotton swabs are available at most counters, but unfortunately they are terrible makeup applicators. Taking your own brushes is an option, but that makes things problematic for the next customer. Regardless of what you choose to do, always ask for clean demo brushes first. If they are not available, then use a cotton ball, cotton swab, or your fingers to apply the makeup so that you can at least get some idea of how the product will look on you. Once home, use a sponge to apply foundation and full-size brushes to apply eyeshadows and blushes.

8. Do not test colors on the back of your hand except when you're comparing colors to narrow down your choices. After selecting the colors that seem to blend well with your skin or look like what you had in mind, take the time to apply them on your face.

9. Always ask if you can have a sample of the product to try at home. More and more frequently, free samples are available at cosmetics counters.

SHOPPING FOR COSMETICS IN A DRUGSTORE

When I started reviewing drugstore cosmetics lines, I was surprised how much I liked the experience of shopping for cosmetics without anyone attempting to sell me products I didn't need or want. That was particularly true for skin care products. The frustration occurred when I was shopping for makeup items. Because of the way drugstore makeup products are displayed and packaged, the colors and textures are difficult to see, so there is no way to know exactly what you're buying.

Many of the drugstore products I tried were excellent, but testers are rarely available and free samples are almost nonexistent, so most of the time you are stuck guessing how a makeup color will look on you. Occasionally, I have seen cosmetics tester units at the drugstore, but they're not used consistently from store to store. Most of the product colors are displayed through clear plastic; seeing the color is helpful, but how it will look on your skin is uncertain. There are also products—lip pencils and eye pencils for example—where you can't see the color at all. In these cases, names or color swatches—and we all know how reliable they are—are the only references you can go by. Even simple names like "brown" or "pink" cover a wide range of variations.

My suggestions in the product review sections in Chapters Seven, Eight, and Nine will help, but in order to know how a product will really look on you, you'll have to wait until you get home. When you consider the expensive department store alternatives, it's often worth the risk. A bag of cosmetics costing $60 at the drugstore could contain 15 or 20 products, while at the department store $60 worth of cosmetics might include three to five. The pros and cons are obvious, but what should you do? My feeling is that there are some products that it makes no sense to buy at the department store, and others it makes no sense to buy at the drugstore.

The most difficult item to buy at the drugstore is foundation. I almost never recommend buying foundation that you can't try on and check in the daylight, but there are some suggestions in Chapter Six that will help if the cosmetics counters are just too expensive for your budget. Lipsticks and eyeshadows can also be tricky items to buy at the drugstore. Although I found that many cosmetics lines at the drugstore had excellent lipstick choices, it is very hard to judge how the color will end up looking on your lips. For those women who already have a good sense of what colors look best on them, the drugstore is a great place to shop for lipstick; those who aren't sure should go back to the department store. The problem with buying eyeshadows at the drugstore is the paltry selection of matte colors; most are just too shiny to recommend. But if you choose to wear shiny eye colors (although by now I hope I've talked you out of that fashion no-no because it makes the skin around the eye look wrinkled and crepy even when it isn't), there is absolutely no reason to pay $15 for them at the department store when you can buy the same thing for $3 at the drugstore.

There is no reason to buy mascara at the department store—the prices are absurd. I found several wonderful mascaras at the drugstore that were as good as, if not superior to, many of the department store brands I tested. This is also true for lip pencils and some eye pencils. The lip pencil colors are fairly standard, as are the textures and wearability. Eye pencils are more problematic, but some of the ones at the drugstore are identical to those at the department store. There is no reason to spend more than $3 to $5 on a pencil; any more is a blatant waste of money. If you follow my advice in the makeup review section you will discover this for yourself.

In terms of skin care, I can't encourage you strongly enough to avoid wasting money on expensive department store skin care items.

There is no reason in the world to believe that the cosmetics counter products are any better for your skin than those you can purchase at the drugstore. Read the ingredient labels and you'll understand why this is true. I know this is hard to swallow. After all, how could a $100 wrinkle cream be as good for your face as a $5 cream? But test this one yourself: use an expensive skin cream on one side of your face and one or two of my inexpensive suggestions (see Chapter Seven) on the other side. I will be surprised if you notice any difference at all, but please let me know if you do.

CAN YOU RETURN COSMETICS?

How many times in your life have you stood in your bathroom looking at all your unsatisfactory, unwanted, or "didn't work out" cosmetics? How many times have you felt guilty because you spent all that money, made the wrong choices, and now think there is nothing you can do about it?

Relax. Your regrettable cosmetics purchase blues can end. You do not have to throw out products that didn't work, turned out to be the wrong color, or caused an allergic reaction. There is another alternative to banishing these pariahs to the top shelf of the medicine cabinet to live out their lives in unused darkness. You do not have to feel guilty. You can be a savvy consumer. The truth of the matter is, *you can return cosmetics.*

Most women assume otherwise and would never think of returning cosmetics. When I began to research this book, I informally polled friends and acquaintances, asking them if they had ever returned any cosmetics. Without exception, every woman said to me, with great assurance, "Of course I've never returned cosmetics. You are not allowed to return them. If I choose the wrong color or if I don't think a product is working on my skin, it's *my* problem, *my* mistake. The cosmetics company is not responsible."

Absolutely not true. In fact, all cosmetics companies will accept returns or exchanges. They want your business, your goodwill, and your loyalty. And they don't want you saying critical things about them to friends. So, purely from a public relations viewpoint, it is in the companies' best interest to keep you happy. And if that means refunding your money, or replacing a defective product, or giving you another product of comparable value, they will do it.

It just makes good business sense, and it is also an ethical way to treat consumers. If a product is defective, certainly it is appropriate to replace it or refund the purchase price. Or, if a customer is dissatisfied with her selection, it is only decent not to make her pay for something she cannot use.

There are many reasons why women don't return cosmetics. Some of us feel that cosmetics are like underwear—nonreturnable once worn. Others assume that because cosmetics purchases involve so much *choice* (indeed, such arbitrary, irrational choices), they are irreversible decisions. Or (think carefully about this one) we feel guilty about the purchase in the first place and therefore would never consider asking for some adjustment (it's our fault we made such a foolish choice, we should have known better). It is also quite likely that we feel so intimidated by the experience of buying products at the cosmetics counters that returning something must be even worse.

All that is incorrect thinking. You can return cosmetics, and if you are returning responsibly and ethically, you *should* return. If you are seriously disappointed (a mascara wasn't supposed to smudge but did; a foundation was supposed to smooth over wrinkles but didn't) or you've have an allergic reaction, companies need to hear that. Simply never buying a company's products again does not help them (or other consumers) understand what they are doing wrong.

RETURNING AT THE STORE

To test my assumption that companies will return, I designed what I considered the ultimate test of a company's cooperativeness. I bought ten lipsticks from ten different companies in a wide range of prices—everything from a $21.50 Yves Saint Laurent lipstick at an elegant department store to a $3.50 Max Factor lipstick at a chain drugstore. After a week or two, I went back to each store, with my lipstick and its sales receipt, explained very simply in one sentence that I was unhappy with the color, and asked for a refund. *In every single case, except one, I was given a full refund, with no questions asked.* In the exceptional case, at YSL, the saleswoman said she could not give me a refund but would give me a replacement lipstick in a different shade. When I repeated the procedure at another YSL counter in a different department store, that store did give me a refund without any fuss.

It was that simple. The only hard part was overcoming my shyness. Basically, we are all too scared to ask for a refund or a replacement or to complain to a company about a product, and we shouldn't be. If you found that a lotion was too greasy or caused an unpleasant skin reaction, a moisturizer didn't moisturize, a color "turned" on you, a lipstick or pencil broke soon after purchase, a fragrance stained your clothes—any legitimate problem—then it is perfectly fair for you to complain and ask for a refund or a replacement.

The store returns the product to the manufacturer, who assumes the loss for the returned product, so don't feel you are hurting the store. Just be polite, clear, and responsible about your returns, and you'll probably be pleasantly surprised by the result. If the clerk refuses to accommodate your request, ask to speak to a manager. More than ever, both the manufacturers and the stores are very anxious to keep you as a customer, so they are usually willing to be cooperative. (And when you're talking about returning a $50 moisturizer that left your skin dry, that is by no means loose change.)

RETURNING TO THE MANUFACTURER

If you don't get satisfactory treatment in the store or if you made your purchase while traveling, write or call the manufacturer directly. The second phase of my research involved calling the cosmetics companies to present the same lipstick color question. (I also made several calls pretending to be unhappy with a "too heavy" moisturizer, and others pretending to be unhappy with a leaking fragrance bottle.) Because the results were so consistent, it is monotonous to report the specifics of those conversations. Rather, I can summarize easily: from Avon to Revlon to Chanel, *every single company responded in exactly the same way*. They will make a refund or replace any product that a customer complains about—whether it is a question of product defectiveness *or* "customer preference." The unequivocal answer is "Yes, we will take it back." (A list of phone numbers for almost all the consumer relations phone numbers of the cosmetics lines reviewed in this book is included in the appendix at the back of the book.)

Most of the companies prefer cleanly typed letters with a detailed explanation of your complaint. They also prefer that you return the product or its packaging with your letter; most will reimburse you for postage. (All cosmetics manufacturers are required to list their city and zip code on either the product or its packaging, so you can write to them even if you don't have a phone number or complete address.)

Every company has a phone number you can call if you would rather speak to someone about your problem. The phone staff can also be helpful if you're trying to track down your favorite discontinued color or looking for a store in your area that carries a particular product. In general, the people on the phones are not particularly informative about ingredients or "controversial" questions (that's why I wrote this book—to provide you with information that is not easily obtainable from the manufacturers), however, I found all the consumer relations representatives extremely polite and willing to listen to my complaints and take action to make me a happy customer.

If we do our part and become informed and assertive (proactive) consumers, manufacturers are more likely to do their part and create the very best products they can. Returning products and explaining our preferences and complaints is actually a way to educate manufacturers. We can tell them what we think, and hope all our talk leads—on their part—to real action.

Facing Skin Care Realistically

SKIN CARE UPDATE

As much as things have changed when it comes to skin care products available from the cosmetics industry, many things remain the same. The good news is such things as alpha hydroxy acids (AHAs), nonchemical sunscreens, gentle water-soluble cleansers, irritant-free toners, and a remarkable array of moisturizers. The bad news is the continuing procession of wrinkle cream products with the most preposterous claims imaginable and the accompanying pitch by the cosmetics salesperson. I almost get tired of reviewing these products. How many times can I say, "This product is an OK moisturizer but it won't prevent or alter a wrinkle on your face," or "This is a very good sunscreen but it won't alter a wrinkle on your face," or "This is an OK eye gel but it won't alter or prevent a wrinkle on your face."

Information about each individual skin care product is important, but it is also crucial to discuss the value of the different types of products and the needs of your particular skin type. I wrote extensively about this entire subject of skin care and skin care routines in *Blue Eyeshadow Should Absolutely Be Illegal.* I will summarize some of what is in that book and update the new developments you need to know about in order to obtain the best care possible for your skin.

Perhaps more than any other question I get asked, women want to know what is the best moisturizer available. Before you can make any skin care decision it is vital for you to understand that there is no "best" product out there. It would be great if I could say X is the absolute best cleanser or Y is the best moisturizer, but that is just not the case. This is particularly true for moisturizers.

The thousands of moisturizers with all sorts of names and descriptions all basically do the same thing: they keep the skin moist, so it isn't possible for there to be a best. There are many bests, and finding out which product is best for your skin takes some experimentation on your part, not mine. Quality comes down to what works for you and not what is the most expensive or reputedly the "best" product. I have talked to hundreds of women who have jumped from one expensive skin care line to another in a desperate search for the perfect routine, only to find that they were never satisfied. What they are looking for— the skin of someone younger or the prevention of what they fear most, wrinkles—is not attainable. You can have moist, soft skin, but it won't change a permanent wrinkle or the wrinkling process one iota. I am only one voice echoing in your ear, telling you to rethink what is truly possible, and that isn't always enough to compete with the glossy presentations the cosmetics companies present to you. If Lancome, Borghese, Estee Lauder, Avon, Revlon, L'Oreal, Orlane, Chanel, La Prairie, Oil of Olay, and the multitude of other cosmetics companies want you to believe that their anti-wrinkle creams, gels, and lotions might work, they can afford to sway you.

Another concept to examine is the basic merchandising premise most cosmetics lines share, and that is the claim of authenticity. Almost without exception every product line makes the same heroic claim about how it was formulated by a chemist, physician, pharmacist, dermatologist, makeup artist, actress or actor, or cancer specialist (and who knows who else?). These concerned professionals have formulated some remarkable, unprecedented skin care product or products that can do what others can't do for your skin. In each case the testimonials flow like water; women who are thrilled with their skin vouch they can hardly believe the difference. All lies or all truth? (Usually half lies, the rest truth.) Are the ultra-expensive products the only ones that really work and are all the rest a sham? (A lot of products in all price ranges work, but not to the degree the cosmetics lines want you to believe.)

Besides "unique" formulations and so-called medical expertise, another thing almost all product lines share in common is their lack of unique ingredients. I have yet to see one that contains anything unusual or rare that can impact the skin in any significant way. All cosmetics products are made from basically the same ingredients, but each has its own intriguing marketing twist to make it sound like you're getting something remarkable. The lists on most cosmetic products contain standard cosmetic ingredients, and then include essential oils, herb extracts, exotic proteins, or the latest water binding ingredient so they read like you are getting an exclusive elixir for your skin. Nothing could be further from the truth. All the herbs (usually in the form of tea), oils (essential or unessential), or any of a dozen wonder ingredients thrown into a cosmetic won't prevent wrinkles or change them. Many herbs and oils have exotic names, but you can extract oil or make a tea from any plant and that doesn't make it beneficial for the skin, particularly after it's been blended and preserved in a cosmetic.

WHAT CAN YOU BELIEVE?

Hopefully by now your skepticism about cosmetics and the cosmetics industry is firmly in place. However, you must be wondering, if you can't trust the cosmetics industry and all of its promises and claims aren't real—then what *is* real? What is and isn't possible when it comes to your skin? If you can ask these questions and accept the following premises, you are much less likely to ever be swayed by miraculous sounding skin care products again.

1. You can clean your skin but you can't "deep clean" it. You can't get inside a pore and clean it out like a dentist drilling. An expensive water-soluble cleanser will not make your face any cleaner nor is it necessarily any more gentle than the less expensive water-soluble cleansers. A gentle cleanser that cleans the face is essential; it should not dry out the skin or leave it feeling greasy. Many cleansers that claim they are water-soluble are really too greasy to rinse off completely and can cause clogged pores.

2. Spending more money does not affect the status of your skin. The amount of money you spend on skin care doesn't have anything to do with how your skin looks. However, what you use does. An expensive soap by Erno Laszlo is no better for your skin than an inexpensive bar soap such as Dove or Cetaphil Bar; an irritant-free toner by L'Oreal is just as good as an irritant-free toner by Lancome. Spending less won't hurt your skin, and spending more won't necessarily help it.

3. Getting a tan is a foolish thing to do and there's no way around this. If you are exposed to the sun, even for only 10 to 20 minutes a day, which includes walking to your car or talking to a neighbor outside, that cumulative exposure over the years will wrinkle your skin and there are no cosmetic products except a sunscreen with a high SPF that can change that. If that minimal exposure can wrinkle the skin, the impact of sunbathing is even more insidious. In short:

There is no such thing as careful tanning, safe tanning, or wrinkle-proof tanning.

4. The time and money spent obtaining perfect skin are damnable. Even the small minority of women who have "normal" skin will eventually have their share of breakouts and wrinkles. Trying to escape wrinkles and blemishes by slathering on facial masks, moisturizers, and other specialty creams (besides avoiding the exposure to the sun's ultraviolet radiation) is a fool's game. Those women who tend to break out will still break out, and those who tend to have oily skin will continue to have oily skin. If you try to "dry up" blemishes or dry up the oil on your skin, all you will have is dried-up skin that is still oily and still breaks out (as anyone with this skin type knows). There isn't anything at the cosmetics counters that can stop this—all the oil-control products in the world won't change a thing. (There are things you can do, but drying up blemishes and zits doesn't work.)

5. Ironically, a great number of skin care problems are caused by the skin care products women use most frequently to prevent them. Overly emollient moisturizers can clog pores, temporary face-lift products can cause wrinkles, and products designed to control oily skin can make skin oilier. Allergic reactions to cosmetics are often caused by using products that are too irritating, too drying, or too thick and creamy.

6. I know I've said this before, but it is a myth that is not going away: dry skin doesn't wrinkle any more or less than oily skin. Oily skin may *look* less dry, which means it can have a smoother appearance, but wrinkles are caused by sun exposure, genetic inheritance, or illness, not dry skin. All the moisturizers in the world won't change a wrinkle.

7. Your skin may become inflamed, dry, and blemished if you use too many scrubs or potentially irritating products at the same time. For example, a granular cleanser used with a loofah, a washcloth used with an abrasive scrub, an alpha hydroxy acid product used with a granular scrub, or an astringent that contains alcohol used with an alpha hydroxy acid product, can hurt the skin. If you use too many irritating products on your face at the same time, you are likely to develop skin irritations or breakouts. **Exfoliating the skin does not regenerate skin or build collagen.** It is good to exfoliate the skin and very important for almost any skin care routine, but exfoliation doesn't create new skin or get rid of wrinkles. It can smooth the skin and help moisturizers absorb better, but the effects are temporary, and it doesn't alter the skin.

8. For the most part, the fewer products you use on your skin, the better for your skin. The more you use the greater your chances of allergic reactions, cosmetic acne, and/or irritation.

9. Do not automatically buy skin care products based on your age. Many products on the market are supposedly designed for women who are 30, 40, or over 50. Before you buy into these arbitrary divisions you should ask yourself why the over-50 group always gets lumped together. Isn't it unlikely that women between the ages of 20 through 49 have skin that requires three categories but women over the age of 50 only need one? There are a lot of years between 50 and 90. According to this logic, someone who is 40 shouldn't be using the same products as someone who is 50, but someone who is 80 should be using the same products as someone who is 50. And what could a 30-year-old woman need different from a woman in her 40s? Age is not the largest influence on your skin. Categorizing products by decades is nothing more than a marketing device that sells products and does not benefit the skin. Skin has different needs based on how dry, sun-damaged, oily, sensitive, thin, blemished, or normal it is, and that has little to do with age. Plenty of young women have severely dry skin and plenty of older women have oily skin. Turning 50 does not mean a woman should assume that her skin is drying up and begin using overly emollient moisturizers or skin creams.

Beauty Note: Age can affect the skin more when a woman is in her middle to late 60s, 70s, and 80s. Skin does becomes thinner, oil production slows down, and cell turnover decreases. But nothing in a cosmetic or prescription drug can change the thinness of the skin, only a moisturizer can handle reduced oil production (and there are already plenty of those on the market), and exfoliation can take care of turnover (but it cannot make skin thicker). Nothing can change wrinkles or prevent the effects of aging, particularly the thinner skin. Hoping for more will only waste money. Why the age differential anyway? Because it sells more products to women who hope to stop age from affecting their skin. Bottom line: Putting an age on the product doesn't affect the ingredient list, which is all that counts in a cosmetic.

10. **Do not automatically buy skin care products based on your skin type.** I know that sounds strange, but there are several reasons for this. It's not that skin type isn't important, but more often than not, your skin type is not what you think it is. Possibly your skin type has been created by the products you are already using. Soap can severely dry the skin; a wrinkle cream can clog pores and cause blemishes; an alcohol-based toner can irritate the skin, causing combination skin. The only way to know what your skin type really is, is to start from square one with the basics: a water-soluble cleanser, irritant-free toner (or disinfectant if you break out), exfoliator, sunscreen for the daytime (which can be included in your moisturizer or foundation), and a moisturizer or alpha hydroxy acid product at night. If your skin is truly dry or you really are prone to breakouts, you can do the extra things, such as using a more emollient moisturizer at night, a more emollient foundation, or moisturizer with sunscreen during the day. For breakouts you may want to try a stronger alpha hydroxy acid product or use 3 percent hydrogen peroxide twice a day over blemishes.

Another problem is that products the cosmetics companies label as designed for a specific skin type might not really be good for your skin type. The way products for different skin types are formulated often can cause problems or make problem skin worse. Most skin care products made for oily skin types contain harsh ingredients that can make the skin oilier or cause breakouts. The same is true for products designed for someone with dry skin; the products can be so greasy they can actually make the skin look dull and also cause breakouts.

A final consideration concerning skin type is that your skin type can fluctuate. Skin care routines based on a specific skin type don't take into consideration that your skin changes according to the season, your emotions, the climate (humidity, dryness, cold, and heat all affect your skin), and your menstrual cycle. Pay attention to what your skin tells you it needs at any given time. This month you might need a moisturizer morning and night, next month only at night. The same is true for oily skin and breakouts. Don't hold fast to the idea of your skin fitting into one group—it changes and so should your skin care routine. That doesn't mean you need new products, it just means you may need to use less of one item or more of another.

11. **There are no products on the market that can close pores or clean them out.** Masks can't extract pores, astringents can't close them, and scrubs can't yank them out. The most coveted skin is that with no visible pores, but that skin type doesn't come in a bottle.

There are no cosmetics available anywhere that can close pores for any longer than a few minutes, after which they return to normal.

12. Teenagers are not the only ones who have acne. One of the biggest fallacies around is that women over the age of 20 should not have blemishes. What a joke. Women in their 30s, 40s, and 50s can have acne just like teenagers. Not everyone who has acne as a teenager will grow out of it, and if you had clear skin as a teenager it doesn't mean that you won't get acne later in life.

13.   One of the best ways to deal with extremely dry skin is to find a gentle skin care routine, not a greasy one. Someone with dry skin readily understands that she shouldn't use anything on her face that is drying or irritating, including washcloths, tissues, hot water, dry saunas, or skin care products with irritating ingredients. But it is equally bad for the skin to use products that are too greasy or thick on the skin. This can make the skin look dull and cause breakouts.

14.   The best way to calm down oily skin is to use a gentle skin care routine. Most skin care products designed for oily skin contain irritating ingredients that cause an increase in oil production, clogging the pores, which in turn may cause blackheads and breakouts.

15.   Oily skin types rarely require the use of a moisturizer. Specialty products such as oil-free moisturizers are not good for someone with oily skin. Most women with oily skin have enough of their own oil so that they don't need to worry about dry skin (unless the skin care products they are using dry out their skin). Oil-free moisturizers can be good for someone with normal to slightly dry skin, but they are a waste for someone with oily skin or someone who tends to break out. And oil is not the only ingredient in skin care products that can cause breakouts. Focusing just on oil narrows an area of concern. When should you consider using an oil-free moisturizer? Only if your skin is oily and truly dry in patches and the dryness isn't caused by other skin care products you may be using.

16. Facial masks, particularly expensive ones, are a waste of money. Facial masks, especially clay masks, simply peel off a layer of skin. That can temporarily make the skin feel smooth. Do you remember putting glue on the back of your hand when you were much younger, letting it dry, and then peeling it off? It made the back of your hand feel silky smooth. There was nothing unique about the glue, it just peeled a layer of dead skin off the hand. Masks work the same way. There is also nothing special about clay, whether it is from Europe, Israel, or Arizona. Minerals in the earth cannot be absorbed into the skin. It all sounds good, but it doesn't change skin for more than a few minutes. Using an exfoliant or an alpha hydroxy acid product on a regular basis can do the same thing without the mess, time, or extra money.

SKIN CARE BASICS—WHAT YOU REALLY NEED

By now you are ready to look more objectively at your skin and what it really needs. There aren't any obscure or miraculous formulas here, just options and some great products that can help you take care of your skin.

Here are the skin care basics: A water-soluble cleanser (never use an eye makeup remover or wipe-off cleanser); an exfoliating product (a scrub such as baking soda or an alpha hydroxy acid product); a disinfectant if you have blemishes, such as 3 percent hydrogen peroxide and/or an irritant-free toner; a moisturizer during the day that contains a sunscreen with an SPF of 15 (or a foundation that contains an SPF of 15 if you don't want to use a moisturizer) if you have dry skin.

If you have dry skin you may want to use a different moisturizer at night, but it isn't essential. The only real reasons to have different daytime and nighttime moisturizers is if your daytime moisturizer contains a sunscreen or if you want to use an alpha hydroxy acid at night only (you can wear an AHA product during the day, but you would still need a sunscreen in a foundation or another moisturizer). It isn't necessary to have a sunscreen in your nighttime moisturizer for obvious reasons. If you have very dry skin you may prefer to use a more emollient moisturizer at night than the one you use during the day, but again that is strictly personal preference.

Skin Care Basics

1. Water-soluble cleanser (no eye makeup removers).
2. Exfoliating product.
3. 3 percent hydrogen peroxide and/or an irritant-free toner.
4. A sunscreen for daytime either in a moisturizer if you have dry skin or in a foundation if you don't want to wear a moisturizer.
5. A moisturizer at night if you have dry skin.

Beauty Note: I recommend only moisturizer-based AHA products. The liquid and most of the gel AHA products contain alcohol, which dries the skin, so I do not recommend them. AHA products are used to exfoliate the skin, but because they are not a scrub they are applied during the moisturizing part of your skin care routine. Most people do not need an additional moisturizer. You can use an AHA product once or twice a day. If you find that the AHA product you are using does not leave your skin moist enough, you can also use a regular moisturizer at night and a regular moisturizer with sunscreen during the day. Apply the AHA product first, then wait 15 minutes before you apply the moisturizer.

Among the vast number of cleansers, toners, exfoliators, moisturizers, and sunscreens on the market are many good products. Yet we agonize over which company has developed the best ones, or which product contains the secret ingredients for procuring a peaches-and-cream complexion. I do not suggest for one moment that some benefit cannot be gained from the use of skin care products. In fact, they are very necessary, especially to women who wear makeup or are concerned about the sun. It's just that perfect skin—that carrot of hope dangled in the form of beautiful, overpriced containers and jars—is not possible. And, more so than any other facet of cosmetics, spending a lot of money to achieve perfect skin is a waste. If I can convince you that there is no reason to spend money on wrinkle creams it will save you vast sums over the long haul. Our concern about wrinkles lasts the longest because it takes quite a while to grow older, and your skin is always there for the ride. If you can stop spending on average $200 a year on expensive wrinkle creams, over a 30-year period that represents a savings of $6,000.

A GOOD REALISTIC SKIN CARE ROUTINE

Most skin care regimes are at best unrealistic. They are either too complicated or too contrived. The following routine is a way to change the unreal into the real. This means letting go of the fantasy and the hype and discovering what is honest and reliable. It isn't about getting back to basics, which is a comment I hear from a lot of cosmetics-weary women. They think soap and water is all they need, but using soap and water dries the skin and offers no protection from the sun. Getting real also doesn't mean mixing honey and avocado together in your kitchen. If it's too complicated you won't do it, because who has time for all that, it isn't convenient, food isn't great for the face, and what about sun protection. Getting real means doing what it takes to be good to your skin without wasting money, even if you have money to waste, and buying only products that live up to their claims.

The following list is a realistic, viable skin care routine free from gimmicks and selling techniques.

Step 1: Even at night, when you're removing makeup, always wash your face with a water-soluble cleanser that rinses off completely and doesn't irritate the eyes. Your eye makeup should come off with the same water-soluble cleanser that cleans your face. It shouldn't be necessary to use an extra product to wipe across the eye, pulling the skin and eyelashes unnecessarily. (Wiping off makeup in general is never good for the skin; wiping pulls at the skin and a tissue or washcloth can irritate it.)

Step 2: Rinse using only tepid to slightly warm water. Hot water burns the skin and cold water shocks it.

Step 3: Exfoliating the skin helps unclog pores and removes dead skin cells, benefitting dry skin and oily skin. If your skin is oily and tends to break out, after you've rinsed off your water-soluble cleanser, and while your face is still wet, pour a scant handful of baking soda into the palm of your hand. Add a small amount of water to the baking soda to create a paste. Gently massage your entire face with this paste, and then rinse generously with tepid water. Be extra careful not to get carried away: overscrubbing can cause more problems than it solves. The operative word for all skin care is "gentle."

You may want to try mixing the baking soda with Cetaphil Lotion, a very good water-soluble cleanser readily available at drugstores and many grocery stores. Any skin type can use Cetaphil Lotion mixed with baking soda instead of using the baking soda on the face alone. Mix 1 or 2 teaspoons of baking soda with 1 or 2 tablespoons of Cetaphil Lotion.

If you have **combination skin**, follow Step 3, but massage only those areas that tend to break out, and avoid the areas that are dry.

If you have **normal skin**, follow Step 3, but only three or four times a week.

If you have **dry skin**, use the baking soda mixed with Cetaphil Lotion only about once or twice a week. Rinse generously with tepid water.

If you have **extremely dry skin**, follow the advice for dry skin, but use even more Cetaphil and just a pinch of baking soda in your mixture and be very, very gentle when massaging your face. Repeat as often as needed.

Alpha hydroxy acid products are another alternative for exfoliating the skin, and many can double as moisturizer. I do not recommend most liquid or gel AHA products because they usually contain alcohol and can irritate the skin. If you use an AHA moisturizer, see Steps 6 and 7. Wait 15 minutes after cleansing your face before you apply the AHA lotion or cream.

Step 4: Now that your face is clean, this is the time to gently squeeze any blackheads or blemishes you want to remove. The only way to get rid of blackheads once you have them is to squeeze them out; they do not often get up and leave on their own. Blemishes can heal on their own, but relieving the pressure and contents can help them heal faster. If you are shocked by this suggestion, that's OK, you don't have to do this, but it does help. This is what most facialists do best for your skin, however, it is cheaper to do it yourself. Many people worry about making matters worse. The only way to prevent that from happening is to NEVER, absolutely NEVER oversqueeze. If the blemish does not respond easily, stop and leave it alone. Squeezing, in and of itself, does not cause problems on the face; in fact, it is one of the best ways to clean out the skin. The problems occur when you massacre the skin by squeezing to the point where you create scabs and sores on the face.

Step 5: When your face is completely rinsed and dried and you've finished any squeezing that you need to do, if you have problems with breakouts take a cotton ball soaked in 3 percent hydrogen peroxide and go over those areas that break out. Hydrogen peroxide works as a disinfectant over blemishes and bleaches the discoloration of black-heads. Do not use this step if you don't break out. You can use the 3 percent hydrogen peroxide in place of an astringent or toner once or twice a day.

If you have **normal to dry skin** that does not break out, rinse your face completely and go over it with a skin freshener or toner that does not contain alcohol or any other irritants. Most of these provide a pleasant sensation, but for the most part the more expensive ones are not worth their exorbitant price tag (especially when you consider that the basic ingredients are usually the same: water, glycerin, polypropy-lene glycol, polysorbate, dimethicone copolyol, and some herb extracts).

If you have **extremely oily skin** or **skin that breaks out frequently**, consider trying a facial mask of plain Phillips' Milk of Magnesia. Milk of Magnesia is a mixture of magnesium and water. Magnesium is a good disinfectant, and it can absorb oil. The clay masks for oily skin have no disinfecting properties, and their ingredients cannot absorb oil as well as magnesium. Your skin type and reaction to the mask will determine how often you can use it. Those with severely oily skin can use it every day; those with slightly oily skin should only need to use it once a week.

Step 6: During the day it is essential to wear a sunscreen with an SPF of 15. If you have normal to dry skin you need to wear a moisturizer. If you have normal to oily skin you do not need to wear a moisturizer. All skin types need to wear a sunscreen with an SPF of 15. Either your foundation or your moisturizer can contain the sunscreen. If you have oily skin a foundation with an SPF of 15 is great. Only one product should contain a sunscreen, not both.

If you want to wear an alpha hydroxy acid product during the day, use it as you would your moisturizer if it is a cream or lotion. Most alpha hydroxy acid products are designed to be moisturizers and can be used as such. (Some AHA products are in the form of astringents and would replace whatever toner you were using, but I do not recommend these because of their alcohol content.) The only difference in using an AHA moisturizer is that you apply it 15 minutes after you cleanse your face. Wait another 15 minutes before you apply your foundation or sunscreen. Be sure to read the section on alpha hydroxy acids following this list carefully before you run out and buy anything.

Step 7: Unless you have dry skin it is not necessary to wear a moisturizer at night. If you do choose to wear a moisturizer at night, apply a light lotion-type moisturizer to your face over a thin layer of water and allow it to be absorbed into your skin rather than rubbing it in. Heavy, creamy moisturizers are best only for extremely dry skin. Try the less expensive moisturizers available in drugstores before you venture into the higher-priced brands. You can use a thicker, more emollient-type moisturizer for the drier areas of your face, but just over those areas and just at night. A pure oil can do the same thing, but a cream may feel better and absorb more readily.

If you want to use an AHA moisturizer at night, it should be the only moisturizer you need. Wait 15 minutes after cleansing before you apply it. If you do choose to use an additional moisturizer or eye cream, wait another 15 minutes before you apply that one.

If you have severely dry, irritated, allergic, or red skin, you may want to consult a dermatologist. The cosmetics industry has limitations and cannot take care of all skin problems. If you have severe acne, consult your dermatologist about the use of Accutane (see Chapter Five). This is a serious, expensive drug to use, but its success rate in curing chronic acne is remarkable.

ALPHA HYDROXY ACIDS: THE NEW SKIN CARE SENSATION

If you haven't heard about alpha hydroxy acid, the latest unofficial skin care wonder ingredient, be patient—you will. Products containing this natural exfoliator are coming to the market fast and furious. The claim from most sources—including dermatologists, cosmetic chemists, and, of course, the companies making AHA products—is that regular AHA use can make the skin smoother, diminish wrinkles, and unclog pores. Quite a lot for one group of ingredients derived from such sources as sugarcane, but more about that later. The bottom line is, do they work? The good news is that most of the AHA products do, to some extent, live up to some of those intriguing claims. But below the bottom line, where the cosmetics companies begin, the whole topic gets exaggerated and quite confusing. It's not easy to undo the pretense, but it can be done.

There are five types of alpha hydroxy acid ingredients on the market: glycolic, lactic, malic, citric, and tartaric acids. The most commonly used are glycolic and lactic acids, because of their special ability to penetrate the skin. All of these are derived from very inexpensive natural sources such as sugarcane, sour milk, citrus fruits, apples, and grapes. Alpha hydroxy acids have been used in cosmetics for quite some time. What these acids can do is "unglue" (or burn off) the outer layer of dead skin cells and help increase cell turnover (exfoliation). As with most types of exfoliators (cosmetic scrubs, baking soda, washcloths, and Retin-A), removing this dead layer of skin can improve skin texture and color, unclog pores, and allow moisturizers to be better absorbed by the skin. The difference is that AHAs have more in common with Retin-A (retinoic acid derived from vitamin A) than with cosmetic scrubs, yet they are *not a drug*, so no prescription is necessary.

AHAs work much the way Retin-A does, in a chemical rather than physical process, by unglueing the skin on a deeper level. That means AHAs can possibly produce better results than cosmetic scrubs (which work only on the surface), and they are more readily available and gentler than Retin-A.

To say that cosmetics companies are jumping on the AHA bandwagon with both feet is an understatement, witness Avon's *Anew*, Biersdorf's *Eucerin Plus*, La Prairie's *Age Management Serum*, Elizabeth Arden's *Ceramide Time Complex Moisture Cream*, Neoteric's *Alpha Hydrox*, Murad's *Skin Smoothing Cream*, Estee Lauder's *Fruition*, and Herald Pharmacal's *Facial Lotion*. Some of these products can be purchased from drugstores and cosmetics counters while others are available through estheticians, physicians, and via mail order. A few companies claim their products contain AHAs, but won't give even basic information as to how much AHA is in the product. Chanel's consumer relations department (which we called several times) first told us their *Day Lifting Refining Complex* contains glycolic acid, but it isn't in the ingredient list; when asked, they said the name of the ingredient and the percentage used are confidential. (For $45 they should come up with some better information.) Elizabeth Arden's *Ceramide Time Complex Moisture Cream* contains HCA (hydroxycaprylic acid), a synthetic form of AHA that does not penetrate the skin the way glycolic or lactic acid can. HCA is good for moisturizing, but not much else. Sodium lactate, another form of AHA, is used in many products, including *Ceramide*. The salespeople will tell you it is the same as lactic acid. It isn't the same at all; it can be a good moisturizing ingredient, but it won't help exfoliate the skin.

Is there a difference between all these products? Yes, but it isn't in the name. The crucial information is the percentage of AHAs used in the formulation. Most important, *none of these products can prevent aging or can change a wrinkle.* They can smooth the skin, improve texture, and unclog pores, but they do not in any way prevent wrinkles or change deep, permanent wrinkles one bit.

What all of these companies would like you to believe is that after a few weeks you can expect a dramatic reduction of wrinkles and clogged pores, and near-flawless skin. Unfortunately, there are some major problems with those claims. All of the studies and clinical observations have been done by dermatologists, pharmacists, and chemists who directly profit from the success of these products. Their claims are impressive and persuasive, but you can't exactly call them objective. Furthermore, the test groups used have been extremely small, with fewer than 30 people, and usually with no established control groups. That is not a scientific base, nor is it enough to extrapolate to millions of women.

Despite the flawed information, there is still enough evidence to suggest that AHA products (depending on the percentage) can work for two main categories of skin problems: sun-damaged skin and skin that breaks out. How can AHAs help such disparate skin conditions as dry skin and acne, generally thought to be at opposite ends of the skin continuum? Good question.

Dry skin suffers from "hyper" skin-cell production that stacks up on the skin's surface, creating a flaky, dull appearance. Oily, acne-prone skin is aggravated by thick dead skin cells that block the pore and trap the oil inside, causing the pore to become clogged. With increased exfoliation, both dry skin and skin that breaks out can improve by removing dead skin cells that block absorption of moisturizers (dry skin) or block pores (oily skin).

The following are the most typical questions I am asked regarding AHA products:

How do you read AHA product labels? You can be sure that many companies are going to make claims about their AHA products. Glycolic acid and lactic acid have been around for some time as moisturizing ingredients or as ingredients used for acid balancing, so they aren't anything out of the ordinary. If a product is 1 percent to 4 percent glycolic or lactic acid, it is little more than a moisturizing ingredient. Less than 1 percent and the AHA works to balance the alkaline/acid level of a product. If a product is 5 percent to 7 percent AHA, there are those who say it is only somewhat effective as an exfoliator. For a very effective exfoliating product, look for one that is between 8 percent and 15 percent AHA. You won't be able to tell the AHA percentage from reading the label; you have to ask for that information specifically. Insist on getting a straight answer or don't buy the product.

There are several ingredient-list synonyms for both glycolic acid and lactic acid that you need to be aware of. The following indredients are different forms of glycolic acid: hydroxyacetic acid or alpha hydroxyacetic acid, hydroxyethanoic acid, ammonium alpha hydroxyethanoate, ammonium glycolate. Lactic acid counterparts are: 2-hydroxypropanoic acid and ammonium lactate. Regardless of the name, the percentage is the key to knowing what you are really buying.

How do you use the products? For most of the products, excluding the new department store cosmetics lines, the general recommended usage is to apply the AHA lotion, cream, or liquid solution to your face or any other area 15 minutes *after cleansing*. You can apply the AHA product *twice a day* if you want after each cleansing, but be sure to wait 15 minutes. (If your cleanser is alkaline it will negate the acid component of the AHA product, making it less effective. Waiting 20 minutes allows your face to return to its own acid balance, which won't affect the AHA product.)

You can apply the AHA product with either your fingers or, if you are using a liquid solution, with a cotton ball. Fifteen minutes after you have applied the AHA product, once it has dried or been absorbed, you can apply a daytime moisturizer and/or foundation (one that contains a sunscreen of SPF 15, of course) or a nighttime moisturizer. It is not essential or required to wear a moisturizer over an AHA product. That totally depends on your type of skin and how it reacts to AHAs. If you find that the AHA product is slightly drying out your skin you will probably want to wear a moisturizer, but the AHA product may be all you need. Of course, the cosmetics salespeople will tell you to use the AHA products along with their complete program, including two or three other moisturizers, but that is definitely not necessary. Be prepared for the hard sell when it comes to AHA products. Many cosmetics companies are treating this like the fountain of youth.

What about using moisturizers? You may be wondering how AHA products differ from a moisturizer or a scrub. Well, that depends on who you talk to and what kind of product you're using. Here's where it can get complicated. Most of the AHA products from cosmetics companies have just a little AHA (usually less than 5 percent), which is placed in a fairly emollient moisturizing base. These products may be all you need as far as a moisturizer is concerned and can be used twice a day, but they won't do much for exfoliating the skin. A product that is 8 percent AHA or more does produce mild exfoliation while you wear it. Remember, the acid unglues the skin through a gentle burn ("gentle" depends on the amount of AHA present and how your skin handles it) while it is on the skin. Some companies deal in specialty AHA products that contain a higher percentage (from 8 percent up to 15 percent), and the suggestion when using them is to continue using your regular moisturizer. Products designed for oily skin may require the use of a moisturizer, but that depends totally on your skin type and what happens your skin when you use an AHA product. In short, watch and listen to your skin; it will tell you what to do and what other products you need. You will not want to use an astringent or toner that contains alcohol or other cosmetic scrubs at the same time you are using an AHA product.

What does the FDA have to say about the AHA products? The majority of AHA products, even the professional-strength versions (except for prescription-only *Lac-Hydrin-5* and *Hydrin-12*), are currently classified as cosmetics, and that's exactly where the manufacturers would like to keep them. Safety review and legal standards for cosmetics manufacturers are almost nonexistent. On the other hand, safety testing for drugs is vastly more stringent. According to Dr. John Bailey, director of colors and cosmetics at the Food and Drug Administration (FDA), his department has an active interest in the AHA products. His main concerns are: (1) What are the effects on people with sensitive skin? (2) Since this is a "controlled burn," what are the long-term side effects? (3) What levels of concentration are safe and effective? These are good questions, but it will take some time before we have all the answers.

So far, the FDA has analyzed about 35 products. While the agency's study isn't complete, a spokesman did tell us that a trend is emerging from research data. "We're looking carefully at alpha hydroxy acid and glycolic acid products made by small entrepreneurial companies that derive authority from 'name' physicians and pharmacists," said Dr. Stanley Milstein, associate director of cosmetics at the FDA. "We're finding products from these sources with up to 70 percent concentration of AHAs, a level that is potentially corrosive to skin." Ouch!

Several brands of alpha hydroxy acid skin treatments are made or marketed by doctors. (They sell the products to salons and other doctors, who in turn sell to clients and patients.) These include Murad Skin Research products (based in California, although their products are manufactured by Connecticut's NeoStrata Company) and M.D. Formulations (made by Herald Pharmacal, Inc., of Virginia). Interesting to note: NeoStrata, which markets glycolic acid formulations to physicians, discontinued sales of its 50 percent and 70 percent glycolic acid just 13 days before the FDA advisory on skin peelers was issued.

What about alpha hydroxy lotions, gels, and creams from major cosmetics houses? Most contain low to moderate (2 percent to 4 percent) concentrations of AHAs, according to Dr. Milstein. This group includes Avon's *Anew Perfecting Complex for the Face,* Chanel's *Day Lift Refining Complex,* Elizabeth Arden's *Ceramides Time Complex,* Estee Lauder's *Fruition,* Guerlain's *Issima Aquaserum,* La Prairie's *Age Management Serum,* and Prescriptives' *All You Need.* None of them are all you need, and none of them are very good strong AHA products either.

Are there any side effects or precautions? Most people have a tingling or slight stinging sensation when they use glycolic acid products with concentrations of 8 percent or greater. Some people have had minor to severe problems with dryness and flaking using glycolic acid products. This is to be expected, given the nature of the ingredient. Most of the products tell you not to use it on your eyelids. Listen to your skin: if it gets dry and flaky, consider using a moisturizer; if it gets red and irritated, consider cutting back the frequency of use; and if your skin gets very dry and irritated, consider stopping altogether.

Severe irritation is not the goal or the desired result. And as you already know, wearing a sunscreen of at least SPF 15 for protection from further sun damage during the day is essential no matter what else you use on your face.

If you want to find out for yourself whether an AHA product can make a difference on your face, you need to know what is available. The prices range from less than $10 for a jar or bottle of Alpha Hydrox at your local drugstore, to $12 to $60 for mail-order products. How do you decide? First, keep in mind that only *one* AHA product is necessary, and it is probably best to start with an 8 percent to 12 percent concentration and see what happens. You do not need two, three, or four more products that contain varying levels of AHA. That is complete overkill. Remember, the percentage is what counts. The following section will give you a good idea of what is presently available and the levels of AHA in the product.

AHA SUMMARY

1. Products that contain high concentrations—8 percent to 15 percent—of AHA can mimic and possibly replace many of the effects of Retin-A.

2. AHA in concentrations of 1 percent to 4 percent is an excellent moisturizing ingredient, prevents moisture loss, and does not mimic Retin-A at all.

3. Most products on the market claiming to contain AHA contain less than a 2 percent concentration.

4. AHA products that contain less than 4 percent should be considered moisturizers and not sloughing agents, although some skin types may experience some peeling and tingling. That is OK and part of what AHAs are supposed to do. In larger concentrations AHA is primarily a peeling agent with some moisturizing effect. However, you should not experience severe irritation or blotching. If you do, discontinue use, return the product, and try one that contains less AHA.

5. Depending on your skin type and on the concentration of AHA in the product you are using (particularly ones containing 8 percent to 15 percent AHA), AHA products can be used once or twice a day. During the day you still need to wear an SPF 15 sunscreen (no one is currently making an SPF 15 sunscreen that also contain AHAs). When you use an AHA product it should be applied at least 15 minutes after cleansing your face. Wait an additional 15 minutes before you apply your sunscreen, foundation with sunscreen, or additional moisturizer.

6. Most AHA products do not require the additional use of a moisturizer. The AHA product already contains moisturizing ingredients. However, some AHA products contain alcohol or lack enough moisturizers for dry skin. In that case, you may need an accompanying moisturizer at night or during the day over drier areas. (I do not recommend any products that contain alcohol, including AHA products.)

7. One AHA product is all you need, used once or twice a day. Do not buy one for daytime and one for nighttime. What counts is the AHA percentage and the way the product feels on your skin.

8. AHA products designed for age spots (sun discoloration) often contain 8 percent AHA and hydroquinone. This is potentially a very drying combination of ingredients, but some women benefit from this type of product. It is worth a try to see if it works for you.

RETIN-A VERSUS ALPHA HYDROXY ACIDS

No more Retin-A? The big question everyone is asking: Are these AHA products a replacement for Retin-A? It depends on who you talk to. Some "experts" recommend AHA products along with Retin-A, while others suggest that it can be used totally alone instead of Retin-A. They do work in similar fashion (both are acids that unglue dead skin cells and encourage new cell growth) and both can help sun-damaged skin as well as skin that breaks out. The major difference, according to some, is simply that one is a relatively expensive prescription drug and the other is a cosmetic available over the counter. Are they interchangeable? That's hard to say. Right now, with all the promotion of AHA going on, it seems the answer is yes, but the proof isn't all in to buy an AHA product. Remember that skin can be sensitive to AHA too and Retin-A may be more effective for you.

Retin-A and alpha hydroxy acids have much in common. Both Retin-A and AHA products (8 percent or greater) can thin the outer layer of skin and, to some extent, improve the appearance of sun-damaged skin by smoothing the outer layer of skin. What is considered much more controversial and not yet proven is whether or not Retin-A or AHA products can stimulate the growth of collagen and elastin in the lower layers of skin. The evidence is meager on this one and is best summed up as "No way," but that doesn't change the positive effects of exfoliating the outer layer of skin.

Retin-A and AHA are both acids. Retin-A is derived from vitamin A and AHA is derived from sugar. Without getting too technical, both work as acids on the skin, causing the skin to shed its dead outer layer and making way for healthier skin to show through and come to the surface. The cycle of cell turnover can be problematic, particularly for those with oily, dry, or sun-damaged skin. Retin-A and AHA products can improve cell turnover. Retin-A is generally considered to be stronger and more irritating than AHA products. Unlike Retin-A, AHAs also have moisturizing properties so the chance of dry, irritated skin is actually much less with an AHA product than it is with Retin-A. The main issue with both of these products is the percentage used. A higher percentage means better results, but it can also mean increased irritation. This you have to monitor for yourself. If your skin becomes irritated you may have to use a lower concentration until the skin adapts to it, and then you can move on to a higher concentration. This is true for both Retin-A and AHA products.

One problem with both of these products is that once you stop using them your skin will revert back to the way it was before. No permanent change is produced or generated from using Retin-A or AHA products. The smooth exterior lasts only as long as you use them. This is one of the major reasons why researchers don't believe that either AHA or Retin-A changes the deeper layer of skin. If they did create more collagen and elastin in the skin the effects wouldn't be quite so temporary.

The FDA still hasn't approved Retin-A for use as an anti-photoaging (anti-sun-damaging) prescription drug. That prospect doesn't change anything for the consumer; it simply gives Johnson & Johnson (the maker of Retin-A) more outlets and gives other pharmaceutical companies room to make their own versions of Retin-A. Already Retin-A, as an FDA-approved acne treatment, can be prescribed for anything a dermatologist or physician deems necessary; the only restriction is that Johnson & Johnson can't market the drug specifically as a wrinkle cream. Obviously, there are immense loopholes in that restriction, or every woman and her sister wouldn't think of Retin-A as a wrinkle cream.

When it comes to Retin-A and AHA products, don't believe any of their wild claims. They are not a cure for wrinkles, and they do not take the place of staying out of the sun or getting a face-lift. But practical benefits can be gained from using Retin-A and AHA products.

Some women find it gives them rosier, smoother skin, diminished acne lesions, a reduction in the amount of superficial wrinkles, or a combination of all the above. The bottom line: Retin-A or AHA products may be worth a try if you are over 30 and have sun-damaged skin, or even if you're not. AHA is easier to get, so you might want to start there and see what happens.

Beauty Note: There is some very inconclusive evidence that Retin-A and possibly AHA products may someday prove useful as a step in combating some forms of skin cancer.

It is important to be careful when using both Retin-A and/or AHA products. This list is very important to review and learn:

1.You cannot tan after you start using Retin-A or an AHA product that contains an 8 percent or greater concentration for several reasons. As the skin peels and becomes somewhat thinner it becomes more sensitive to sunlight and is therefore more subject to serious sunburn. Also, tanning will negate any positive effects you hoped to gain from using Retin-A or AHAs.

2. Please remember that Retin-A and AHA products can irritate the skin, particularly Retin-A. If you use any other irritant on the skin at the same time you are using Retin-A, you will exacerbate the initial negative side effects of the drug. You must eliminate all of the following from your skin care routine during your first months of using Retin-A: washcloths, hot water, cold water, all astringents, toners, fresheners, clarifying lotions, refining lotions and the like, scrubs, facial masks, bar soaps, skin care products that contain fragrance or strong preservatives, saunas, steam rooms, and any and all products that contain alcohol. It is essential that you continue to use a fragrance-free moisturizer. This is not as urgent for AHA products because the concentration is not as potent as Retin-A. It is still best to stay away from many of the things listed above and to follow the skin care routine I laid out in the preceding section.

3.Many of the studies you read about Retin-A or AHA products are sponsored by the companies that make them such as Johnson & Johnson, the manufacturer of Retin-A, or Murad and NeoStrata, makers of AHA products. Obviously, these companies have a vested interest in proving that Retin-A and AHA products are indeed a treatment for wrinkles.

4. Do not think of Retin-A as a cosmetic. Do not borrow a tube of it from a friend or ask your children's pediatrician or your gynecologist for a prescription. Although I disagree with some of the things dermatologists recommend for skin care, I believe that they are the best source for Retin-A therapy.

5. If you want Retin-A or AHA products to work, you must use them regularly. To sustain the results, you must continue using them for the rest of your life. The changes that take place on the skin are not permanent. Once you stop using the product, the skin slowly reverts to its original condition. Using something forever is a scary proposition and a tremendous commitment. According to the women I've interviewed and who have written to me, the difference is positive enough to warrant the long-term relationship.

SUNSCREENS: THE ONLY REAL ANTI-WRINKLE CREAMS

As the sun rises on yet another day, summer or winter, you can be assured of at least one thing: confusion about what kind of sunscreen you need to adequately protect your skin from the sun's damaging rays. Many warm-weather enthusiasts apply sunscreen only to prevent sunburns (by now we all know sunburns are bad in addition to being painful), but what about getting a tan slowly without burning and what about sun exposure of any kind even if you don't get a tan? Is there such a thing as a safe tan? Is there such a thing as any safe sun exposure? If you use a sunscreen with an SPF of 8, is that good enough as long as you reapply it often? What if you try to avoid tanning at all costs and are absolutely diligent about using sunscreens, yet still get some color? How can that be when the sunscreen was applied just as the directions indicated and it had an SPF of 25 to boot? And what about the depletion of the ozone layer? How does that affect your skin? And last, in spite of the warnings, how can you really want to keep the sun off your skin when all the ads show beautifully tanned bodies having so much fun in the sun? After all, isn't that what summer or escaping to a tropic hideaway during the winter is all about: shedding the white pallor of winter for the glow of a radiant summer tan? Well, it may have been once, but it isn't anymore.

Important questions abound when it comes to sun safety, yet the answers are not always easy to come by. Understanding sun protection is clouded by complex technical information, an excess of products that promise all types of immunity, and, most disturbingly, the media's constant reminder that obtaining a golden brown tan is the beautiful thing to do. This is why things get complicated. The technical information involves understanding what the SPF number means, what the term "broad spectrum protection" represents, and what the differences are between chemical and nonchemical sunscreen ingredients. Add to that a huge number of sunscreen products, from gels and creams to oils and cosmetic products that contain sunscreen, and you should be getting lost by now.

First things first. There is no such thing as a safe tan or safe sun exposure. Ultraviolet (UV) radiation from the sun, in the form of UVA and UVB rays, are dangerous to the health of your skin. UVA rays penetrate the skin deeply and cause the skin to age, while UVB rays are responsible for sunburns and pose a long-term cancer risk. Due to the world's thinning ozone layer, which lets more of the sun's harmful rays break through the earth's atmosphere, concern about skin cancer is at an all-time high. There's no way around this, either. You are not taking good care of your skin if you prevent sunburn while still tanning slowly. A sunburn is only one form of sun damage; the other is a suntan. The effects of both are cumulative and insidious. Those of us who never wore sunscreen in our youth are seeing the damage of all those sun-baking years now, in our 30s, 40s, and 50s.

The price of unprotected sun exposure is wrinkles and possible skin cancer. To avoid paying it, keep the sun off your face as much as possible and as early as possible, even during the seasons when you think it doesn't count. *Ultraviolet radiation is present all year long, fall, winter, and spring. Wearing sunscreen every day, as you would wear a moisturizer, is the key, and the only way to adequately stop the sun from damaging your skin.* It doesn't help to think: "I'm not in the sun that much, I don't have to worry." Damage begins in the first 10 to 30 minutes of exposure.

Sunscreens are a remarkable invention. More than 30 chemical sunscreen ingredients have been approved by the FDA for use in a wide variety of products that can, to some extent, keep the sun off the face. These chemicals are rated by sun protection factor (SPF) numbers that start with 2 and go on up to 50. These SPF numbers are of the utmost importance. No other information on a product has meaning. A product can claim to prevent exposure to ultraviolet radiation, reduce sun damage, or eliminate environmental damage, and none of that information is reliable unless it is accompanied by an SPF number. Only products with an SPF number have complied with the FDA's regulations regarding efficacy.

One of the many approved chemical sunscreens on the market is PABA [paraaminobenzoic acid]. You may have noticed several sunscreen products labeled as PABA-free. Although highly effective as a sunscreen, PABA also caused a high percentage of allergic reactions. Dermatologists and other physicians began recommending that their patients avoid PABA, and its harmful reputation eventually became well established. Most companies no longer use PABA, but it is still wise to check the ingredient list of the product you're considering and be sure it isn't there. PABA is not the only culprit when it comes to allergic reactions. Many people have trouble finding a sunscreen they aren't allergic to. Be patient and keep experimenting—there is one out there with the right combination of ingredients for you.

Understanding sunscreens is probably the most essential component of good skin care. If you don't want wrinkles you must learn the truth about sunscreens. The following answers will help you do just that.

What's the difference between expensive and inexpensive sunscreens if their SPF number is the same? Regardless of the price or promises, all SPF-rated products are created equal as long as the SPF numbers are the same. There is positively no difference between an expensive sunscreen with an SPF of 15 and an inexpensive sunscreen with an SPF of 15. Price has nothing to do with it. In fact, because liberal application is a major element of correctly applying a sunscreen, you are more likely to use the proper amount with a less expensive product than you are with a more expensive one, which means you will get more protection from the bargain brand. Sunscreens purchased at the drugstore will provide your skin with the exact same protection as department store sunscreen if the SPF number is the same.

Does the kind of base the sunscreen comes in make a difference? Not one little bit. Cream, lotion, gel, oil, and oil-free products all provide equal protection under the sun as long as the SPF numbers are the same. Deciding which one to use depends only on what you prefer having on your skin.

What, exactly, does the SPF number mean? Unfortunately, sunscreens were designed to protect the skin from UVB rays only and not UVA rays. *All SPF numbers refer to how long you can stay in the sun before you get burned by UVB rays. They don't tell you how long you can stay in the sun before you will be adversely affected by UVA rays.* This is where "broad spectrum protection" comes into play. Many products use this term because they want you to believe that their product can protect against both UVA and UVB rays, but that simply is not the case. There are no reliable tests presently available that prove a sunscreen can stop UVA rays from infiltrating the skin's exterior. Photoplex and Filteray, which have the blessing of many dermatologists and the FDA for being strong sunscreens, have a higher risk of irritation then most.

If you can't believe claims about broad spectrum protection, why should you bother wearing a sunscreen? Because it is still essential to prevent a sunburn caused by UVB rays.

What SPF number is best for you? The SPF number indicates the length of time someone can be in the sun without getting a burn while wearing that specific SPF-rated sunscreen. Let's say that normally after 20 minutes in the sun you get a burn. If you apply a sunscreen with an SPF of 8, you can stay in the sun eight times longer than if you weren't wearing a sunscreen before you burn (approximately two and a half hours). If you wear a sunscreen with an SPF of 15, you can stay in the sun 15 times longer before you begin to burn (approximately five hours). Keep in mind that everyone's complexion is different, and circumstances—skin type, time of day, time of year, and altitude—vary greatly. A fair-skinned Caucasian who goes out in the sun at 12 P.M. at a 5,000-foot elevation stands a good chance of beginning to burn within 10 minutes of exposure. Take that same person but change the time of day to 10 A.M. and the elevation to sea level and it may take 25 minutes before the skin begins to be affected.

What if you don't know how long it takes you to burn? Dermatologists use a standard six-point scale to determine skin type and response to sun exposure. This isn't an exact measurement, but it should help give you an idea of how much protection you may really need.

Type 1 has fair skin with blue or green eyes and light blond or red hair; typical time for skin to burn—10 to 20 minutes.

Type 2 has fair skin with ash blond, deep red, or light brown hair, and deep blue, hazel, or brown eyes; typical time for skin to burn—15 to 30 minutes.

Type 3 has medium skin with brown hair and brown eyes; typical time for skin to burn—20 to 40 minutes.

Type 4 has medium to light brown skin, dark brown hair and eyes; typical time for skin to burn—25 to 50 minutes.

Type 5 has light to medium golden brown skin, black hair, and dark brown eyes; typical time for skin to burn—30 to 60 minutes.

Type 6 has brown to deepest brown skin, black hair, and dark brown eyes; typical time for skin to burn—40 to 75 minutes.

One of the critical aspects of sunscreen is frequent reapplication when you are active or swimming. (Important reminder: Be sure to apply sunscreen to your lips, ears, back of neck, hairline, and tops of feet. The places you miss can get badly burned if they are exposed to the light of the summer sun.)

The American Academy of Dermatology and the Skin Cancer Foundation recommend the use of products with an SPF of at least 15 or higher. Complete protection is the goal because that is the only way to stop the adverse effects of the sun.

What about sunscreens rated SPF 25 to 50? Are they the ultimate in sun protection? Many experts say there is no reason to use a sunscreen with an SPF greater than 20 because there just isn't enough daylight to warrant a larger number. Remember, a larger number doesn't mean greater protection, it only means *longer* protection. If there aren't that many hours of sunlight in a day, the protection is wasted. The higher the number also means the greater the amount of sunscreen chemicals in the product, with a stronger likelihood of an allergic reaction or at least a more sticky-feeling product.

Why might you still be getting tan if you are diligent about applying liberal amounts of sunscreen with a high SPF number? Part of the problem, which is not in your control, is the lack of protection chemical sunscreens provide against UVA rays, which can cause the skin to tan. What is in your control, but you may not be doing, is reapplying your sunscreen frequently if you perspire or swim. Also, be sure to apply sunscreen at least 20 minutes before you expose your skin to the sun. Waiting until you get to your destination allows plenty of time for sun damage to start taking place.

Consumers have definitely become more aware over the past ten years of the hazards of sun exposure. As a result, in a relatively short period of time we've radically changed the way we look at the sun. Where once we purchased oils and aluminum sun-reflectors to increase the sun's potency, we now look for sunscreens with higher SPF numbers to reduce the possible consequences. Johnson & Johnson's Consumer Information Department said they are selling more sunscreen products with an SPF 15 than ever before. That's the good news. However, according to the American Academy of Dermatology, statistics indicate that skin cancer is still on the increase. Hopefully, as we become more educated about sun protection and young consumers start using them it earlier, our skin can beat the odds.

THE NEW BARRIER TECHNOLOGY

If you feel that it is more complicated to go out in the sun than it should be, you'd be absolutely justified in your frustration. Be patient. It is about to get simpler. The best current news in the sunscreen world is the arrival of products containing a nonchemical sunscreen that works as a physical barrier against the sun instead of absorbing the rays as all the other existing chemical sunscreens do. These nonchemical sunscreens contain the rather mundane cosmetic ingredient titanium dioxide. In the FDA's original guidelines for sunscreens back in 1978, titanium dioxide was approved as a "blocker" screen that "scatters" or deflects the rays before they can damage skin cells. Because it works as a block, forming an opaque blanket over the skin much as its sister ingredient, zinc oxide, does (zinc oxide is the thick white stuff you often see smeared over sun-weary noses and cheeks at the beach), many experts believe that titanium dioxide-based sunscreens protect skin from UVA as well as UVB rays. Not only does it seem to provide complete sun protection, but it doesn't cause any of the irritation chemical sunscreens do. Titanium dioxide-based sunscreens also won't burn eyes. What took so long to bring this nonchemical wonder to the attention of sunscreen makers everywhere?

While some sunscreens in the past have combined conventional chemical ("absorber") screens with titanium dioxide, until the past year none have relied solely on their blocking substance. The problem with titanium dioxide is it can leave a white film on the face, making the skin look slightly chalky. It also has a greasy feel, much like zinc oxide. Happily, titanium dioxide can be micronized to the point where it can protect from the sun and not look white. This technology is still in its infancy, so you won't find many of these nonchemical sunscreens presently on the market, and of those that are available some can leave a slight to noticeable white cast to your skin. Almay's *Eye Protector SPF 15*, Clinique's *Cityblock SPF 13*, Johnson & Johnson's *Baby Sunblock No More Tears Formula SPF 20*, Physicians Formula's *Non-Chemical Sunscreen SPF 15*, Neutrogena's *Chemical Free Sun Blocker SPF 17*, and Origins' *Let the Sun Shine SPF 14 Non-Chemical Sunscreen* all have varying degrees of clarity on the skin. Elizabeth Arden and Estee Lauder both have several different nonchemical sunscreens available in different strengths.

SUNSCREENS AT THE COSMETICS COUNTER

Everything from foundations and moisturizers to lipsticks and face powder contain sunscreens nowadays. In all price ranges, from Coppertone to Bain de Soleil, L'Oreal to Clarion, and Physicians Formula at the drugstore to Lancome, Prescriptives, and Estee Lauder at the department store, you can hardly avoid the onslaught of sunscreens in cosmetics. Is there any difference between a cosmetic (i.e., a moisturizer or foundation) that contains a sunscreen versus a sunscreen designed for the beach or all over the body, and does price make a difference? As I've said before, as long as the products sport the same SPF number (preferably an SPF of 15 or greater), there is no difference whatsoever between the protection the products impart. The cosmetics industry has actually provided a wonderful service by introducing much-needed sunscreens into women's daily skin care or makeup routines. Women with oily skin who dislike the feel of a cream, lotion, or gel-type product on their skin, even one that claims to be oil-free, will love the advantage of an oil-free, nonchemical, titanium dioxide-based foundation that contains an SPF of 15 such as the one Clinique makes.

Unfortunately, many skin care and makeup products contain only minimal sunscreen, usually less than SPF 8 and often less than SPF 4, which isn't considered adequate protection. If you are careful about watching numbers and remember that all the sunscreen rules mentioned above apply equally in the world of cosmetics (such as a foundation with sunscreen must be reapplied if you perspire), you will do fine with all cosmetic products that contain sunscreens of SPF 15 or greater.

Fashion Warning: All the cautions and information about the sun and its ill effects have little meaning, particularly for teenagers, when ads parade deeply tanned men and women in skimpy bathing suits glorifying a bronze veneer. You can't hope to educate young people (or adults for that matter) about the risks of prematurely wrinkled skin and, even worse, skin cancer, if the media continually tempts them to tan.

And it isn't enough to have a terrific tan only during the summer when tanning salons sell "fake" year-round tans. Consumers are often misled into believing that tanning machines somehow use only "safe" ultraviolet radiation. Nothing could be further from the truth. *There is no such thing as safe ultraviolet radiation.* Maintaining a year-round tan only increases the risk of sun damage, and there is nothing fake about that. Yes, tanned skin can look beautiful, but it can also cause skin cancer and wrinkles—and that's something the ads don't show.

FREE RADICALS—THE NEXT (AND POSSIBLY FINAL) STEP IN COMBATING WRINKLES

Stories in all types of media have heralded the elimination of free-radical damage as the fountain of youth for the '90s. According to many skin experts, all aspects of aging, including wrinkling, are caused by free-radical damage. Vitamin companies and cosmetics companies alike use the term and want you to believe that they can eliminate it. The evidence is fairly convincing that free-radical damage is an insidious "natural" process that causes the body to break down. What isn't known is whether or not you can really stop free-radical damage from taking place.

Explaining free-radical damage is like trying to explain how television works. No matter how many times I've heard how transmission happens, all I know is that I can watch television whenever I turn it on. Nevertheless, here's a simplified explanation of free-radical damage.

Free-radical damage has to do with oxygen and ultraviolet radiation. Oxygen molecules are generally stable, but when they become unstable, due primarily to the presence of ultraviolet radiation and other unspecified molecules, the unstable oxygen molecules run around and grab other molecules as a way to become stabilized. What happens then is that those other molecules also become unstable and grab other molecules to become stabilized. This chain reaction can go on indefinitely. There seems to be primarily one way to stop it, but I'll get to that in a minute.

A good example of how free-radical damage takes place is paint. When paint is shut off from air in a sealed container it remains liquid. When it is exposed to air (oxygen) it hardens. What takes place is that an unstable oxygen molecule gets into the exposed paint and goes to work on the paint's molecules, changing their form. These molecules also become unstable and in turn run around grabbing all the other molecules, resulting in solid paint. Actually, to refer to this process as damaging can be misleading. Free-radical damage is a major life function of things such plants as well as the human body. Immune systems, metabolism, cells communicating with each other, and collagen production are all affected by the presence of free-radical damage. So what does that have to do with aging? When the free-radical process continues unrestrained it can cause systems to break down. Instead of building collagen, free-radical damage can destroy it, and the same is true for all aspects of human physiology. How can you control free-radical damage so you only get the good results and none of the bad? That's the $64,000 question.

What stops free-radical damage from going too far is the presence of free-radical scavengers. As silly as that sounds, they really do exist, and they stop or, a better term, eat free radicals. These scavengers are better known as antioxidants. Antioxidants keep air (specifically, the unstable oxygen molecule) from interacting with other molecules and causing them to degenerate. What kind of antioxidants does it take to do the job? Most forms of vitamin E (tocopherol), vitamin C (ascorbic acid), and vitamin A (retinyl palmitate). Whether you take these orally or apply them in your moisturizer, they supposedly can reduce free-radical damage. The only problem with this theory is that free-radical damage is constant and extensive. How could you ever use enough moisturizer or take enough vitamins to stop it? Conversely, you would never want to stop all of it. Scientists have no idea how much is too much free-radical damage.

Major research is yet to be done in this fascinating area of human aging, but a lot of people are working on it. In the meantime, if you want to get a jump on things, check the back of your moisturizer and see if it contains any free-radical scavengers. Almost every company from Avon to Lancome makes moisturizers that contain antioxidants, so they aren't hard to find. You won't see any difference in your skin, but if free-radical damage can be slowed and the destruction of collagen and elastin can be prevented, this should help. It's a long shot, but many scientists think if there is a fountain of youth, this could be it.

Beauty Note: Because of its composition, hydrogen peroxide is considered a free radical and there are those who think it has negative side effects on the skin. Their point is well taken, but I don't agree that the negative impact is significant and I still consider 3 percent hydrogen an effective disinfectant for acne lesions. There are also those experts who consider soap and water as effective a disinfectant as 3 percent hydrogen peroxide. Again I disagree (as do some physicians), but you should know this so you can make the best decision for your skin. If you have acne I encourage you to try the 3 percent hydrogen peroxide and see if it works for you.

Clearing the Air— Acne Products

OVER-THE-COUNTER ACNE PRODUCTS

Horror of horrors! Another blemish. Why me? I'd give anything for clear skin. Blackheads abound and you could drill for oil on my face. I thought I had outgrown this stuff; doesn't it ever end?

Does this sound familiar? It has happened to a lot of us at one time or another; to many of us it happens all the time, as it does to me, and it doesn't go away at 20 or 30. It can even start at 40. Whenever endless breakouts besiege the face, a defensive counterattack begins almost immediately. The first line of assault is more often than not the drugstore shelves where the acne products reside.

In our search for relief from the emotional and physical discomfort that often accompanies acne, we turn to the myriad products that promise to "zap zits" and give us clear skin. The commercials and ads sound fairly convincing, but a closer look reveals that these products can't zap zits or even stop them from occurring, and the irritation they cause can create more problems than they clear up.

These products claim they are designed for skin that breaks out, offering choices for oily, dry, and sensitive skin. But read the label, where the real information is, and you'll find an array of ingredients that can often make acne worse and cause problems for sensitive skin. Several main ingredients show up repeatedly: salicylic acid (a peeling agent); benzoyl peroxide (a disinfectant); sulfur (a mild antiseptic); boric acid (a toxic antiseptic); and camphor, menthol, eucalyptus, and clove oil (all skin irritants). Including some of these ingredients does make sense. Sulfur and benzoyl peroxide help to disinfect skin that breaks out, and salicylic acid can peel the skin, which can possibly keep pores from getting clogged. My concern is that almost all of these ingredients are too strong for the face and end up overly irritating the skin, making things worse than before. There are gentler ways to do the same things. For example, alpha hydroxy acid products can do the same thing as salicylic acid, and with much less irritation.

And what are menthol, camphor, eucalyptus, clove oil, and boric acid used for in acne products? They have no positive effect on acne whatsoever. They only irritate the skin, which serves no purpose on any skin type and makes oily skin more oily. Alcohol is also used in almost all of the products listed below. It is very irritating and drying. It is not even a good disinfectant, because the products don't include enough of it. Alcohol is something every skin type should avoid. Bottom line: If an acne product is working for you, stay with it. If your skin is red and irritated, still oily, and you still have blemishes, reconsider what you are doing. And don't assume that because one or two acne products didn't work, that you should continue looking for another product that might work. As you read the product reviews below, notice how similar they all are. Bouncing from one product to another won't help when they all contain basically the same things.

Beauty note: Benzoyl peroxide has been a major player in the fight against acne for both prescription and over-the-counter acne products. It is indeed a good disinfectant and can be helpful for some types of acne, even though it is potentially quite irritating. Studies in the recent past have suggested that benzoyl peroxide is a possible carcinogen. There is significant research that also indicates the opposite is true. Most dermatologists still recommend benzoyl peroxide and contend that the evidence is on the side of it being safe to use. However, a small number of dermatologists also recommend 3 percent hydrogen peroxide solution. As you know, I also encourage the latter.

Adult Care Medicated Blemish Cream (*0.6 ounce for $3.40*) contains sulfur (an antiseptic), resorcinol (an antiseptic), water, clay, thickeners, preservatives, fragrance, and coloring agent. There is nothing particularly adult about this product, but it can be quite irritating to the skin.

Adult Care Medicated Cover Stick (*0.125 ounce for $3.43*) contains ingredients similar to those in the cream, only in a stick form. The same caution applies.

Apri Apricot Facial Scrub, Gentle Formula (*2 ounces for $4.29*) contains mostly water, walnut shell powder, detergent cleansers, apricot seeds, thickeners, more detergent cleansers, apricot oil, lanolin oil (can cause breakouts and allergic reactions), magnesium powder (can absorb oil), water binding agent, thickener, preservatives, allantoin (can help skin to heal), glycerin, tocopherol (vitamin E oil), and aloe extract. The aloe and tocopherol are too far down in the ingredient list to have much effect and the lanolin oil isn't great for someone who has problems with breakouts.

Apri Apricot Facial Scrub, Original Formula *(2 ounces for $4.29)* has almost the exact same ingredient list as the scrub above minus the oils, which makes it much better for the skin. As an exfoliant this isn't bad, but Cetaphil Lotion mixed with baking soda is much better and doesn't contain so many wax thickeners, which can clog pores.

Aveeno Natural Colloidal Oatmeal Cleansing Bar for Dry Skin *(3 ounces for $2.99)* is about 50 percent oatmeal, along with detergent cleanser, vegetable oil, vegetable shortening, glycerin, thickener, detergent cleanser, humectants, preservative, and thickener. This is a fairly gentle bar soap. Chances of irritation are minimal, but oatmeal can't do anything to change acne or oily skin.

Aveeno Natural Colloidal Oatmeal Cleansing Bar for Combination Skin *(3 ounces for $2.99)* is almost identical to the one above except for the addition of petrolatum. Fairly gentle.

Aveeno Natural Colloidal Oatmeal Cleansing Bar for Acne *(3 ounces for $2.99)* is almost identical to the other two Aveeno soaps, but this one contains salicylic acid, which can be very irritating to the skin and should not be used near the eyes.

Aveeno Acne-Aid Cleansing Bar *(4 ounces for $3.29)* is a more traditional bar soap made out of sodium tallowate (can cause blackheads and irritation), detergent cleanser, mineral oil, salt (can be an irritant), lye cleanser (irritating to skin), and quaternium-15 (considered one of the most irritating preservatives used in cosmetics). This not only won't aid acne, it will make the skin quite irritated and possibly worse.

Avon Clearskin Antibacterial Scrub *(2.5 ounces for $2.99)* contains mostly water, slip agent, vegetable oil, mineral oil, thickener, glycerin, more thickener, alcohol, detergent cleanser, menthol, and a blue salt coloring agent. As a scrub it is OK, but the oils are not great for anyone with oily skin, and the menthol and alcohol are irritating.

Avon Clearskin Maximum Strength Cleansing Pads *(42 pads for $3.49)* contains salicylic acid (skin irritant and peeling agent), water, alcohol, witch hazel (skin irritant), an antiseptic, preservative, fragrance, menthol (skin irritant), aloe, and tocopherol. Too strong and drying for most skin types, particularly in association with any of the other Clearskin products.

Avon Clearskin Astringent Cleansing Lotion *(8 ounces for*

$3.49) contains alcohol, antiseptic (can be irritating), water, slip agents, antiseptic (can be irritating), isopropyl myristate (can cause breakouts), and coloring agent. This is too drying and irritating for most skin types; the inclusion of isopropyl myristate is a mystery.

Avon Clearskin Foaming Facial Cleanser *(4 ounces for $3.29)* contains water, detergent cleansers, coloring agent, preservatives, salt (skin irritant), and menthol (skin irritant). Can be irritating for most skin types, but may be OK for younger skin.

Avon Clearskin Clarifying Mask *(4 ounces for $3.49)* contains water, a cosmetic plastic, alcohol, an ingredient that turns the mask hard, preservative, and coloring agent. Just a drying mask that can cause more problems for skin.

Avon Clearskin Vanishing Cream *(0.75 ounce for $3.39)* contains water, slip agent, thickener, preservative, sodium hydroxide (caustic detergent), and benzoyl peroxide (possible irritant). Too strong for most skin types, and I do not recommend using benzoyl peroxide.

Avon Clearskin Overnight Acne Treatment *(2 ounces for $3.49)* contains salicylic acid (skin irritant and peeling agent), water, alcohol, and thickeners. It will peel the skin and dry it out terribly. Not a great thing to wake up to in the morning.

Basis Soap for Sensitive Skin *(3 ounces for $2.69 or 5 ounces for $3.69)* contains sodium tallowate (can cause acne or blackheads), detergent cleanser, glycerin (skin softener), petrolatum, thickener, salt (can be an irritant), water, preservatives, a form of lanolin (can be irritating to sensitive skin), and thickeners (including beeswax, which can also be irritating to sensitive skin). Not a product for sensitive skin: it contains too many ingredients that can cause sensitive skin to react.

Basis Soap for Combination Skin *(3 ounces for $2.69 or 5 ounces for $3.69)* contains sodium tallowate (can cause acne or blackheads), detergent cleanser, glycerin (skin softener), clay, petrolatum, thickener, salt (can be an irritant), water, preservatives, a form of lanolin (can be irritating to sensitive skin), and beeswax (can be irritating to sensitive skin). Combination skin will probably get drier and oilier using this product.

Basis Soap for Extra Dry Skin *(3 ounces for $2.69 or 5 ounces for $3.69)* contains sodium tallowate (can cause acne or blackheads), detergent cleanser, glycerin (skin softener), petrolatum, almond oil, thickener, salt (can be an irritant), water, preservatives, a form of lanolin (can be irritating to sensitive skin), and beeswax (can be irritating to sensitive skin). Too drying; even with the oils it won't prevent dry skin or irritation.

Benoxyl 10 Lotion *(1 ounce for $7.29)* contains mostly benzoyl peroxide, thickeners, and preservatives. Benzoyl peroxide can disinfect, but it can also be an irritant.

Brasivol, Medium *(6 ounces for $8.19)* contains aluminum oxide (scrubbing particles), water, detergent cleanser, thickener, clay, foaming agent, glycerin, thickener, sodium hydroxide (lye cleanser, can be very irritating), fragrance, quaternium-15 (considered one of the most irritating preservatives used in cosmetics), and coloring agent. This is fairly drying and irritating.

Brasivol, Fine *(5.1 ounces for $8.19)* is virtually identical to the Brasivol Medium. The size of the particles is what sets them apart.

Buf-Puf's Daily Cleanser for Normal to Dry Skin *(2.5 ounces for $4.79)* contains mostly water, several detergent cleansers, formaldehyde (very irritating), thickener, shea butter (can be greasy), and preservatives. This very drying and irritating cleanser would be harmful for anyone with normal to dry skin.

Buf-Puf's Daily Cleanser for Normal to Oily Skin *(2.5 ounces for $4.29)* contains mostly water, soap texturizer (can be irritating), detergent cleansers, thickeners, preservatives, an irritating thickener, and ammonium hydroxide (an irritant). In some ways it is less irritating than the cleanser for normal to dry skin, but it is still irritating and should not be used near the eye area.

Buf-Puf Singles/Skin Conditioning Cleanser *(40 sponges for $4.69)* contains soft fabric sponges soaked in a solution of detergent cleansers, thickeners, a preservative, and coloring agents. It is OK as a cleanser, although it tends to be drying and the pads are a waste of money. If "conditioning" means good for dry skin, it isn't. Plus, wiping off makeup is the long way to get your face clean.

Buf-Puf Singles/Oil-Free Cleanser *(40 sponges for $4.69)* is similar to the Skin Conditioning Cleanser, containing mostly detergent cleansers, thickeners, and a preservative. Both are oil-free, so the distinction between the two is unclear, but the comments about dryness, wasting money, and wiping off makeup apply here too.

Clean & Clear Blemish Fighting Pads *(50 pads for $3.69)* contains salicylic acid (skin irritant and peeling agent); preservative; camphor, clove oil, eucalyptus oil, and peppermint oil (all skin irritants); alcohol; and water. This won't fight anything, but it will cause irritation.

Clean & Clear Blemish Fighting Stick *(1 ounce for $3.99)* contains the same ingredients as the pads and the same warning applies.

Clean & Clear Bar & Buff *(3 ounces for $2.69)* contains sodium tallowate (can cause blackheads and irritation), water, glycerin, alcohol, thickeners, detergent cleansers, slip agent, preservatives, and coloring agents. It's a standard bar soap, although the alcohol can make it particularly drying.

Clean & Clear Bar, Regular *(3.75 ounces for $2.19)* contains ingredients similar to those in the Bar & Buff except that it also has a mild antiseptic and no alcohol. Drying on the skin.

Clean & Clear Bar, Sensitive *(3 ounces for $2.19)* also contains almost the same ingredients as the Bar & Buff. Too irritating for anyone with sensitive skin.

Clean & Clear Moisturizer, Sensitive *(4 ounces for $2.69)* contains salicylic acid (skin irritant and peeling agent), thickeners, coloring agent, more thickeners, preservatives, a long list of thickeners, and water. I wouldn't recommend salicylic acid for anyone with sensitive skin.

Clean & Clear Moisturizer, Regular *(4 ounces for $2.69)* contains almost the same ingredients as the moisturizer for sensitive skin. The same warnings apply.

Clean & Clear Foaming Facial Cleanser, Regular *(8 ounces for $2.69)* contains a small amount of antiseptic, water, detergent cleanser, salt (can be a skin irritant), thickeners, fragrance, coloring agent, quaternium-15 (considered one of the most irritating preservatives used in cosmetics), coloring agents, and preservative. Too irritating for most skin types.

Clean & Clear Foaming Facial Cleanser *(8 ounces for $2.69)* contains water, detergent cleansers, thickeners, fragrance, and quaternium-15 (considered one of the most irritating preservatives used in cosmetics). I would not recommend this to anyone with sensitive skin.

Clean & Clear Oil Controlling Astringent, Regular *(8 ounces for $2.69)* contains salicylic acid (skin irritant and peeling agent); an antiseptic; camphor, clove oil, and eucalyptus oil (all skin irritants); coloring agent; peppermint oil (skin irritant); alcohol; and water. If anything, skin will be irritated uncontrollably.

Clean & Clear Oil Controlling Astringent, Sensitive *(8 ounces for $2.69)* contains almost the exact same ingredients as the regular astringent, with less salicylic acid. The same warnings apply.

Clearasil Daily Face Wash *(3.5 ounces for $4.99)* contains mostly water, glycerin, a foaming agent, a defoaming agent (I know it doesn't make sense, but that's what's on the ingredient list), detergent cleanser, thickeners, detergent cleanser, preservative (can be irritating), an antiseptic, aloe vera, and fragrance. This is actually not a bad facial cleanser for someone with oily skin, although it can be drying and irritating to the eyes.

Clearasil Vanishing Lotion, Maximum Strength *(1 ounce for $5.29)* contains benzoyl peroxide (possible irritant), water, an antiseptic, thickeners, glycerin, citric acid (for pH balance), preservatives, and fragrance. Can cause irritation.

Clearasil Vanishing Cream, Maximum Strength *(0.65 ounce for $4.19 or 1 ounce for $5.29)* contains almost the exact same ingredients as the lotion. Can cause irritation.

Clearasil Tinted Cream, Maximum Strength *(0.65 ounce for $4.19 or 1 ounce for $5.29)* contains almost the exact same ingredients as the cream and lotion plus a light foundation tint. The same warnings apply, along with a recommendation not to stick this stuff over a blemish. It almost always looks like you've stuck a patch of dried orange stuff over a blemish, and it never hides anything.

Clearstick, Regular Strength *(1.2 ounces for $5.19)* contains salicylic acid (skin irritant and peeling agent), alcohol, water, witch hazel (can be irritating), thickener, aloe vera gel, menthol (skin irritant), preservative, and fragrance. This won't clear anything, but it can definitely irritate the skin.

Clearstick, Maximum Strength *(1.2 ounces for $5.19)* contains almost the exact same ingredients as the regular strength, but more salicylic acid. The same warnings apply.

Fostex Bar, Regular Strength *(3.75 ounces for $4.79)* contains sulfur (an antiseptic and possible skin irritant, although it can promote healing), salicylic acid (a strong irritant and peeling agent), boric acid (despite warnings from the American Medical Association in regard to severe irritation), thickener, coloring agent, fragrance, water binding agent, thickener, detergent cleansers, preservatives, and water. For "regular strength" this is pretty strong, and it will irritate most skin types.

Fostex Bar, Super Strength *(3.75 ounces for $5.49)* contains benzoyl peroxide, boric acid (despite warnings from the American Medical Association in regard to severe irritation), thickener, coloring agent, water binding agent, thickener, detergent cleansers, thickener, and preservative. This is too irritating for most skin types, particularly with the boric acid, and should be avoided.

Fostex Wash, Super Strength *(5 ounces for $8.49)* contains benzoyl peroxide, citric acid (can be an irritant), coloring agent, a powder that can absorb oil, thickener, salt (can be an irritant), detergent cleanser, and water. This is more of a toner than a wash, and it can be very irritating.

Fostex Vanishing Lotion *(1.5 ounces for $6.99)* contains benzoyl peroxide (possible irritant), thickeners, coloring agent, detergent cleanser, and water. This can be very drying and irritating to the skin.

Fostex Medicated Cleansing Cream, Regular Strength *(4 ounces for $9.99)* contains sulfur (an antiseptic and possible skin irritant, although it can promote healing), salicylic acid (a strong irritant and peeling agent), an emollient, coloring agent, thickener, fragrance, more thickeners, salt (can be an irritant), detergent cleanser, thickener, and water. Don't use this anywhere near your eyes, as it is potentially very irritating and drying.

Hibiclens Antiseptic, Antimicrobial Skin Cleanser *(4 ounces for $4.69 or 8 ounces for $6.99)* contains a mild antiseptic, fragrance, alcohol, water, and coloring agent. Without the fragrance, coloring agent, and alcohol, the antiseptic would be fine, but those are too irritating or unnecessary on the skin.

Ionax Scrub *(4 ounces for $13.99)* contains a binding agent (holds the product together), water, detergent cleanser, alcohol, slip agent, detergent cleanser, an abrasive (similar to sand), detergent cleanser, preservative, coloring agent, and fragrance. This fairly expensive scrub is OK, but no better than mixing Cetaphil Lotion with baking soda.

Jergens Bar for Oily Skin *(3.25 ounces for $2.09)* contains a mild antiseptic, water, alcohol, detergent cleansers, glycerin, thickener, fragrance, lanolin (can cause skin allergies), preservative, allantoin, and coloring agent. The alcohol makes this product very drying, and the lanolin makes it awful for oily or acne-prone skin.

Listerex Golden Scrub, Medicated Lotion *(8 ounces for $7.29)* contains salicylic acid (skin irritant and peeling agent), slip agent, coloring agents, detergent cleanser (possible skin irritant), another coloring agent, fragrance, preservatives, water, and thickener. Fairly irritating; there is nothing "medicated" about this product.

Listerex Herbal Scrub, Medicated Lotion *(8 ounces for $7.29)* contains almost the exact same ingredients as the Golden Listerex. The same warnings apply. By the way, it has no herbs.

Mudd Deep Cleansing Treatment *(2 ounces for $4.19)* contains fuller's earth, a clay that according to my sources is no longer permitted in cosmetics. All of the Mudd products contain fuller's earth. These products should not be used by anyone. I am checking into why these products are still on the market.

Noxzema Anti-Acne Lotion, Maximum Strength *(1 ounce for $5.29)* contains benzoyl peroxide, a slip agent, several thickeners, preservative (may release formaldehyde), glycerin, a mineral that can absorb oil, preservative, thickeners, water, and thickener. The only ingredient in here that would make this product anti-acne is the benzoyl peroxide, which I do not recommend because it can cause irritation..

Noxzema 2-1 Pads, Regular Strength *(50 pads for $3.49 or 75 pads for $3.79)* contains mostly alcohol; salicylic acid (a strong irritant and skin peeler); water; thickener; and clove oil, camphor, eucalyptus oil, and menthol (all skin irritants). This product is very drying and irritating for almost all skin types.

Noxzema 2-1 Pads, Maximum Strength *(75 pads for $4.29)* contains salicylic acid (a strong irritant and skin peeler); camphor, clove oil, eucalyptus oil, and menthol (all skin irritants); thickeners; alcohol; and water. Maximum strength in this case means maximum irritation.

Noxzema Astringent for Normal Skin *(4 ounces for $2.29 or 8 ounces for $3.79)* contains mostly alcohol, benzoic acid (an antiseptic and possible skin irritant), coloring agent, camphor (a skin irritant), a preservative (can release formaldehyde), fragrance, menthol (a skin irritant), castor oil, and water. Extremely drying for almost all skin types.

Noxzema Astringent for Sensitive Skin *(8 ounces for $3.79)* contains mostly water, alcohol, glycerin, camphor (can be a skin irritant), eucalyptol (a skin irritant), eugenol (a strong skin irritant), fragrance, menthol (a skin irritant), benzoic acid (an antiseptic and possible skin irritant), a preservative (can release formaldehyde), castor oil, and coloring agents. No one with sensitive skin could survive this product for very long.

Noxzema Astringent for Oily Skin *(8 ounces for $3.79)* contains mostly alcohol; benzoic acid (an antiseptic); coloring agent; camphor, eucalyptol, eugenol (can release formaldehyde), and menthol (all can irritate the skin); castor oil; water; and coloring agent. Like the astringent above, it will not help oily skin, but can irritate it and make it worse.

Noxzema Medicated Deep Cleanser *(7.75 ounces for $5.35)* contains salicylic acid (skin irritant and peeling agent), alcohol, water, witch hazel (can be an irritant), aloe vera, menthol (skin irritant), allantoin (can help heal skin), fragrance, thickener, water binding agent, thickener, and preservative. This isn't much of a cleanser; it can irritate the skin and should be kept away from the eyes.

Oxy Facial Scrub *(2.65 ounces for $4.94)* contains antiseptic (can be irritating), peeling agent, detergent cleansers, thickeners, fragrance, thickeners, and antiseptic. A mediocre scrub, more of a peel than anything else. Can be irritating to the skin.

Oxy Medicated Cleanser *(4 ounces for $2.59)* contains alcohol, salicylic acid (skin irritant and peeling agent), citric acid (possible skin irritant), menthol (skin irritant), slip agent, and detergent cleanser. Extremely irritating for most skin types.

Oxy Medicated Pads for Regular Skin *(90 pads for $3.94)* contains alcohol, detergent cleanser, citric acid (possible skin irritant), fragrance, menthol (skin irritant), slip agent, and water. Very drying and irritating for most skin types.

Oxy Medicated Pads for Sensitive Skin *(90 pads for $4.53)* contains mostly salicylic acid (skin irritant and peeling agent), alcohol, detergent cleanser, fragrance, menthol (skin irritant), thickener, detergent cleanser, water binding agent, and water. Irritating for almost any skin, especially sensitive skin.

Oxy 5 Pimple Medication *(1 ounce for $4.39)* contains benzoyl peroxide, thickener, citric acid (possible skin irritant), coloring agent, preservatives, scrub agent, detergent cleanser, thickener, water binding agent, thickener, and water. Can be irritating to the skin; benzoyl peroxide is a problem for all skin types.

Oxy Daily Face Wash *(4 ounces for $4.44)* is almost identical to the pimple medication except it contains more benzoyl peroxide. The same warnings apply.

Oxy Night Watch, Maximum Strength *(2 ounces for $4.44)* contains mostly salicylic acid (skin irritant and peeling agent), thickener, coloring agent, preservatives, slip agent, preservative, scrub agent, detergent cleanser, thickener, and water. Can be irritating for most skin types.

Oxy Night Watch for Sensitive Skin *(2 ounces for $4.55)* contains almost the exact same ingredients as the maximum strength except for a smaller amount of salicylic acid. This would irritate even nonsensitive skin.

Pan Oxyl Bar *(4 ounces for $6.79)* contains 10 percent benzoyl peroxide, thickeners, cornstarch, glycerin, castor oil, and more thickeners. Benzoyl peroxide is a skin irritant, and the castor oil won't make women with oily skin very happy.

pHresh *(6 ounces for $4.99)* contains water, detergent cleanser, AHA, thickeners, foaming agent, preservative, and fragrance. One of the least irritating cleansers in this entire list. Worth considering.

PropapH for Sensitive Skin *(6 ounces for $3.49)* contains salicylic acid (skin irritant and peeling agent), aloe vera gel, a sunscreen, fragrance, menthol (a skin irritant), water, alcohol, detergent cleanser, and an antiseptic. This isn't a product for anyone with sensitive skin.

PropapH for Normal/Combination Skin *(6 ounces for $3.49)* contains ingredients almost identical to the one for sensitive skin; the same warning applies.

SalAc Acne Medicated Cleanser *(6 ounces for $8.79)* contains salicylic acid (skin irritant and peeling agent), benzyl alcohol (mostly a preservative and very irritating), detergent cleansers, thickener, water, thickener, and salt (can be an irritant). Irritating and drying on the skin; keep away from eyes or open wounds.

Sayman Soap, Cleansing Bar with Lanolin, for Dry Skin (*3.5 ounces for $1.69*) contains sodium tallowate (can cause acne or black-heads), detergent cleanser, fragrance, oil, lanolin, thickener, more oil, water binding agent, preservatives, and coloring agent. The oils should soothe dry skin after washing, but if you tend to break out this will only make things worse.

Sayman Soap, Cleansing Bar with Witch Hazel, for Oily Skin (*3.5 ounces for $1.69*) contains sodium tallowate (can cause acne or blackheads), detergent cleanser, thickener, fragrance, skin softeners (a form of lanolin that can cause blackheads or acne), a form of witch hazel, preservatives, and allantoin. It's drying, and the skin softeners can cause breakouts.

Sea Breeze Facial Scrub (*2.5 ounces for $2.59 or 4 ounces for $3.69*) contains mostly water, thickeners, alpha hydroxy acid, stabilizer, thickener, glycerin, camphor (skin irritant), and preservatives (one of these may release formaldehyde). Worth a try except for the camphor and formaldehyde releaser.

Sea Breeze Towelettes (*20 towelettes for $4.19*) are soft cloth-like towels soaked in alcohol; camphor (skin irritant); water; peppermint oil, clove oil, and eucalyptus oil (all skin irritants); antiseptic; and coloring agents. Very irritating and drying.

Sea Breeze Antiseptic (*4 ounces for $2.49 or 10 ounces for $4.39*) is identical to Sea Breeze towelettes; the same warning pertains.

Sea Breeze Astringent for Sensitive Skin (*4 ounces for $2.49 or 10 ounces for $4.39*) contains mostly water; alcohol; glycerin; preservative; camphor, clove oil, and eucalyptus oil (all skin irritants); fragrance; and coloring agent. Sensitive skin would not survive even one application.

Sea Breeze Antiseptic (*4 ounces for $2.49 or 10 ounces for $4.39*) contains almost identical ingredients to the Sea Breeze Astringent and the same warnings apply.

Sea Breeze Daily Cleansing Wash for Normal/Combination Skin (*5.5 ounces for $4.49*) contains mostly water, detergent cleanser, slip agent, thickeners, detergent cleanser, fragrance, citric acid (for pH balance), coloring agent, preservative, and more coloring agents. In some ways, surprisingly, a fairly gentle cleanser. Worth a try.

Stridex Antibacterial Cleansing Bar with Glycerin (*3.5 ounces for $1.85*) contains sodium tallowate (can cause blackheads and skin irrita-tion), detergent cleansers, water, glycerin, thickeners, a lanolin derivative (can cause allergies and breakouts), preservatives, an antiseptic, and coloring agents. Not much antiseptic in this bar, and the lanolin and sodium tallowate make it a problem for someone who has acne.

Stridex Dual Textured Pads, Extra Strength *(32 pads for $2.85)* contains salicylic acid (skin irritant and peeling agent), alcohol, nail polish solvent (like acetone), citric acid (possible skin irritant), fragrance, menthol (skin irritant), water, slip agent, and detergent cleanser (possible skin irritant). Extra strength is an understatement; nail polish solvent sends this beyond strong, all the way to detrimental.

Stridex Dual Textured Pads, Oil Fighting Formula *(32 pads for $3.10)* contains salicylic acid (skin irritant and peeling agent), alcohol, water, nail polish solvent, citric acid (skin irritant), detergent cleanser, thickener, menthol (skin irritant), and fragrance. Same warning as above.

SEEING A DERMATOLOGIST

Although at times I disagree with dermatologists on the subject of daily skin care, when it comes to chronic acne or serious skin problems there is absolutely no other option but to see a dermatologist. The general rule of thumb is that daily skin care for someone with minor or normal skin problems such as occasional breakouts or dry skin is best handled with cosmetic cleansing routines. Of course, you should be cautious of what you buy. Generally, the products I recommend are safe for the millions of women who have normal skin that happens to not always be flawless.

However, if your skin burns, itches, swells, or is constantly red, if you have skin discolorations that are not normal and do not go away, or if you have acne that is chronic, causing scarring or disfigurement, then it is imperative that you make an appointment immediately to see a dermatologist. I also advise seeking a dermatologist if you are fair-skinned and have spent a great deal of time in the sun getting a tan; the chances are fairly high that you may start showing signs of skin cancer sooner than you think. I know several women in their early 30s who are sun worshippers and already have uneven brown patches on their skin.

Chronic or serious skin problems are not ever to be handled at the cosmetics counters or the drugstore. That is when it is essential to consult a dermatologist.

ACCUTANE—A CURE FOR ACNE?

Have you patiently waited for your skin to clear up? Spent untold dollars on dermatologists and followed their instructions, diligently wiping antibiotic lotions over your face and taking oral antibiotics for years? For most of that time your skin may have improved, but it probably never really stopped breaking out. In spite of the improvement from using antibiotics, you probably don't want to stay on them permanently. The negative side effects of chronic low-grade stomach problems and adapting to the antibiotics are risks you may not be willing to live with forever. Who knows how long your skin will continue breaking out? But with Accutane this persistent cycle can be over in four months. Sounds unbelievable, doesn't it? Well, it isn't.

Most dermatologists will tell you that it is possible, in fact highly probable, that Accutane can cure acne. Accutane, which has been around for more than ten years, is a synthetic drug made to resemble the molecules in vitamin A, and it is taken orally. It essentially stops the oil production in your sebaceous glands (the oil-producing structures of the skin) and literally shrinks these glands to the size of a baby's. This prevents sebum (oil) from clogging the hair follicle, mixing with dead skin cells, rupturing the follicle wall, and creating pimples or cysts. Oil production resumes when treatment is completed and the sebaceous glands slowly begin to grow larger again, but never (or at least rarely) as large as they were before treatment.

Are you ready for this? In 85 percent of patients who complete a four-month treatment with Accutane, acne is no longer considered to be clinically significant. In other words, for all intents and purposes, *their acne is cured!* Does this mean you'll never break out again? Once in a while, but an occasional pimple here and there is hardly anyone's definition of acne. Especially anyone who has, on a daily basis, many breakouts on her face and body.

What about the remaining 15 percent of patients who do experience recurrences? When the breakouts return, three to six months after treatment, they are typically milder, easier to treat, and can generally be cured with a second treatment. Yes, cured. I have to keep repeating that to myself just to comprehend the significance of this drug. But not to have oily acned skin anymore is a miracle for anyone who's been suffering with problem skin.

By the way, dosage and duration depend on the severity of the patient's acne, but treatments generally last 16 weeks. If a second treatment is necessary, an eight-week rest period is required in between. Interestingly, acne continues to improve even after the course of treatment is completed, although doctors do not know exactly why this happens.

So what's the catch with this "miracle" drug and why don't doctors prescribe it to everyone? How come no one has told you about it sooner? If you've been seeing a dermatologist for acne, the prescriptions are always the same, everything but Accutane, and the acne never really goes away.

Accutane is a controversial drug for many reasons, but principally because of its most insidious side effect: *it has been proven to cause severe birth defects in nearly 90 percent of the babies born to women who were pregnant while taking it.* Before physicians knew about this alarming hazard, when it was first prescribed in France back in the 1970s, before enough research had been conducted to establish its safety, more than 800 babies out of 1,000 births were born seriously deformed.

Roche Dermatologics, the company that produces Accutane, has launched a fervent campaign to inform doctors and patients about the risks involved for pregnant women. Female patients of child-bearing age are required to use effective birth control (which includes abstinence) for one month before, during, and one month after treatment, in addition to having regular pregnancy tests during treatment.

If you aren't pregnant, are there still risks? Yes, but for many reasons, they are only somewhat more serious than taking antibiotics for 10, 20, or 30 years, which for many women is how long their acne lasts.

Other commonly reported, although temporary, side effects are dry skin and lips, mild nosebleeds (your nose can get really dry for the first few days), aches and pains, itching, rash, skin fragility, increased sensitivity to the sun, and peeling of palms and hands. More serious, although much less common, side effects can include headaches, nausea, vomiting, blurred vision, changes in mood, depression, severe stomach pain, diarrhea, decreased night vision, bowel problems, persistent dryness of eyes, calcium deposits in tendons (doctors don't know yet whether or not this is significant), an increase in cholesterol levels, and yellowing of the skin. However, as scary as all that sounds, *the majority of patients tolerate Accutane very well.* One dermatologist reported that over the past 15 years he has prescribed Accutane to thousands of patients and only five have had to stop because of negative side effects.

Understandably, most people, doctors included, are scared off by the side effects alone, above and beyond the risk to pregnant women. Most dermatologists will only recommend Accutane to patients with chronic acne (large, recurring cysts or blemishes that can permanently distort the shape and appearance of the skin), or sometimes to people with less severe acne that has not responded successfully to other forms of treatment. Doctors are hesitant to prescribe Accutane liberally, largely because of fears of malpractice suits in cases where a patient does experience serious negative side effects or accidentally becomes pregnant. Many doctors won't prescribe Accutane at all.

Although the high risk of birth defects and the other side effects should be taken seriously, it seems a shame that Accutane has been kept secret from many acne patients. Without much, if any, argument, it is the most effective drug for acne available today. The public is largely misinformed about its potential dangers as well as its potential benefits. Many doctors believe that if it weren't for proven birth defects, Accutane would be prescribed almost as frequently as antibiotics. Not surprisingly, it has been prescribed much more frequently to men.

Given what I have learned, I wish somebody had told me about Accutane ten years ago! It would have saved me a lot of time, money, and heartache. Although oral and topical antibiotics can work successfully for people who eventually outgrow their acne, the question remains, When are you going to outgrow it? How do you know if you're *ever* going to outgrow it? People who don't are looking at years of antibiotics and topical solutions that sometimes work and sometimes don't. Plus, antibiotics can negatively affect the digestive system and can create further complications over long periods of time, which are also risky side effects. Accutane seems to be a practical and equally important option. (Although I am certain some dermatologists would not agree with that assessment, there are just as many who do.)

How do you determine whether or not your acne is short-term or long-term, or, better yet, whether or not your acne is severe enough to merit taking Accutane? Men often have more severe acne as adolescents, but also have a better chance of outgrowing their acne in adulthood. Many women never outgrow it, while others develop adult-onset acne that can last for years. If you have had acne for five or more years or if you have acne on your face, chest, and back, it is likely your acne will continue to be a problem. Even if you won't have acne forever, it could continue for another three to five years and up to ten. If your skin is manageable or breakouts are infrequent and minimal, Accutane is probably not necessary for you. You need to assess how much of a problem acne is in your life, what kind of treatment it presently requires, whether or not the treatment is working to your satisfaction, and whether you are willing to put up with the potential side effects that go along with Accutane. If you have been on antibiotics for several years and don't foresee that changing, if your acne is not responding to current treatments, or if your acne is severe cystic acne, you might want to ask your doctor about Accutane. Doctors, like anybody, have their biases, so try not to be swayed by one doctor's opinion. I spoke with several dermatologists about Accutane, and their opinions varied. Some felt strongly that Accutane should be taken off the market, while others felt that it was a safe and valuable drug that should be recommended for use more often.

WHEN IS ACNE NOT ACNE?

Many women and men suffer from a skin condition that closely resembles acne but isn't. The condition is called acne rosacea, but using the word acne is actually quite misleading, because it isn't acne nor is it treated like acne. Rosacea is distinguished by redness and inflammation over the nose and cheek area of the face, similar to a butterfly pattern. The redness is often ignored by women as being just a skin color problem and not a disease. Another problem with identifying rosacea is that pustules and papules (pimples) are often present, also resembling acne. Perhaps one of the most distinguishing characteristics is that rosacea is rarely if ever associated with blackheads.

Several factors can make rosacea worse. These catalysts include hot liquids, spicy foods, exposure to extreme temperatures (including cooking over a hot stove), alcohol consumption, sunlight, stress, saunas, or hot tubs. Another characteristic of rosacea is dry, highly sensitive skin. Skin care products must be selected very carefully. No irritants of any kind should be used. As important as it is for those with typical acne cases to stay away from irritating skin care products, it is doubly important for those women with rosacea. Avoid all products that contain alcohol, boric acid, acetone, menthol, camphor, eucalyptus, lemon oil, herbs, clay masks, and/or anything that stings or burns the skin.

Because blemishes can make rosacea look like acne, many doctors misdiagnose it, prescribing everything but the one course of treatment that can cure rosacea. Only two drugs on the market can successfully treat rosacea: a topical drug called Metro Gel and oral tetracycline. Using both together can be effective in almost all rosacea cases. But first you and your doctor need to know what you are dealing with. Knowing the difference between acne and acne rosacea can mean a definite difference in the health of your skin.

Putting On Your Best Face

STEP-BY-STEP MAKEUP APPLICATION

All those creamy potions, luscious colors, and dazzling promises of instant, or almost instant, beauty are lying before you at cosmetics counters and drugstores, on television, or at in-home demonstrations. What do you buy? If you choose to wear makeup (and it is a choice), how do you get your face on efficiently and beautifully?

There is an order to dressing your face just as there is an order to dressing your body. Getting dressed involves a progression and an array of options, and so does wearing makeup. When you get dressed in the morning, even though it seems automatic, there are a series of choices you make so that you can leave the house feeling and looking great. No one part is necessarily any more important than any other, but the ones you choose definitely impact the way you look: bra and underpants first, then nylons, pants, shirt, and jacket; or no bra and underpants, just nylons, pants, shirt, and no jacket; or bra, underpants, no nylons, skirt, blouse, jacket, scarf, and belt; and the variations go on and on from there. The same sorts of decisions apply to wearing makeup.

For example, I prefer to apply the foundation first (powder is optional and I often don't use it at all), then the concealer, contour, blush, and finally the eye design, or sometimes I put on the contour color after the eyeshadows are applied. Some makeup artists start with the foundation only over the eye area, follow with the eye design, and then apply the rest of the foundation, concealer, powder, blush, and contour. This way any drips from the eyeshadow won't become a permanent part of the makeup. Although I think this approach is too time-consuming, it can work. You may want to experiment to see which order works best for you. Throughout this chapter I will proceed in the order I customarily use, pointing out exceptions and options along the way.

The following list describes possible steps for applying makeup. Which ones you choose are up to you. I think the nuances and permutations are intriguing and part of what makes wearing makeup so much fun. The other part is the fashionable looks you can achieve when it all goes on the way it is supposed to.

STEP 1—FOUNDATION

Foundation, as the name implies, is the base for the rest of your makeup. It actually involves two options: foundation and concealer. (Concealer is sometimes called under-eye highlighter or corrector, depending on the company. The name is irrelevant; both do the same thing.) The order in which you put on the concealer and the foundation is up to you. Some people apply the concealer first and then the foundation, while others put on the foundation and then the concealer. The main rule is that *the foundation should never be obviously pink, green, orange, peach, rose, ash, or true yellow.* From the lightest shade of Caucasian skin to the deepest shade of African-American skin, the foundation should always be a neutral shade of beige to tan to dark brown to ebony, with no overtones of the aforementioned colors. Please follow carefully my recommendations regarding color in Chapter Nine. There are a lot of pink-, peach-, and ash-colored foundations out there from many cosmetics lines, both expensive and inexpensive. Don't get this one wrong. Your face is a very central focus point, and wearing a color that doesn't match your skin will make you look overly made-up no matter how sheer the foundation is.

Foundation is supposed to match exactly. If you see a color difference between you neck and the foundation it is the wrong color. A foundation that is a different color then than your neck will look like a mask on your face.

When it comes to foundations, almost every cosmetics line has several styles for you to choose from. The general rule here is to choose a lightweight foundation that provides even coverage but that absolutely never looks like foundation. Avoid heavy-duty foundations like the plague. There is almost never a reason to hide your skin under a thick layer of makeup. It always looks artificial. Unless it is your goal to look overly made-up, stay away from thick foundations.

Foundation can be broken down into the following groups: oil-free liquid foundation for oily skin (including glycerin-based or alcohol-based foundations); water-based (meaning the first ingredient is water and the second or third is oil) liquid foundation for normal to dry skin; water-based liquid foundation with extra emollients or thicker coverage for dry skin; traditional cream foundation that comes in a stick, pot, or compact for extremely dry skin; and cream-to-powder compact foundation.

The popularity of cream-to-powder compact foundations continues, and many cosmetics lines, from the department store to the drugstore, offer them. This interesting product goes on smooth and creamy, then dries to a powder, usually providing light to medium coverage. The texture is lovely. The only negative note is that this product works best on normal skin types. Dry skin can look chalky and parched with this type of foundation and oily skin can become streaky and caked.

The search for good oil-free foundations is a problem for many women. It's not that you can't find a wide selection of lightweight oil-free foundations, but none of them will stop your oily skin from being oily. Don't be lured by claims of oil-control. What these foundations do provide is wonderful, light, uniform coverage. As a general precaution, steer away from foundations that you have to shake before applying. If the color and liquid separate in the bottle they can tend to separate on your skin.

Once you've narrowed down the color and coverage, the only way to tell whether a foundation is the right one for you is to wear it and see how it feels and check the color frequently in the daylight (along the jawline) to be sure it is an exact match. Texture preference is very subjective. Only you can make that final decision. It has to feel comfortable on your skin. Choose carefully; if you get the foundation wrong, the chances are all other aspects of the makeup will be wrong too. For this reason I always recommend purchasing a foundation that you can try on. That makes shopping at the drugstore for foundation almost impossible (except in Canada, where a few of the higher-priced cosmetics lines are available at the drugstore and have testers for all their products). L'Oreal is one of the few drugstore lines that consistently offers testers for its foundations. Maybelline and Revlon offer testers for some of their products, but not consistently, although they do have great testers for their products designed specifically for women of color. If you can't test a foundation, it is probably best not to buy it.

STEP 2—CONCEALER

Apply the concealer next to the inside corner of the eye and gently blend it out along the lower lashes, avoiding the top of the cheek. The goal here is to not see where the concealer stops and starts. Blending is the best way to prevent lines of demarcation for this step. Use your foundation to help soften obvious edges. To help prevent the concealer from slipping into the lines around the eyes, avoid greasy or thick products, and apply only a thin layer; it also helps to refrain from using heavy, greasy, or very emollient moisturizers around the eyes. A light (and I mean light) dusting of powder over the face after you apply your foundation will also make a difference, but don't overdo the powder.

Considering the array of concealers and highlighter on the market, you might think that none of us would have a dark circle to worry about. Unfortunately, in spite of this whopping selection of shades and consistencies, many of the colors are either too dark, too orange, too peach, too yellow, too rose, too pink, too greasy (filling in the lines around the eye), too dry, too thick, or too thin. I can understand the different textures—something for every preference—but the strange assortment of shades is beyond me. There is no way a concealer that is darker than your foundation, darker than your skin tone, or tinted peach or pink can make any dark area lighter. If you want to lighten a dark area, you must put a light color on it—something that matches the foundation or, at the very least, doesn't darken the color of the foundation. Concealers in non-neutral tones will alter the shade of the foundation around the eye; the result is an odd color wherever the concealer and the foundation merge, and they must merge in order to look blended. I recommend concealers in neutral tones that are at least one or two shades lighter than the foundation, and there are plenty of those on the market.

I think it is fairly safe to shop for a concealer at the drugstore. The color choices offered there are about the same as at the cosmetics counters, with a good range of consistencies in a handful of shades. Follow my color suggestions before you buy, because there are some strange colors out there.

Although I only use concealers under the eye, most cosmetics companies also recommend using concealers to cover blemishes. Covering a blemish with an extra product in addition to the foundation usually builds up too much makeup over the blemish and actually makes it look more obvious.

Beauty Note: I never recommend color correctors under foundation. I'm sure you've seen those pink, yellow, mauve, or green concealers that are supposed to go on under your foundation to change the color of your skin before you apply foundation. If your skin is red you're supposed to put on yellow or green, and if your skin is yellow you're supposed to put on mauve. I consider this unnecessary because it doesn't change the skin tone all that well, at least not by my standards, and definitely no better than the foundation can by all itself. You also end up feeling like you have too much makeup on the skin. The foundation should be enough if it is the right color.

If you insist on checking out color correctors, apply the corrector to one side of your face and then apply foundation all over; if you don't see an improvement, it isn't worth it.

STEP 3—POWDER

After your foundation and concealer are blended on evenly, with no lines or edges anywhere on the face, you can apply your loose or pressed powder. I generally do not use this step first thing in the morning; instead, I save it for touching up as the day goes by. I prefer the dewy look foundation leaves on the face to the matte, opaque look of powder, but this choice is completely up to you. Powder one side of your face and leave the foundation alone on the other, and see which you prefer.

Some makeup artists work only with loose powder and some work only with pressed powder. Because loose powder is lighter and doesn't contain waxes, it is preferred over pressed powder, but there is no getting around the fact that loose powder is also messy. Pressed powder is preferred by consumers for just that reason—it is easier to use. Whichever you choose, be sure to apply it only with a full brush and never a sponge or puff (that technique is reserved for television). Never build up too much powder and always knock the excess off the brush before applying it to your face. Too much powder can make the face look chalky, so be careful not to overpowder. For the most part you can only get away with powdering two or three times a day before the face starts looking thick and heavy.

Beauty Note: Excellent professional makeup brushes are available at most department stores. Please make this a priority. You can buy the most exceptional products in the world, but they won't look right without the right applicators. Many pressed powders, particularly at the drugstore, come packaged with powder puffs. Throw these away and use a brush. Puffs lay too much powder on the skin, making it look thick and overly madeup.

I guess it isn't surprising that a product as simple and basic as pressed and loose powder can end up with as much marketing hype as any wrinkle cream or skin treatment. The best thing about "setting" or "finishing" powders is that they come in a wider range of color choices than ever before, in consistencies ranging from silky to sheer. (The more expensive powders do tend to have a silkier feel, but not always.) Surprisingly, the texture does not affect the performance. A drier-feeling powder works just as well as a silkier one. Also, no matter how silky it is, if you build too much powder on the skin it will look caked. Many of the expensive cosmetics lines have replaced talc with a range of other absorbant powders, but none of them is any more effective than talc, and some people feel talc is better. There is absolutely no reason to spend a lot of money on pressed or loose powders. This is one area where it is best to shop at the drugstore or in-home sales.

STEP 4—EYESHADOW

Eyeshadow application is probably the most challenging facet of wearing makeup, and the one where you can display the most creativity. Applying foundation is fairly straightforward: match your skin color exactly and blend smooth; blush goes only on the cheek area, not too close to the nose or eyes or below the cheekbone; and lipstick speaks for itself—just apply it to the lips, with or without a lip liner. Eyeshadow, in contrast, has almost unlimited choices, more than I care to count or can summarize here. Lids can be any color (well, not *any*, according to me, but the options do exist) in a spectrum of shades from light to medium to dark; under-brow color can be light, medium, or dark; crease color can be medium to dark; and shading at the back corner of the eye can be any rich color or basic black. Eye lining is also complicated: it can be a thick, medium, or thin line, smudged or exact, and done with a powder, pencil, or liquid liner. To fully discuss all these options would take a separate book, and it just so happens that I wrote extensively about this very subject in *Blue Eyeshadow Should Absolutely Be Illegal.* What I will summarize here are some of the basic rules to be aware of when shopping for and applying eyeshadow.

While color placement offers myriad possibilities, as a general rule the lighter color goes all over the eyelid, from the lashes to the eyebrow, and a deeper color follows the crease and back corner of the eye. You might want to use a third, highlighter color under the eyebrow, which is a fine option, but don't make the entire under-eyebrow area light. Placing a very light or whitish color under the eyebrow makes it look puffy. The under-eyebrow highlighter should only follow a small area just under the eyebrow itself.

Avoid shiny eyeshadows. Shiny eyeshadows are still around but the cosmetics companies have finally caught on, and it is almost impossible to find a cosmetics line that doesn't have at least a few matte eyeshadows. Sometimes they throw in a little shine, which I still suggest you avoid, but is isn't as bad as it used to be. Just to remind you, the major reasons to avoid shiny eyeshadows are: (1) they make the skin on the lid look wrinkly, and (2) they are as inappropriate for daytime wear as a sequined evening gown.

Unless you are wearing a specific evening look, you should also avoid pastel or vibrant-colored eyeshadows. Stick to neutral shades such as tan, beige, brown, sable, chestnut, camel, mahogany, hazel, gray, charcoal, slate, mauve, plum, navy, and the list goes on and on and on. The variations on the neutral theme are endless. Keep in mind that the purpose of eyeshadow is to shade the eye, not color it. Color for the face is carried by the blush and lipstick. You do not want to overcolor the face. Colored eyeshadow creates too obvious a look and doesn't define the eye. Neutral colors can be worn with just about everything and look extremely sophisticated. Greens, blues, lavenders, and bright pinks are best left out of your eye design.

Finally, never use sponge-tip applicators: use only eyeshadow brushes. Sponge-tip applicators pack the makeup on in a layer and they tend to drag along the skin making the powder streak. Brushes pick up a lighter layer of powder and can better glide over the skin.

STEP 5—EYE LINING

You might think that selecting an eyeliner is easy—just choose brown or black. But if you want to get creative, the number of options for lining the eye can be astounding: liquid liners in a tube, thin eye pencils, fat eye pencils, automatic eye pencils, eye pencils designed like felt-tip pens, pencils that don't have to be sharpened because the material around the tip peels away, pencils with sponges at one end, pencils with a powder eyeshadow and applicator at one end, waterproof pencils for those who want their eyes to stay lined while they jog in the rain. The different textures produce a wide assortment of looks, from subtle to exotic. Liquid liners or felt-tip pen eyeliners tend to create a more dramatic, obvious line, while thin pencils or automatic pencils can look either soft or obvious. Many pencils come packaged with a sponge tip at one end for blending (to soften the line) or for shading at the back corner of the eye. How do you choose? It depends on the look you want. Experimentation is the only way to know which ones you prefer. Bottom line: Here is yet another area where it doesn't make much sense to spend a lot of money, since there is little difference between brands. Regardless of type, consider using only automatic pencils. They cost more money than regular pencils but don't require sharpening, which is extremely convenient.

Beauty Note: I prefer lining the eye with powders instead of pencils. All I do is use a dark shade of eyeshadow with a tiny eyeliner brush and line my eyes. The line can be made to look soft or dark and stays particularly well under the lower lashes. This look is also less expensive, because all of your eyeshadows can double as eyeliners and you won't need to buy an additional product. For a more dramatic look, wet the powder. No pencils, no liquids, no tubes, just one eyeshadow that can perform several functions just by changing the shape of the brush. I usually use various shades of brown or black eyeshadow to do my eye lining. It always works great.

STEP 6—EYEBROWS

Filling in eyebrows is tricky because nothing can make a face look more artificial or dated than "drawn-on" brows. An eyebrow pencil is a good choice if you know how to feather it on so it doesn't look heavy or like a line above the eye. Some brow pencils come with a brush at one end, thus encouraging the user to comb through the line and soften it once the color has been drawn into place. Alternatives include eyebrow powders or an eyeshadow that matches your brow color. Although these can look soft, they have never really replaced brow pencils.

My favorite products for the brows are brow gels, both with or without color. These mascara-like products are brushed on through the brow much the way mascara is brushed on through the eyelashes, making the existing brow hair look fuller, thicker, and darker. Only a few women are used to using the gels, but they do a remarkable job and can even be used in addition to a brow powder. Using the gel and powder together can create a very full, thick brow and, if done carefully, can create a remarkably natural look. Most lines don't include brow gels, but the few that do—Chanel, Borghese, and Lancome—are worth testing for yourself. I prefer Borghese's Brow Milano, but the others aren't bad either.

STEP 7—CONTOUR

Contouring the face is basic for a full makeup application, yet it is one of the most frequently left-out steps. Contouring creates a balance, adding definition with color. For all skin tones the contour is always some shade of brown never—rose, pink, plum, or red. Contour is not blush. The color should be similar to what your skin would look like if it were tan; for women of color with dark skin tones, the contour color can be a deep mahogany or even ebony. Keep this guideline in mind and you won't go wrong.

Contour is used at the back corner of the eye, going out to the temple area and up. Placing a contour color here helps blend out the edge of the eyeshadows you applied. You can also place contour under the cheekbone and along the sides of the nose. Some artists choose to apply the blush and then the cheek contour. I apply the contour first, which defines the cheek area, and then apply the blush by blending down onto the cheekbone. Apply contour with a blush brush, and never stripe the color on.

STEP 8—BLUSH

We all know where our cheeks are and we all want to have a soft blushed look after we apply what was once called rouge, but why does it so often look like stripes, smudges, or patches of color? Applying blush correctly is even trickier than choosing the right color. One of the first mistakes most women make is not using a full-enough brush. The brushes that come with most blushes are garbage and should not be used. You must purchase a good blush brush in order to do this step correctly. Brush down as you proceed straight back; do not brush in a straight line or it will look like a line. If you do these two things your cheeks will look blushed and not striped or smudged. The way to choose the right blush color is to coordinate it with the color tone of your lipstick. If your lipstick is plum your blush should be plum or a mauve-pink. The other consideration is to always choose a color that provides the softest application. Stay away from obvious blush colors.

Almost every cosmetics line now carries several types of blush: standard powder blush, gel blush, and cream-to-powder blush. The cream-to-powder blushes are an interesting alternative for most skin types. They tend to blend easily and merge well with the skin. Borghese's liquid version of the cream-to-powder blush is unique and worth a test to see if you like it, but only if it's in your budget.

Beauty Note: Many makeup artists choose blush colors in the peach, tan, or almost beige color families. To me this is not blush, and the results look a little too "Vogue" and mask-like. Blush should be a soft pastel color such as rose, pink, mauve, coral, or plum. All skin types look more alive and tasteful with a blush that is neither too vivid or too pale.

STEP 9—LIPSTICK

The colossal range of available lipstick colors is nothing less than outstanding, and the textures are, for the most part, nothing less than sublime. Choosing the color is actually more difficult than choosing the cosmetics line you want to buy it from. I often hear women say that one particular company or another has the best lipsticks on the market. The truth is that most cosmetics companies get this one right. Most lipsticks are creamy and moist with some amount of staying power. Only one or two companies have really awful lip products. The worst assumption a woman could make is that expensive lipsticks are somehow superior to inexpensive lipsticks. That just isn't the case.

Lipstick texture can be creamy, greasy, matte, powdery, and everything in between. Some lipsticks are tinted, which makes the color hang around longer after the creamy part is gone. Avoid shiny, luminous, luster, and pearl lipsticks; they tend to look whitish and even dry as they wear off. Creamy lipstick has enough shine on its own—you don't need to add any more. You should also avoid greasy lipsticks. These are OK for teens, but they simply don't last long enough or have enough color for someone who wants a more sophisticated look.

Many of the matte lipsticks on the market claim to tackle the problem of lip color bleeding or feathering into the lines around the mouth. Many cosmetics lines have lipsticks that contain powder (usually talc or kaolin) or are somewhat creamy powders to supposedly prevent this problem. These options are worth a try, but most of them are not reliable. Some colors bleed while others do not. Also, I am not fond of the lipsticks that contain powder: they tend to dry out the lips and their appearance is rather severe (some women love this look). Do not expect these lipsticks to absolutely not bleed if this tends to be your problem. There are only a few products available that really keep lipstick from feathering, and some of them work very well; this isn't one of them. I list the ones that really do work in Chapter Nine.

Most makeup artists will tell you that lip lining is an essential part of getting your lipstick on correctly. I won't argue that lip lining is helpful; I just wouldn't call it indispensable. Unless you have difficulty putting lipstick on evenly, it is only an option—a good option, but nothing more. There are a handful of lip-lining products around, including waterproof lip pencils (if having red lips while swimming is important to you), lip pencils that incorporate a lip brush at one end of the pencil, and automatic lip pencils that conveniently eliminate the need for sharpening. All of these pencils, regardless of their price tag, do essentially the same job. There is little to no difference between a

$3 lip pencil and a $22 lip pencil. Most lip pencils come from Germany, regardless of the company, so spending more dollars here will not improve the look of your mouth.

STEP 10—MASCARA

Most makeup artists leave mascara application to the very end. This way they can blend and add to the eye design, powder, and touch up under-eye concealers without wrecking the mascara and causing it to flake. I also leave mascara to the end. If I wear nothing else, I wear mascara. A good mascara goes on fast and easily and doesn't flake, smudge, wear off, or clump. If there is one thing that has changed dramatically in the world of cosmetics, it is the quality of mascaras. There are many available in all price ranges, particularly the inexpensive ones, that go on beautifully without clumping or smearing. Buying an expensive mascara ever again simply does not make sense.

Speaking of mascaras, waterproof mascaras do not stay on any better than water-soluble mascaras. Both will smudge and smear if your eyes tend to get oily during the day or if you wear a moisturizer or a moisture-rich foundation. Waterproof mascaras are also hard on the lashes because they can only be removed with a greasy cleanser that is wiped off. Such wiping can easily pull out delicate lashes. But don't worry, I have found a great assortment of water-soluble mascaras to recommend, and you will find them all in Chapter Seven.

MAKEUP FASHION

Is blue eyeshadow coming back? Should I tweeze my eyebrows thin like the women on the cover of Harpers Bazaar *or leave them thick? What about Madonna's latest look; should I try that?*

This is where the subject of makeup application gets tricky and where I get very conservative. There is every reason in the world to be both circumspect and knowledgeable about what is going on in the world of fashion. Mind you, I'm not talking about what is trendy or chic, I am talking about what is currently fashionable. Fortunately, "fashionable" is no longer as narrowly defined as it once was. Actually, in some regards that makes getting dressed that much harder. Deciding what to wear used to be rather straightforward. When bell-bottom pants were "in," that's what you wore. Now every length and width is fashionable, so what do you choose?

Well, you could opt for the good old standby "I only wear what looks good on me and damn the fashion world." But to suggest in the same breath that false eyelashes, bright blue eyeshadow, dark brown lipstick, or peach-colored foundation looks good on you is missing the point. I would be the last person to suggest that we should be controlled by the dictates of Madison Avenue and the subsequent pronouncements of the fashion magazines, yet I'm not going to work in go-go boots or Nehru jackets. This is where I start to sound contradictory.

There is a difference between utilizing fashion and being a slave to it. I do want to be fashionable, after all, that's part of being attractive, but when fashion starts working against me, that's where fashion stops and I start. Fashion works against women when it takes away their power, when it makes them little more than made-up dolls with four-inch high heels that are harmful to the back and feet. This book is about having both beauty and power at the same time. Any fashion statement that looks exaggerated, contrived, overdone, or that wears you instead of the other way around, is not a reliable or even a healthy option for most women. It's not that you can't do what you want, but you may want to think about what it's doing to your opinion of yourself.

So should you overly tweeze your eyebrows or wear blue eyeshadow because it is supposedly coming back in fashion or imitate Madonna or whoever is currently hot? The answer is decidedly no. Many fads in the fashion and entertainment world are better ignored or left to rock stars and wannabes who have nothing better to do.

I always assume no one is really going to take seriously many of the fashion statements I see in the fashion magazines. But then I saw it. A friend of mine had plucked her beautiful, full, expressive eyebrows down to one line of hair across her brow bone. It looked dreadful. Her face seemed constantly surprised, not to mention the after-five shadow and irritation spots from all that plucking. When I asked her what had provoked her into such a rash decision, she said, "But that's all they're showing in the fashion magazines now." I said, "Yes, it's true, but they show a lot of things in the fashion magazines, like five-inch platform shoes, see-through blouses sans bras, and $2,000 blazers. You can't do everything the fashion magazines consider important. Particularly when it hurts, takes too much time, and is blatantly a trend that won't last."

Please, no overly tweezed eyebrows. Natural growth with a slight arch only. Why go back to all that tweezing and pain? The grow-back alone makes it too time-consuming to even consider.

How do you choose what to follow and what to ignore? Great question, hard answer. Frequently, it is just a gut feeling, a sense that trendy isn't the direction you want to go. Another good guideline is to ask whether it will make you look elegant and sophisticated or just showy and conspicuous. True style isn't about blending into a crowd nor is it about standing out because you look strange. Finding a compromise between those two extremes isn't easy, but it is the essence of combining power and glamour for every woman.

CHOOSING WHAT LOOKS GOOD ON YOU

This is the hardest thing to write about. Unfortunately, I would need to see you personally in order to help you evaluate how something looks on you. If you're blonde and fair-skinned, a soft bronze lipstick might look beautiful on you, but if your blonde hair comes from a bottle and you have sallow skin, bronze lipstick could make you look sick. If you have vibrant red hair and classic white skin, magenta lipstick or pink eyeshadow could make your face look inflamed and swollen. Once you've established what colors look best on you, you must also consider your own life-style, the colors in your wardrobe, the look you want to achieve at work and at play, how much makeup you feel comfortable wearing, and what is an appropriate amount of makeup for each occasion. All of these factors should influence what makeup shades you choose to wear.

There is also the question of taste, individuality, and the degree of effort you're willing to expend on your looks. Besides, if you have a very specific notion of what makes you look good and what works for you, there is almost nothing anyone can do to change that opinion. Nothing is as difficult for women as the challenge of self-objectivity. One of the most entertaining portrayals of this was shown in the movie *Working Girl* with Melanie Griffith and Sigourney Weaver. Weaver plays a successful businesswoman, and Griffith is her overly made-up, rather gauche assistant who desperately wants to move ahead in her career. Part of the assistant's game plan involves acquiring a more sophisticated hairdo and wardrobe and more subtle, less obvious makeup. Then, along with her natural drive and brains, she makes it to the top. Could she have done the same thing if she looked the way she did at the beginning of the movie? It would be highly unlikely. How we look affects the way others see us, and that affects what we achieve in life.

Choosing what looks good when it comes to makeup colors is just like shopping for clothes. It requires patience and trial and error. Find a look in a fashion magazine that you are attracted to and try it on for size at the makeup counters. This is when getting your makeup done can be so wonderful. The makeup artist might get it wrong, but remember that you are just experimenting, trying things on to see what looks good.

"What a strange illusion it is to suppose that beauty is goodness or worthwhile."
Leo Tolstoy

Simply Makeup: A Product-by-Product Review

THE PROCESS

Tackling the cosmetics counters is never effortless. I thought it would be infinitely simpler this time out, given my previous experience and the number of products I was familiar with, but the number of new lines I wanted to add and the number of old products to rereview made researching this new edition a fairly awesome pursuit. I kept wondering, as I waded through the colors, creams, and never-ending ingredient lists, how the average consumer makes any sense out of all of this. Perhaps she can't. That's why I continue doing what I do.

I tried to approach the cosmetics counters with conviction and purpose. If they were going to kick me out, give me strange looks, or give me a hard time, I was ready. Well, almost ready. The work my research assistants and I do was still considered inappropriate investigation at the cosmetics counters. Writing down names of colors and copying ingredient lists was seen as improper and irksome, and asking for prices was annoying. More times than I care to remember we were told to stop, asked to leave, talked about (while we were standing there they would say things like "They say they're doing research, but it's just wasting my time"), and generally given a hard time. That doesn't mean there weren't exceptionally helpful salespeople, because there were. Some were so helpful it was almost amazing. A handful of salespeople took pen in hand and began helping us write down ingredients, and a few even let us Xerox some of their lists, but those were exceptions, not the rule.

In spite of the hassles, we did get it all done, and that felt good. As expected, there are some great products out there and, as expected, there are some mediocre, poor, and rotten ones too. All price categories contain products that work exceptionally well, if you know what to select.

For the most part my evaluation process remained the same. I reviewed each cosmetics line for several different elements. The first consideration was overall presentation and how user-friendly the displays were. Many display units had convenient color groupings that divided a majority of the makeup products into yellow and blue tones; this was always considered a line asset. All of the individual product categories—blushes, eyeshadows, concealers, foundations, and specialty items such as brushes or eyeshadow bases—were assessed on the basis of texture (did it feel silky smooth or was it grainy and hard), color (how large a range of colors was available and was there a selection for women of color), application (could it be applied easily to the skin or was it difficult to spread or blend), ease of use (was the container tricky to control, such as eyeshadow sets with colors placed too close together or foundations in pump containers that squirted too much product), and price (which speaks for itself).

I also asked myself the following questions when I was finalizing my critique: (1) Given what was described on the label, could the product do what it promised? (2) How did the product differ from other products? (3) How intense was the fragrance? (4) How absurd were the products' claims? (5) Would I want to use or recommend this product again?

I wish I had the space to challenge and explain every single exaggerated claim and lofty explanation that accompanies each product listed in this book. But there is just not enough room (or time) to tackle that Herculean task. A book that big would be impossible to lift, let alone read. Hopefully, the introduction will provide you with all the information you need to surmount the sales and advertising language and dwell on a product's quality alone.

Each product group had different elements that I considered essential for establishing a single product's desirability. These criteria were very specific and not something everyone would automatically agree with, particularly the people who sell the makeup. But then again, I don't expect them to agree with me very often anyway. Although they do tend to strongly agree with me when I recommend one of their products, they vehemently disagree when I suggest that one of their products doesn't live up to its claims. I feel strongly that most professional makeup artists, especially the ones who don't work for a specific cosmetics line or the ones I can get to talk with me off the record, would concur with almost everything I've delineated and specified.

Foundations: The fundamental expectation for any foundation I tested was that it not be any shade or tone of orange, peach, pink, rose, green, or ash. Consistency, coverage, and feel were also important factors for finding a foundation to be a good investment.

Concealers: Two major problems with any under-eye concealer were color and consistency. Concealers should never be any shade of orange, peach, pink, rose, green, or ash, and they should not slip into the lines around the eye. I was looking for creamy smooth textures that went on easily without pulling the skin and did not crease into lines.

Powders: Finishing powders come in two basic forms: pressed and loose. They were evaluated on the basis of whether or not they went on chalky, sheer, or heavy, and whether they were too pink, peach, ash, or rose. I consistently gave higher marks to powders that went on sheer with a natural beige, tan, or rich brown finish.

When it comes to bronzing powders, I generally suggest using them as a contour color and not an all-over face color. Trying to darken the face almost always looks overdone. After all, if a foundation is supposed to match the skin, exactly how can the use of a powder that darkens the skin be rationalized? It will look like the face is a decidedly different color than the neck, and there will be a line of demarcation where the color starts and stops.

Eyeshadows: Obviously I didn't recommend shades that were too shiny or vivid colors of blue, violet, green, or red. Choosing an intense color may be a personal preference, but I don't want to encourage anyone to imitate that style. Texture and ease of application also played a large part in my determination of shadow preference. Colors with heavy, grainy textures were pointed out because they can be hard to blend. Eyeshadows that were too sheer were also a problem because the color tended to fade as the day wore on. I was also leery of eyeshadow sets that included difficult-to-use color combinations. Many lines have duo, trio, quad, and quint sets of shadows with the most bizarre colors imaginable. Sets of colors must be usable as a set, coordinated in complementary color patterns; they can never be used to paint a rainbow across the eye.

Blushes: Shiny blushes were not on my list of recommendations. Although they don't make the cheek look crepy or wrinkly like shiny eyeshadows do to the eyes, it still looks out of place to have sparkling cheeks during the day. Blushes that went on with a sheen or shine but did not sparkle received a warning, but were not rated as high as matte blushes. This is more of a personal preference than a problem. You should just know exactly what you are buying and what you can and cannot expect from any product. It was essential for blushes to have a smooth texture and blend on easily, however, the silkier the feel, the better the rating.

Lipsticks: The hardest products to review were lipsticks. Each woman has her own needs and preferences. Some women like more sheer applications; others prefer glossy or matte finishes. Color is also difficult to recommend because of the wide variation in taste and wardrobe colors. When it came to appraising lipstick, I primarily reviewed the range of color selection and textures available, citing my personal preferences for creamy lipsticks that went on evenly and weren't glossy or sticky. I overlooked lip glosses unless they were unique in some way, as I usually don't recommend them. Lip glosses don't stay on longer than an hour or two, and most lipsticks nowadays are creamy enough to make the lips feel moist without looking wet and greasy.

Eye, Brow, and Lip Liners: These products had so many variations that it is hard to sum them up, but basically all pencils, regardless of brand, have more in common than not. Most eye pencils, lip pencils, and eyebrow pencils are manufactured in Germany, and whether they cost $20 from Chanel or $4 from Almay, they are likely to be exactly the same. Some pencils are greasier or drier than others, but for the most part there are not marked differences between pencils. Eye pencils that smudged and smeared, lip pencils that were greasy and wouldn't last, and eyebrow pencils that went on like a crayon were all rated as ineffective. Keep in mind that whether or not an eye pencil smears along the lower eyelashes depends to a large extent on the number of lines around your eye, how much moisturizer you use around the eye area, the type of under-eye concealer you use, and how greasy the pencil is. The greasier the moisturizer or the under-eye concealer, the more likely any pencil will smear, and that you can't blame on the pencil.

As a general rule I never recommend pencils for filling in the brow. I only use powder, and I encourage you to do the same. Any eyeshadow color that matches your eyebrow color *exactly* can do the trick with either a tiny eyeliner or angle brush. Brow gel and eyeshadow or brow shadow work superbly together to fill in the brow. There are a handful of companies that make a clear brow gel meant to keep eyebrows in place without adding color or thickness. These work well, but no better than hairspray on a toothbrush brushed through the brow.

Mascara: I reviewed mascaras based on their ability to go on easily and quickly while building length and thickness. Brush shape has improved drastically over the years and definitely makes a difference to the application of mascara. A brush can be awkward to use if it is too big or too small. Mascara should never smear or flake, regardless of price. A $4 mascara is no bargain if it doesn't go on well, smears, or flakes. However, no mascara on the market can hold up to a heavy layer of moisturizer around the eyes. If you pile on any kind of moisturizer, whether it be oil-free, a gel, or designed especially for the eyes, your mascara will be affected.

I did not include waterproof mascaras in the previous edition of *Don't Go To The Cosmetics Counter Without Me*. This purposeful exclusion was because I don't recommend using them. Trying to remove waterproof mascara is awful for the eyes and worse for the lashes. All that pulling and wiping isn't good for the skin and tends to pull out lashes. That has not changed, but this time I did decide to include these for review. Many women, including myself, when swimming or attending a special occasion that may produce tears, choose to wear waterproof mascara to prevent black streaks from lining the face. There are dozens of waterproof mascaras out there, but only a handful are truly reliable. If you're going to wear a waterproof mascara, you should at least buy one that works.

Brushes: The search for brushes was an important one because they are so essential to applying makeup correctly and beautifully. Blush and eyeshadow brushes are carried by some of the major cosmetics lines, and most department stores sell brush sets of some kind. Brush quality was rated on overall shape and function as well as the softness and density of the bristles. An eyeshadow or blush brush that had scratchy, stiff, or loose bristles was not recommended. Let me warn you against buying brush sets. Brush sets are almost always packaged with brushes you don't need or can't use. It is best to buy brushes individually so you can select the best ones for your needs and the shape of your face and eyes.

YOU DON'T HAVE TO AGREE

As you read my comments, you may find yourself disagreeing with me. That's OK, because the criteria you use to evaluate cosmetics may differ from mine. Or, for any one of a dozen reasons, a product I hate may work well for you. What I present are merely guidelines, my point of view, about what works and what doesn't. If you decide to follow any of my suggestions, be sure to try the specific product if you can before you buy it. My recommendation is not a guarantee. But at least I may have sent you down the path of discovering what does and doesn't work for you.

I want to make a few more points about these reviews. Neither the information nor the evaluations are endorsements, nor do they represent a particular company's sponsorship. Believe me, none of the cosmetics companies paid me for my remarks or time; in fact, I think most would prefer to lock me up! Many wouldn't even grant me telephone interviews when I enquired about rationales for product formulations and ingredients.

The following list of brand names is alphabetical, so the order in which they appear does not represent my preference. There is no implied winner among any of the cosmetics companies I included; no one line had all the answers or had a majority of great products. Almost every line had its strong and weak points.

I would encourage you to take this book with you on shopping trips to the cosmetics counters or the drugstore. Then you will have all the information you'll need readily at hand. There is no way you can remember the details of each product, color, and brand. Do try to be discreet at the department store cosmetics counters—don't be surprised if you find that using the book in clear view of the salespeople makes them defensive or irritated. There are always risks when a consumer comes prepared with information. I urge you to persevere. Nothing will change at the cosmetics counters if you don't change first.

Warning: All prices and products listed are subject to change. Prices go up and products are discontinued and replaced without notice. Prices of cosmetics sold in drugstores can vary from store to store, and they often go on sale. In spite of the erratic pricing of cosmetics, I included this information to give you a basic guideline for comparison. Color suggestions were based either on tester units available at the makeup cosmetics counter, samples (including gifts with a purchase or discounted promotions), and products that were purchased. The color, shade, or tone of a particular product can fluctuate for a number of reasons. If I refer to a particular foundation as being "too peach" and you find that it's just right, it may be that we simply disagree or it may be that the product I tested is different from the one you used.

Adrien Arpel

Adrien Arpel needs a face-lift, but that doesn't seem to be happening anytime in the near future. Very little has changed since I reviewed this line more than two years ago. Skin care seems to be the main focus of this company, and they have added some new wrinkle erasers and moisturizers with colorful-sounding names. The color line remains stagnant. Regrettably, many of the products are still too thick and heavy, too out of date, or don't work well. For example, all the foundations in this line are supposed to be applied over a mauve "primer" called Porcelain Coverbase, which goes on rather lavender white. That extra layer feels uncomfortable, so if you like a light makeup application this is not the line to try. Two of the foundation types have colors I don't recommend, and their consistencies are not the best. (Even the salespeople at the Adrien Arpel counters confided that the color choices were poor.) But the Two-In-One Creme Powder Makeup is quite good and can definitely be used by itself. The eyeshadows in this line are almost all too shiny, which is unfortunate, since you can choose any two or three colors for their duo or trio containers. (The concept is nice because, in theory, you shouldn't end up buying a color you won't use). The blushes are also problematic; they are all rather dull mauve tones, which might be all right for some skin tones, but not if you want a soft, pastel look. Actually the entire color line is, at best, sparse. The lipsticks were good, but the selection was also small.

On the other hand, the service at the Adrien Arpel counters I visited was among the best, with salespeople eager to give you mini-facials (most Arpel counters even have private facial rooms right there in the store) and apply makeup. Service is the focus here and it shows. Now if only the products could live up to the sales force.

Foundation: Adrien Arpel has four types. **Sheer Souffle** *($24)* is hardly sheer; rather, it can go on heavy and greasy unless you really know how to blend. This would only be for someone with extremely dry skin except that the colors are all too peach for most skin tones. **Glycerin Liquid** *($24)* has an unusual slippery texture, gives light to medium coverage, is tricky to blend, and might take a bit of getting used to; it is recommended for oily or combination skin, and most of the colors are for women with darker skin tones. **Powdery Creme Foundation** *($25)* has a wonderful consistency and goes on smoothly; it comes packaged with an under-eye concealer, which would be more impressive if the concealer weren't so dark and yellow. **SPF 15 Total Sunblock Creme Makeup** *($30)* has a rich creamy texture and provides medium to almost thick coverage. The SPF is great but there are only four colors, leaving a lot of women out in the cold.

Foundation Colors to Try
Glycerin Liquid *($24)*
Sable may be a good color for women of color with dark skin tones.
Two-In-One Creme Powder Makeup *($25)*
All of these are great color choices: Naturelle (slightly peach), Flesh, Nude, Flesh, Bare, and Buff.
SPF 15 Total Sunblock Creme Makeup *($30)*
All of these colors are great: Bisque, Beige Silk, Tawny Beige, and Midnight Suntan.

Foundation Colors to Avoid
Sheer Souffle *($24)*
All of these colors are either too orange or too pink: Ivory, Fair, Basic, and Tan.
Glycerin Liquid Powder *($24)*
All of these colors are too orange: Wheat, Cashmere, Honey, and Maple.
Color Tint Sport Moisturizer *($20.50)*
All of these colors are too peach: Light, Medium, Dark, and Bronzer. (The bronzer is too shiny, but may be OK for darker skin tones for evening wear.)

Concealer: Adrien Arpel has a unique concealer system called **Moisturizing Undereye Concealer** *($17)*. It is a yellow-orange color too dark for most fair, light, and medium skin tones, and tends to crease under the eye. It is not meant to be worn alone, but blended over a product called **Coveraway** *($17)*. Coveraway is blue in color and goes on blue. The explanation Arpel gives for this strange color is that blue deflects shadows better than white or light beige. I disagree. **Moisturizing Shadow Undercoat** *($15)* for the eyelid is an unnecessary product because foundation and powder essentially do the same thing. One of the inherent problems with this line, and many other lines, is the ludicrous number of products they want you to use. Case in point: If you use the Shadow Undercoat, the **Porcelain Coverbase** *($23)*, the Coveraway, the Undereye Concealer, *and* foundation, it's quite likely that your face will feel weighed down with makeup because it is.

Powder: Adrien Arpel has three good shades of pressed powder called **Real Silk Powder** *($20)*. You aren't getting any serious amount of real silk although this product does have a soft texture. The **Silk Bronzing Powder** *($22.50)* shades are all shiny and not recommended.

Eyeshadow: Much like the blush, **Mix & Match Eyeshadows** *(two shades plus compact, $20.50; refills, $7 per color)* are a great idea, but again the color selection is poor—they're all too shiny to recommend. The **Powdery Creme Eyeshadow** *($15)* stays well, but is difficult for me to recommend because I personally find it inconvenient to use. The colors are all matte but go on dry, are difficult to blend, and have a tendency to crease.

Blush: I like Adrien Arpel's concept of offering the consumer an empty container with two sections into which you fit individually packaged tins of blush and contour color. It is a cost-effective idea that prevents you from having to buy a color you won't use in order to get a shade you will. The problem is that the selection is limited to darker blush colors and many of them are shiny. You can also choose from a selection of pressed powders that come in a nice array of colors. But it isn't very convenient to buy a compact with two pressed powder colors. The **Powdery Creme Blush** *($18.50)* also comes in a limited range of colors, but the shades are softer and brighter.

Blush Colors to Try
Mix & Match Cheek Color
(two shades plus compact, $20.50; refills, $7 per color)
> All of these colors are OK: Contour, Ginger, Apricot, Azalea, Natural Pink (more mauve than pink), Pink Mauve, and Strawberry.

Powdery Creme Blush ($18.50)
> All of these are a good color choice: Aubergine, Pink, Chocolate (good contour color), and Rouge.

Lipstick: Adrien Arpel makes a product called **Lipstick Lock** *($12.50)* that is supposed to prevent lipstick from bleeding into the lines around the mouth and keep the color the same all day. I found that it did not keep the color from shifting and it definitely did not prevent my lipstick from bleeding. There are three types of lipstick in this line: **Matte Powder Creme** *($15.50)*, which contains kaolin (clay), goes on almost like a powder, and has a tendency to dry out the lips; **Cream Lipstick** *($15.50)*, which has a nice consistency but a small selection of colors; and **Sheer Lipstick** *($10.50)*, which is really a lip gloss in a tube.

Eye, Brow, and Lip Liners: Two-Tone Brow Pencil *($12.50)* goes on very dry and hard across the brow and the two colors are not necessary. There are only four shades of **Kohl Eye Rimmer Pencils** *($11.50)*, each with a slick, almost greasy texture that smears. There is also a selection of fat eye pencils called **Eye Trimmers** *($11)*. These are difficult to sharpen and can smear during the day. The **Lip Liner Pencils** *($12.50)* come with a lipstick brush on one end—a nice idea and somewhat convenient, but a decent pencil with a separate lipstick brush would be just as effective and less expensive. Adrien Arpel also makes a brow gel, but it comes in only one shade and, obviously, that color isn't going to suit everyone.

Mascara: I am sorry to say that the **Super Brush Mascara** *($14)* wasn't all that super. It smudged and flaked off by the end of a long day and didn't build very thick lashes. **Every Other Layer Lash Thickener and Conditioner & Separating Creme** *($16)* can't "condition" the lashes, but if used before you apply the mascara it can help make thicker lashes. Of course, the mascara should do that on its own without the need for an additional product to help.

Almay

Almay has a long-standing reputation as one of the few lines, whether sold at the drugstore or at cosmetics counters, that is 100 percent hypoallergenic. Given that there are no specific guidelines about what ingredients are less likely to cause allergic reactions, this is an admirable feat. For the most part, Almay does a good job of eliminating well-known irritants such as fragrance, formaldehyde compounds, lanolin, and lauryl sulfate compounds. But those may not be the ingredients that cause your particular skin problems. Almay has some excellent products worth considering. Though the color selection is a bit sparse, there are several areas in which Almay excels. They make some of the best mascaras, blushes, and lipsticks I've tested, and they also have a superior under-eye concealer that comes in a tube and has a creamy, soft texture.

Foundation: Almay has over six different foundations but testers are not available for any of these. The **Cream Powder Makeup** with SPF 15 *($5.25)* is packaged in such a way that you can't even see the actual color at all. None of the foundations are being included in this review because you can't make a discriminating consumer decision about which color would be best for you.

Concealer: Almay's **Cover-Up Stick** *($3.95)* is a good concealer that comes in three workable shades: Light, Medium, and Dark. The lipstick-like applicator helps it to go on creamy, but not greasy, and it tends not to crease in the lines around the eye. This one is definitely worth looking into, although the consistency may be too moist for oily skin types. There is also an **Undereye Cover Cream** *($3.95)* that comes in a pot in three excellent shades: Light, Medium, and Dark. It is somewhat greasy, although it is good for dry skin and doesn't crease in the lines around the eye. Almay's **Waterproof Extra Protection Concealer** *($4.50)* also comes in three shades: Ivory, Light, and Medium. These are not great colors; they are all fairly peachy plus I don't recommend using anything that's waterproof for everyday use.

Powder: Almay has three types of powder: **Luxury Finish Loose Powder** *($5.73)* and **Matte Finish Pressed Powder** *($5.23)*. They are almost identical; all are talc-based, although the Matte Finish does not contain mineral oil and the **Blotting Powder** also contains clay. Most of the colors are neutral, without peach or pink overtones. Unfortunately, the way the colors are packaged you can't see the colors so there is no way to be certain you are getting the right color.

Eyeshadow: Almay has recently introduced a matte selection of eyeshadows that are quite lovely. **Matte Classic Duo** *($3.95)* has a small but good color selection. The rest of the eyeshadow selections are not the best I've seen on the market. The colors are too shiny and the selection is extremely limited. Their **8-Hour Color** *($4.95)* eyeshadows lasted longer than eight hours, yet I wonder why Almay markets an eyeshadow that lasts less time than most women would consider reasonable; nevertheless they are all shiny and not recommended. Their **Waterproof Shadow Pencil** *($4)* comes in colors that are too shiny to recommend or too difficult to use—tones such as Marine Blue, Yellow, and Bright Teal. The waterproofing is also a problem because of the difficulty in removing it when you cleanse your face. **Liquid to Powder Eye Tint** *($4.25)* comes in a tube with a sponge-tip applicator. It goes on slightly wet and then dries to a powder. For an overall eye color it isn't bad and it does stay on well, but it would be hard to control for specific shading or placement. Almay also makes a **Wear Extending Eyeshadow Primer** *($3.95)* that is basically just talc and mineral oil. It doesn't work any better than using your foundation over the eyelid followed by a light dusting of powder.

Eyeshadow Colors to Try
Singles ($2.75)
> Both Fawn and African Violet are good color choices.

Matte Classic Duo ($3.95)
> All of these colors are wonderful and blend easily: Soft Suede, Neo Classic, Honey Plum, Lilac Confetti, Paradise (difficult combination of colors), Painted Desert, Wall Street, and Rainforest (can be too green for most skin tones.)

Eyeshadow Colors to Avoid
Singles ($2.75)
> All of these colors are extremely shiny: Topaz, Tapestry, Platinum, Pebble Beach, Rose Fresco, Island Breeze, Champagne, Organdy, Sherbet, and Batik (too blue).

8-Hour Color ($4.95)
> All of these colors are extremely shiny: Crystal Violet, Sunset, Night Sky, Moonrose, Thunderstorm, and Tradewind.

Blush: Almay has a small but excellent selection of blushes. There is little difference between the **Cheek Color Blush** *($3.95)* and the **Brush-On Blush** *($6.50)* except that the latter has an attractive mirror compact. The **Cream To Powder Blush** *($3.95)* is outstanding and the colors go on very soft.

Blush Colors to Try
Cheek Color ($3.95)
> All of these colors are beautiful: Mauve, Rose, Soft Pink, Peach, Fuchsia, Plum, Cherry, Mid Pink, Apricot, Blush, and Soft Bronze (good contour color).

Brush-On Blush ($6.50)
> All of these colors are beautiful: Tawny Rose, Dune Blossom, Sunlit Peach,

Hint of Mauve, Pure Pinkberry, Soft Apricot, Damask Rose, and Silkberry.
Cream to Powder Blush ($3.95)
All of these colors are great: Rosewood, Crystal Mauve, Pink Sand, Primrose, Fresh Peach, Berry Mauve, Tender Pink, and Terra Rose.

Blush Colors to Avoid
Brush-On Blush ($6.50)
Shimmering Pink is the only color to avoid.

Lipstick: Almay has a small but attractive selection of lip colors called Color Protective Lipstick *($4.95)* that go on soft and perfectly creamy, but be careful: some are shiny. They also have an **SPF 15 Lip Color** *($4.95)* that is more of a sheer gloss and doesn't stay on very well, although the SPF 15 provides good protection from the sun.

Eye, Brow, and Lip Liners: Almay has an excellent, albeit small, selection of automatic **Lipcolor Pencils** *($4.95)* with a dry but smooth texture. There are several eyelining products: **All Day Shadow Liner** *($4.50)* comes in colors that are too bright to recommend; **Kohl-Formula Eye Pencil** *($4.75)* has a sponge tip at one end and, in spite of the limited color selection, it is a good basic pencil; **Skip Proof Eye Lining Pen** *($4.95)* is a felt-tip liquid liner that comes in navy, black, and brown. **Eye Defining Liquid Liner** *($4.79)* is a standard liquid liner in a tube that can create a very dramatic line around the eye. **Soft Brow Color** *($3.13)* is a standard pencil with a brow brush at one end. If you're going to wear eye pencil a brow brush is essential to soften the line.

Mascara: Almay makes some of the best mascaras on the market. Both **One Coat Mascara** *($4.95)* and **Mascara Plus** *($4.95)* create beautiful lashes without clumping or smearing, and the price is right! **Triple Thick Mascara** *($3.99)* and **Perfect Definition Mascara** *($4.79)* both build long thick lashes that don't clump or smear. What a find! **Longest Lashes Mascara** *($4.75)* is a good mascara, but in comparison to the others it is not the one to choose. **Wetproof Mascara** *($4.95)* doesn't build much length, but it definitely stays on underwater.

Avon

I wish I could say I liked Avon's products better than I did, but, sad to say, I didn't. As far as price, variety of products, and convenience are concerned, this is one of the best, but that is pretty much where it starts and stops. The mascaras tended to smear, almost all the eyeshadows are shiny, even the so-called matte ones, and the lipsticks have little to no staying power. One of the other major complaints I have about Avon is their sales force. Although these women try hard, most of them are little more than order takers. In fact, most of the representatives I talked to were quite honest about how much they didn't know about makeup or skin care. Obviously, Avon does not offer much in the way of education about makeup or skin care, the individual products, or the line itself.

The lack of product information is quite understandable: Avon has more products than almost any other line I've reviewed. It would be a wonder if any salesperson could keep track of it all. In addition, most of the women who work for Avon do it less than part-time, to earn extra money, not as a major source of income. (The average sales representative earns about $5,000 a year, top sellers earn about $10,000, and the rare exceptions earn more than $20,000 a year.) That constitutes a sales force whose main interest is not necessarily Avon. For me this meant many failed attempts to find reliable information or sales representatives who had enough product samples so I could make a complete evaluation without having to buy every single product.

One of Avon's major sales tools is their catalog, which comes out every other week (26 times a year). These slick, rather copious compendiums make for some intense retailing and consumer browsing. Jewelry, fragrances, clothing, knickknacks, date books, video tapes, gift items, shampoos, men's grooming products, bath accessories, and toys are within the diverse range of merchandise that fills these mini-books. How do you make a decision about what to buy? It is simply beyond me. When it came to skin care and makeup, none of the sales representatives I talked to had demos of all the products or knew what to recommend. None of them could identify what colors I should wear or why one product would be better for me than another. That means you have to go by the pictures in the product book and your own impressions. Not a great way to decide.

There are some definite bargains to be found here, but not everything is worth recommending. By the way, Avon deserves a lot of credit for using women of all ages and colors in their catalogs. What a refreshing change from the sterile, overly pubescent mainstream fashion magazines. One more point of interest: **Tones of Beauty** is Avon's attempt to have a selection of color tones suited to ethnic women. It is a nice effort, but the selection of eyeshadow and blush colors is disappointing. Almost all of the shades are intensely shiny. The foundations are quite good, but the selection is limited. The rest of the products apply to all women, regardless of skin tone.

Beauty Note: In Canada some of the products have different names; in particular, Avon's Anew is called Nova.

Foundation: Avon has five types of foundation that are remarkably good. The color selection is neutral, with only a few shades that are too pink or orange. That is a strong positive. Each of the five foundations contains sunscreen with an SPF of 6. Not great, but better than nothing. **Natural Finish Creme Powder** *($6.49)* has an excellent texture, and is recommended for normal to dry skin. However, dry skin will have a rough time with this product; because of the powder finish, dry skin will tend to look drier. It is best for normal to slightly oily skin with no visible pores. **Perfecting Creme** *($4.49)* is a very emollient foundation that goes on smoothly, providing medium coverage. It is recommended for very dry skin, but it isn't emollient enough to fit that category. The ingredients actually make it quite matte. It would be great for someone with normal to dry skin who is looking for better coverage. **Oil-Free Liquid** *($4.49)* provides lightweight coverage and a matte finish. It is good for someone with normal to oily skin. **Enhancing Liquid** *($4.49)* goes on smoothly and provides medium coverage. It feels quite emollient on the skin and is actually good for normal to dry skin. **Pure Care Gentle Liquid Makeup** *($4.49)* is also oil-free and provides light to medium coverage. Glycerin is its second ingredient, so it tends to feel more dewy on the skin. The claims for this one are endless, everything from hypoallergenic to nonstinging and nonburning. Any foundation that contains a chemical sunscreen, as this one does, runs the risk of causing an allergic reaction and burning the eyes. The same color names are used for all the various types of foundation and the colors are equivalent.

Foundation Colors to Try Regardless of Product Type

All of these colors are very good to excellent: Porcelain Beige, Blush Beige (may turn pink on some skin tones), Almond Beige, Honey Beige (may turn peach on some skin tones), Spiced Amber (may turn peach), Sunny Beige (may turn peach), Tawny Beige (may be good for very olive skin tones, but may be too ashen for most skin types), Golden Bronze, Rich Copper (may turn orange on some skin tones), and Rich Mahogany.

Foundation Colors to Avoid Regardless of Product Type

Rose Beige is too pink for most skin tones and True Beige is too orange for most skin tones.

Concealer: Avon makes three types of concealing products that come in four shades: White, Light, Medium, and Dark. The Light and Medium are fairly pink and the Dark can be too orange for most skin types. The White is a good possibility, but you have to blend your foundation over it carefully so you don't end up with white circles around your eyes. Unfortunately, these concealers tend to crease easily into the lines around the eye. This is true for the **Ultimate Coverage Concealer** *($4.49)*, which is fairly greasy, and for the **Pure Care Concealer** *($2.99)* and **Concealing Stick** *($2.99)*, which are both somewhat waxy. Concealing Stick and Ultimate Coverage Concealer both contain quaternium-15, a preservative that is considered very irritating, and the Pure Care Concealer contains phenoxyethanol, also considered a very irritating preservative.

Avon also offers **Hide 'N Perfect Correcting Creme** *($2.99)*, lavender and green cover liquids that are supposed to even out sallow or red skin, respectively. This type of product doesn't work and is never recommended by professional makeup artists. Foundation is all the coverage any women needs. One unnecessary product is their **Hide 'N Prime Eyeshadow Base** *($3.99)*; too much wax in this product makes it hard to blend without getting dry skin, and I saw no difference in the way my makeup went on or lasted. Foundation on the lid followed by powder provides the same base without the extra step.

Powder: The five shades of face powder, ranging from light to dark, come as **Translucent Face Powder Pressed** *($5.99)*, **Oil-Control Powder** *($5.99)*, which contains no oil, and **Translucent Face Powder Loose** *($5.99)*. These basic talc powders would work well if the colors were more neutral, but all are a bit on the pink or peach side for most skin types. Be careful.

Eyeshadow: Avon's **Silk Finish** eyeshadow collection is quite extensive. All of the shades come in varying combinations of **Silk Finish Singles** *($2.29)*, **Duos** *($3.49)*, and **Quads** *($4.49)*, which are conveniently broken up into cool and warm tones, and there are some attractive, soft neutrals. (I recommend buying single shades because with quads you end up using only one or two and the other two are wasted.) What also appears convenient is the identification of which colors are shiny and which are matte. Yet almost all of the colors designated matte turned out to be shiny. I *never* recommend shiny eyeshadow because it makes skin look wrinkly, it looks whitish as it wears off, and it is unsuitable for daytime wear. That was very disappointing.

Blush: The same caveat is true for the blushes. The colors for the two different types of blush—**Color Release** *($5.99)* and **Natural Radiance** *($4.99)* (they actually have very similar ingredient lists and aren't that different except for the name and the price)—are conveniently broken down into warm and cool colors. The texture is quite nice, but the ones identified as matte turned out to be shiny. Like shiny eyeshadow, shiny blush is a problem. You might consider buying it for the evening, but this would be the only reason to. And remember: shiny products are never suitable for women with oily skin.

Avon also offers a blush cream stick called **Natural Radiance Blush Stick** *($3.99)*. Cream blushes do not last as long as powder blushes and are difficult to blend on most skin types; they go on choppy unless you are very good with makeup.

Lipstick: With four types of lipstick and Avon's broad color selection, you would think lips are well covered, but that is not the case. While the color selection is good, it tends mostly toward softer pastel tones, and the textures are all fairly similar. The **Color Rich Lipstick** *($3.49)*, **Satin Smooth Lipstick** *($3.75)*, **Unlimited Moisture Lipstick** *($3.49)*, and **Color Release Long-Wearing Lipstick** *($3.79)* all go on sheer and slightly greasy (as opposed to opaque and creamy), which means the color doesn't last all that long and it takes a lot of swipes to build up any color at all. They do keep lips moist and provide a softer, more natural look, but except for the Color Release

Long-Wearing Lipstick, the color just doesn't last long enough. The Color Release Lipstick leaves a subtle tint on the lips after the lipstick is gone, keeping the appearance of color longer than the others. All of the lipsticks have a small amount of sunscreen, and the Unlimited Moisture Lipstick has an SPF of 15. The colors are divided between cool and warm shades, although this time the delineation between frost and matte seems to be dependable.

Eye, Brow, and Lip Liners: Avon's **Lip Lining Pencil** *($1.99)* and **Eye Lining Pencil** *($1.99)* are both excellent. They go on soft, are not greasy, only a few shades have shine, and they stay on well. Now that's my kind of pencil, and at these prices you can buy one of each. (Stay away from the Ocean Blue, Aquamarine, and Blazer Blue eye pencils.) The colors are divided into cool and warm tones. All of the lip liners except the frosts are fine. **The Lip Coloring Pencil**s *($2.49)* go on thicker and creamier than the Lip Lining Pencils, but many shades are shiny. I would recommend giving them a try, but shiny lip color isn't the best; it tends to look whitish after an hour or two. **Glimmersticks** for eyes, lips, and brows *($2.49 and $3.79)* go on too greasy and also have too much shine.

Mascara: At these prices I wish could say these are wonderful mascaras, but they aren't. They aren't terrible, but they don't build up well and can't compare to some of my favorites at the drugstore. A positive is that they don't smear and they wash off easily. Try them if you aren't looking for a mascara that builds up long and thick. An interesting touch, although one I consider unnecessary, is the date dial on the cap. If you set the dial for the month you start using it, it tells you when three months are up so you know to purchase another. I think three months is too short, plus the dial comes loose easily and then you're stuck guessing. Mascara generally gets used up or dried up in three to four months anyway. When it gets dry, throw it out and get another. **Model Perfect Mascara** *($3.29)* builds up the thickest of all the mascaras. **Body Workout Mascara** *($3.29)*, which supposedly stays on better while you exercise, is just the same as the other mascaras. **Pure Care Mascara** *($3.29)* claims to be designed for contact wearers, but there seems to be no difference in how it goes on, wears, or washes off. **Wash-Off Waterproof Mascara** *($3.29)* has the most confusing name, although it does wash off just fine. **Advanced Wear Waterproof Mascara** *($3.29)* is very stubborn, just what you want in a waterproof mascara. No matter how much water you throw on it or how hard you rub, this stuff won't come off. It will only budge with a generous dousing of oil and wiping. It's messy and it pulls at the lashes, but then this is only for water activity and not for every day, right?

Brushes: Avon often sells a small collection of brushes *($19.95)*. The set comes with a blush and powder brush and a lip or eyeliner brush, a small eyeshadow brush, and an eyebrow or lash comb. The blush and powder brush are quite good, but the eyeliner brush is too thick and the eyeshadow brush is too flimsy. The set looks like a deal, but you would be better off buying brushes individually elsewhere.

The Body Shop

Walking into this store can be a bit confusing at first. Instead of being greeted by elegantly dressed salespeople you are likely to find a young, enthusiastic staff wearing jeans and T-shirts that say "CRUELTY-FREE." Brochures describing the horrors of animal testing, the efforts of Amnesty International, the educational impact of The Body Shop in Harlem, and the beauty philosophy of the Woodabe Tribe of Africa are more prominent than any information about makeup and skin care. Yet this is indeed a makeup and skin care boutique, imported directly from England. Starting with only one small storefront in London, it has grown to hundreds of shops all over America, Europe, and Australia. Actually, the London papers have been reporting recently on The Body Shop's financial problems as a result of overexpansion and increased competition from an amazing number of Body Shop clones.

What a unique experience it is to shop these affectionate, unassuming shops. Sad to say, as was true when I first reviewed The Body Shop, I wish I could say only wonderful things about this company, because their philosophy and efforts to live up to that philosophy are quite impressive. But that isn't the case. Although many of their products are good, they aren't as exceptional as the company's outlook, and they have their share of cleansers that dry the skin and toners that can irritate the skin. The products boast a great deal of food, herbs, and vitamins, which are great for those who are interested in that sort of thing (a lot of people are), and the prices aren't bad. The skin care products do come in small trial sizes, so if you disagree with me or want to explore on your own, you can try them for a minimal amount of money.

Colourings is the name of The Body Shop's color line. The small cosmetics display area in the stores is quite accessible and you are free to play with the demos all you want, which is nice, but there isn't any convenient shelving where you can put your things down and the mirrors aren't the best. There is no sales pressure here, which may be company policy or the consequence of hiring store personnel who are not trained to be makeup or skin care experts. There are no sales speeches, but there is also no "expertise." to If you know what you're looking for, it's a wonderful way to shop, although you have to be very careful. Most of the eyeshadows are shiny, the foundation colors are limited, and the mascaras are just average.

Foundation: The Body Shop has two types of foundation. **All-In-One Face Base** ($14.95) can go on either wet or dry, but either way it can look somewhat powdery. It is like a powdery cake foundation, which can be OK for normal to slightly oily skin types. **Liquid Foundation** *($5.95)* goes on light, with a smooth texture. The problem with both of these foundations isn't quality, but the limited number of colors. The nice colors merit a try: 02, 03, and 05. The Liquid Foundation in particular is definitely worth the cost. There is also a **Tinted Moisturizer SPF 12** *($6.95)* that comes in two shades: Fair to Medium (which is fairly pink) and Medium to Dark. These go on very sheer but can give the skin a strange color. **Translucent Bronzer** *($5.35)* has a small amount of shine and can be a bit on the orange side.

Concealer: The **Concealer** *($4.50)* goes on smooth with a dry, thick texture, but it tends to crease into the lines around the eye. The colors are OK but not the best; 001 and 03 are too pinky peach, but 01, 02, and 04 are good choices. **Extra Cover Concealer** *($6.95)* is very heavy and greasy. It comes in two color choices that are both too yellow for most skin types. **Color Balance Fluid** *($8.50)* comes in two colors: Green and Rose-Pink. Both are supposed to change the underlying skin color, but they only leave a strange tint behind that is then covered up by the foundation. This step is best left out of all makeup routines.

Powder: There are two **Pressed Powder** *($6.95)* colors. Both are OK but may go on chalky. The **Tinted Bronzing Powder** *($6.95)* is a great color, but that is the only color, so it isn't for everyone.

Eyeshadow: Unfortunately, almost all of the eyeshadows *($4.95)* are too shiny and not worth recommending except for two: 02 is a nice rose-peach color and 06 is a soft plum. Just before this book went to press The Body Shop discontinued these dated colors and introduced 16 new matte shades of eyeshadow *($4.95)* that looked quite promising. We were unable to evaluate them properly, so you might want to test the neutral shades in this collection yourself. They are not only reasonably priced, they seem to be quite good. The **Eyeshadow Pencils** *($7.15)* look more convenient to use than they are. The color glides on easily, but the tips are difficult to keep sharpened. They are also too shiny to recommend. **Complete Colour** *($9.95)* is an interesting product that comes in a tube applicator and can supposedly be used for eyes, lips, and cheeks. It has a cream-to-powder consistency and is fun to use, but not very practical; it feels too dry on the lips, the colors aren't the best for the eyes, and the tube applicator is hard to use on the cheeks.

Blush: Both **Cream Blush** *($5.25)*, which comes in only two colors, and **Powder Blush** *($5.25)* are definite possibilities; the color choices are limited but very good. **Brush-On Rose** *($10.95)* and **Brush-On Bronze** *($12.95)* are containers of beaded powders. I find this a messy and inconvenient way to apply a product that is nothing more than blush, but it is eye-catching; the colors are shiny.

Lipstick: The Body Shop has a small selection of lip glosses in a tube called **Liptints** *($5.95)*. They stain the lips with a slight color that remains once the gloss part wears off. They are too greasy-looking for me to recommend for a daytime business look, but they can be acceptable if you blot after you apply the

Liptint. The lipsticks *($5.95)* are OK, fairly creamy, but come in a small range of colors and don't last very long.

Eye, Brow, and Lip Liners: The **Double Ended Eye Definer** *($4.50)* eye pencils are matte at one end and shiny at the other. Several of the colors are intensely blue. It's a good idea, but these colors aren't worth it. The **Lip Liners** *($4.15)* are quite good, with basic soft colors that have a nice, smooth texture. The **Eyebrow Makeup** *($7.55)* comes with two colors in one container—a light brown and a dark brown. If you only have one eyebrow color, it is a waste to buy both colors.

Mascara: Colourings Mascara *($4.95)* is not a very good mascara. It goes on poorly, spikes the lashes, and has a tendency to flake.

Brushes: These are some of the nicest brushes *($2.95 to $5.95)* on the market. The blush brush is soft and a perfect size, as are the eyeshadow brushes. The only brushes I don't recommend are the lip brush and the foam applicator stick.

Bonne Bell

Only in Canada, Bonne Bell has an unexpectedly large selection of testers for almost every product. The convenience is appreciated, and it would be great if all the other drugstore lines would follow their lead. However, other than accessibility to testers in Canada, there isn't much to praise in this line. Bonne Bell has come a long way since I was a teenager, when this was the youthful, hot line of the '60s, with an emphasis on blue eyeshadows and pink lipsticks. The flagship of the line back then was Bonne Bell's Ten-O-Six Lotion for acne. It was a standard alcohol-based toner that burned like hell on the skin, but those were the days when we thought that if it didn't burn or hurt it couldn't be working. Bonne Bell now has a totally contemporary feel and their products have improved, but not enough to give them a high rating. The eyeshadows are all shiny and the texture is poor, the foundations are all fairly pink, and the lipsticks are on the greasy side. Even the mascaras come up short on length and thickness. With just a few adjustments Bonne Bell could be a contender with L'Oreal and Revlon, but it still has some work to do to get up to their league.

Foundation: Bonne Bell sells two types of foundation with OK textures but terrible color choices. **Sheer Radiance** *($5.99)*, which is very sheer and has a soft texture, and **Matte Radiance** *($5.99)*, which has a good matte finish, both have a preponderance of peach, pink, and rose colors. As a result, neither foundation can be recommended.

Concealer: Color Care Concealer *($5.79)* has a poor color selection and tends to move right into the lines around the eyes no matter how much you blend. There is also a **Coverstick** *($3.99)* that has a rather heavy texture and a poor color selection.

Powder: Because of the way the **Natural Radiance Pressed Powder** *($4.99)* is packaged, you cannot see the shade. Without any visual reference (a color swatch on paper doesn't cut it), there is no way to make a wise color choice.

Eyeshadow: Bonne Bell has a surprisingly large selection of eyeshadows, called **Stay True Eyeshadows, Singles** *($2.99)*, **Duos** *($3.99)*, and **Quads** *($4.99)*; they are all shiny and the texture is choppy and dry. What a shame, because there are some great neutral shades here.

Blush: Stay True Cheek Color *($5.99)* has a dry, somewhat choppy texture, but the colors are great. I recommend Tea Rose, Rich Berry, Smoky Plum, Purple Plum, Bordeaux, Rosewood, Nude, Bronze, Sweet Cinnamon, and Terra Cotta. Only Pink Parfait and Desert Spice are somewhat shiny.

Lipstick: There's only one kind of lipstick, called **Stay True Lip Colors** *($4.99)* and nicely divided into matte and shiny. Of course you should avoid the shiny ones for daytime. The texture could be better; they are almost too greasy and don't last very long.

Eye, Brow, and Lip Liners: There's a nice array of standard eye pencils in this line.

Mascara: Unlimited Lengths Mascara *($4.99)* won't produce unlimited lengths at all and tends to smear. **Smudge Proof Mascara** *($4.99)* is also a disappointment because it does tend to smudge, the curved brush is hard to use, and it doesn't build much length or thickness.

Borghese

I have to admit that I like many things about Borghese. Its singularly Italian flavor stands out in the midst of so many French and American lines. Borghese is also one of the more expensive product lines. Regardless of the price tag, the products I liked, I really liked, and the ones I disliked, I really disliked. For example, Borghese has some of the most velvety smooth foundations—particularly Milano 2000 (samples are often available), Lumina Compact Foundation, and Liquid Powder Foundation—although they tend to be too fragrant. Their Liquid Powder Blush is also quite remarkable. The eyeshadows, on the other hand, are beautiful to look at in the container but are mostly too shiny to recommend, as are the regular blushes, although they do go on smoothly. Be careful with all of the Borghese products; many of them are overly fragranced.

Borghese has huge, very attractive, and inaccessible counter displays that are organized loosely into three color groupings: Oro (yellow-based), Rosso (pink-based), and Neutrale (neutral/beige). These groupings are helpful but a bit more confusing than some of the other cosmetic lines that divide their colors into the traditional four color families.

Foundation: Borghese has several types of foundation that are outstanding, although the color selection could be better. **Effetto Immediato Spa Firming Makeup SPF 8** *($35)* is a superlative foundation for dry skin. It won't firm anything on your face, even though it is supposed to contain some fancy protein complex; protein can't be absorbed into the skin to do anything except keep it moist. The strongest, or at least the most realistic, selling point is that for about the same price as other high-end foundation you get almost twice as much product. Not a bad deal. I wish the container wasn't a pump bottle, but I guess you can't have everything. **Milano 2000** *($35)* is a wonderful liquid foundation that goes on smooth and velvety and works well for dry skin, although it does have a strong fragrance. It contains a small amount of sunscreen that is not adequate to protect from the sun. **Molta Bella Liquid Powder Makeup SPF 8** *($35)* works well on somewhat flawless, normal skin. If you have any dry skin at all, you may find that this foundation, which goes on wet and dries to a powder, looks tight and flaky. The SPF is low but better than nothing. **Lumina Compact Foundation** *($42.50)* is quite light, although it looks as if it would go on heavy and thick. This is a nice, convenient way to put on foundation and would work well for women with normal skin who want a matte but moist look to their makeup. **Hydro Minerali Natural Finish Makeup with SPF 4** *($27.50)* doesn't contain much of a sunscreen but this is a good, lightweight, very sheer foundation that actually has better colors for darker skin tones than it does for lighter ones. This is supposed to blot oil all day; it won't. In fact, Hydro Minerali has a slight amount of shine. It's not all that noticeable, but someone with oily skin who wants their oil shine absorbed won't be thrilled with the sparkle. **Effetto Bellezza Targeted Treatment Makeup SPF 8** *($35)* is a very creamy, although surprisingly light, foundation that feels great on the skin. The claim is that it can improve the skin's condition in ten days. If you have dry skin, it can help because it contains emollients but that's about it; there are no wonder ingredients in here.

Foundation Colors to Try
Effetto Immediato Spa Firming Makeup SPF 8 ($35)
All of these colors are excellent; Alabaster, Buffed Beige (slightly peach), Golden Beige (slightly ash), Natural Beige, Pale Beige, Richest Beige (slightly peach), and True Beige.
Milano 2000 ($35)
All of these colors are very good, with a silky consistency: Rosso 1 (may turn pink), Rosso 4 (may turn orange), Rosso 5 (may turn slightly orange), Oro 1, Oro 2, Oro 3 (may turn orange), Oro 4, Oro 5, Neutrale 1, Neutrale 2, Neutrale 3, Neutrale 4 (may turn pink or rose), and Neutrale 5 (may turn orange).

Molta Bella Liquid Powder Makeup ($35)
All of the shades are excellent; there's not a bad one in the bunch.

Lumina Compact Foundation ($42.50)
All of these colors are excellent; unfortunately, they are also somewhat shiny, although not enough to be that noticeable: Peretta Beige, Peretta Fresco, Soft Bronzed, Solari Beige, Alabastro, Ivory Lustro, Beige D'Oro, and Golden Biscotti (which may be too ashy for most skin tones). Use these cautiously.

Hydro Minerali Natural Finish Makeup with SPF 4 ($27.50)
All of these colors are good color choices and the texture is soft and sheer: 5, 6, 7, 8 (slightly orange), and 9 (slightly ash).

Effetto Bellezza Targeted Treatment Makeup SPF 8 ($35)
All of these colors are great: Alabaster Beige (slightly peach), Natural Beige, Buffed Beige, Golden Beige (slightly peach), True Beige (slightly peach), and Richest Beige.

Foundation Colors to Avoid

Effetto Immediato Spa Firming Makeup SPF 8 ($35)
Healthy Beige is too peach to recommend.

Milano 2000 ($35)
Rosso 2 and Rosso 3 are too pink for anyone's skin tone.

Molta Bella Liquid Powder Makeup ($35)
Rosso 1 and Rosso 2 are too orange for most skin tones and Neutrale 4 is too ashy for most skin tones.

Hydro Minerali Natural Finish Makeup with SPF 4 ($27.50)
All of these colors are too peach or pink to recommend; 1, 2, 3, and 4.

Effetto Bellezza Targeted Treatment Makeup SPF 8 ($35)
Healthy Beige is too pink to recommend.

Concealer: Absolute Concealer ($25) has a soft, creamy texture and only two good colors to choose from; Ideal Light is fairly pink, but Ideal Medium is a good neutral (slightly peach), and Ideal Deep would be good on darker skin tones. Borghese also makes a concealer and eyeshadow primer in one called **Eye Duetta ($20)**. This two-ended product is a bit of a waste because the eyeshadow primer side is essentially talc and mineral oil and doesn't help the eyeshadow to stay on any longer than your foundation and a light dusting of powder would. The under-eye concealer side is actually quite good, goes on softly, and tends not to crease. However, if you want to give this a try and not waste any product, the eye primer actually works quite well as an under-eye coverup as well.

Powder: Borghese makes a titanium dioxide (opaque white mineral) and talc-based pressed powder called **Powder Milano ($28.50)**. It goes on very soft and comes in excellent colors: Rosso, Neutrale 1 (may be slightly pink), Neutrale 2, and Neutrale 3 are all nice; Oro may look a bit peach on some skin tones. The **Loose Powder Milano ($37.50)** also contains titanium dioxide and talc and is a good, although expensive, powder.

Eyeshadow: Borghese makes an appealing assortment of eyeshadow colors, but almost all have too much shine. I've been told they are working on deshining many of these colors, which would be smashing. Most of the eyeshadows have a great silky texture and go on soft, while others feel very heavy and go on quite thick. The matte shades however, are excellent and worth testing for yourself.

Eyeshadow Colors to Try
Singles, Duales, and Trios ($27/$32)
All of these colors are great velvety matte shades: Lucca Spices, Aida (tricky color combination), La Boheme, Modernist, Roma Charcoal/Roma Ivory, Tuscan Tabac/Tuscan Beige, Amalfi Coastal Plums, and Amalfi Sandstones.

Eyeshadow Colors to Avoid
Singles, Duales, and Trios ($27/$32)
All of these colors are too shiny: Immaginario, Amalfi Teal/Amalfi Violet, Como Moss Green/Como Ecru, La Scala Orchid/La Scala Rose, Capri Chocolate/Carpri Cream, Firenze Pink/Firenze Taupe, Palermo Plum/Palermo Plum Mist, Titian Taupe, Solare, Barocco, Innocente, Neo Classico, Minima, Tempestosa, Venezia, Boldini Berry, Solare, Florentine, and Sonata.

Blush: Borghese makes a unique blush called **Liquid Powder Blush** *($30)* that is one of my favorites. It is similar to the cream-to-powder-type blushes, only softer. It doesn't work well over dry skin and is best suited for someone with normal or oily skin. The Liquid Powder Blush goes on wet, dries to a powder with a rather smooth matte appearance, and the color stays on well. The product comes packaged with a brush and small sponge; the brush is easy to use, as is the sponge. All the colors are worth a try, particularly if you are looking for something different in a blusher. Unfortunately, most of the colors are slightly shiny, although not shiny enough to make a noticeable difference on the skin. **Blush Milano** *($28)* is a very satiny regular powder blush that also has lovely colors. This one feels great but on oily skin types it can wear poorly. By the end of the day it can look choppy and uneven.

Blush Colors to Try
Liquid Powder Blush ($30)
All of these colors are excellent, even though they contain a slight amount of shine: Milano Tulle, Milano Rossore, Milano Vino, and Milano Terrecotte.
Blush Milano ($28)
All of these colors are superior: Coralino, Rose Brillante, Rosetto, Pesca, Peach Biscotti, Frascati (great contour color), Coral Eletrico (can be too orange for most skin tones), Ametista, Pink Marabue (slightly shiny), Peonia, Coral Aida, Garnet Boheme, Botticelli Pink, Plumage, Plum Rosa, Vino, Raphael, Titian, Tangerine, Prato Peach, and Amalfi Suntan and Natural Finish Bronzer (best used as a contour and not an all-over face color).

Blush Colors to Avoid

Blush Milano *($28)*

Terracotta, Pelates, Plumage, Petallo, Pisa Rosewood, and Abbronzato are all too shiny to recommend.

Lipstick: Borghese sells three types of lipstick in a limited selection of colors. **Lip Treatment Moisturizer** *($17)*, with a moisturizing center, is very greasy and more like a lip gloss than a lipstick. **Superiore State-of-the-Art** *($17)* is a set of shiny lipsticks that go on rather dry and iridescent. Last is a matte lipstick called **La Moda Concentrate** *($17)* that goes on matte and rather dry. La Moda wears well, yet although the claim on the package says it won't feather (bleed into the lines around the mouth), it did for me. It didn't feather as much as some lipsticks I've worn, but it definitely did bleed some, plus the dry texture isn't the most comfortable on the lips. Borghese also sells powder lip colors called **Lip Colour Superlativo** *($17)*. Even if I liked the concept of powder lip colors, and I don't, all of these shades are intensely shiny and make the mouth look rather wrinkled.

Eye, Brow, and Lip Liners: The eye and lip pencils *($17)* are basic pencils made in Germany, just like a dozen other lines. They come in a good array of colors, although some are shiny. One end of the eye pencils has a sponge tip to blend the color. Borghese also has an excellent brow gel, called **Brow Milano** *($17)*, with a fantastic brush (which is so important for getting this on right), Unfortunately, the color selection is limited (there are no shades for ash or black brows), but what there is is great.

Mascara: Borghese's **Volumina Luxuriant Mascara** *($15.50)* has a wand unlike most others on the market. One side is smooth with grooves, and the other has small stiff bristles. I didn't care for this product at all: I found it hard to use, it did not lengthen my lashes, and it flaked and smeared as the day went by. **Maximum Mascara for Sensitive Eyes** *($17)* is an excellent mascara, but it isn't any better for sensitive eyes than any other mascara on the market. It builds beautifully and doesn't clump or smear.

Chanel

The people at Chanel counters across the country really have their acts together. I guess when your cosmetics are this expensive, you have no other choice. The salespeople dress in a Chanel uniform and are very enthusiastic about the fact that Chanel has its origins in France (never mind that none of the products seems to be manufactured there). For the most part, I did not find Chanel to be an exceptional product line. None of the Chanel products impressed me as being worth the expense. The foundations were OK and the mascara was good, but not great; the lipsticks were quite good and the way they were arranged by color was very helpful, but, again, I'm not convinced they're worth the steep price. Chanel is definitely a prestige line, and most of the women I interviewed believed that they got something special for their money, though none were exactly sure what that something special was.

Chanel's counter displays are set up in such a way that you need a salesperson to help you test the products. All of their blushes, lipsticks, and eye and lip pencils are attractively divided into very helpful color groupings called Les Violettes (pink/plum), Les Rose Bleus (red/blue), Les Naturels (soft tones of brown/peach), and Les Soleils (yellow/coral). These are then subdivided by intensity. The eyeshadows are grouped similarly, but I was confused about how some of the shades relate to their color groups. Some Chanel counters have a device that asks you questions about your hair and eye color; this is to help place you within a set range of foundation choices. When I tried it, the foundation suggestion was much too dark for my skin tone.

Based on their color groupings and intensity categories, Chanel claims that any woman can wear any color group (yellow tones, blue tones, pink tones, and natural tones, according to their charts) as long as she wears the correct intensity of the color. That may be a valid theory, but most women who know their colors would disagree. If you are interested in trying a different color palette, you may be curious enough to give this a try, but be very skeptical. I think it's just another angle to sell more products.

Chanel eyeshadows tend to be too shiny and too intense—they don't produce what I would call a subtle look at all. The consistency of their eyeshadows and blushes, however, is sensational. The eyeshadows have the new quilted texture that is supposed to prevent cracking and flaking. Many companies use this pressing pattern, but it makes no difference in their products' duration or strength. At almost $50 each, I find Chanel eyeshadows too expensive to even look at, especially when part of what you're buying is crepy-looking eyes.

Foundation: Chanel's foundations have great textures and all have an SPF of 8, which is OK, but SPF 15 is better. Some of the foundation types have an extremely limited and poor color selection, so it almost isn't worthwhile to complain about the cost because there is so little you would want to purchase. However, there are exceptions, and some foundation colors are worth the stretch in budget. The relatively new oil-free foundation **Teint Pur Matte** *($40)* has a medicinal smell, plus it contains aluminum starch, which can be an irritant for some skin types. It also comes in a pump bottle, which is not a container I prefer. Two other foundations, **Teint Naturel** *($48.50)* for normal to

dry skin and **Teint Creme** *($55)* for dry skin, are a better bet, although I defi-
nitely prefer the colors and texture of the Teint Naturel. All of these foundations contain much too much fragrance for my taste. **Teint Essential** *($38.50)*
is an ultra-sheer tint that comes in three shades: Natural, Beige, and Bronze.
These have too much shine to recommend. They also contain honey, which is
supposed to be a good free-radical scavenger. It may be, but there are other
ingredients, such as vitamins A, C, and E, that can do the job just as well and
are found in many moisturizers and foundations. **Teint Facettes** *($40)* is a
cream-to-powder foundation that has a very silky feel and goes on very sheer.
This is actually a wonderful product and the color selection is excellent.

Chanel sells an under-makeup base called **Perfect Colour Matte**, **Perfect
Colour Creme**, and **Perfect Colour Pearle** *($50 each)*. These semi-opaque
tints lay a sheer white or colored layer over the face, supposedly to make the
skin look fair and flawless. It's hard for me to understand this one. In my
opinion these undercoats make the skin look chalky or give it a strange color
that you then cover up with foundation. **Perfect Colour Bronze** and **Perfect
Colour Blush** *($50 each)* are two of the sheerest face tints you'll find on the
market—best for fair to medium skin tones only. All these products contain an
SPF of 8, which is nice but not enough to protect the face from the sun.

Foundation Colors to Try
Teint Pur ($40)
> All of these colors are great: Porcelain, Soft Bisque, Natural Beige (can
> turn pink), Warm Beige (can turn peach), and Golden Beige (a good
> color, but can turn orange on some skin tones).

Teint Pur Matte ($40)
> All of these colors are excellent and incredibly neutral: Opale, Porcelain,
> Ivory, Soft Bisque, Natural Beige, Tawny Beige, and Golden Beige.

Teint Naturel ($48.50)
> All of these colors are great: Natural Beige, Golden Beige, Tawny Beige,
> Soft Bisque, Alabaster, and Porcelain.

Teint Creme ($55)
> All of these colors are great: Tawny Beige, Golden Beige, Soft Bisque, and
> Alabaster.

Teint Facettes ($40)
> All of these colors are excellent: Alabaster, Ivory, Soft Bisque, Natural
> Beige, Warm Beige, Tawny Beige, and Golden Beige.

Foundation Colors to Avoid
Teint Pur ($40)
> All of these colors are either too pink or too peach to be recommended:
> Alabaster, Ivory, and Tawny Beige.

Teint Pur Matte ($55)
> There is only one color in this foundation group to avoid and that's Warm
> Beige, which may be too orange for most skin tones.

Teint Creme ($55)

Natural Beige is too peach for most skin tones and Pale Ivory is too pink for most skin tones.

Concealer: Chanel's under-eye **Corrective Concealer** *($23.50)* has a slightly greasy texture and the colors are not the best. Professional is too blue and combines poorly with the foundation. Light is slightly pink, but may be acceptable for some skin tones. Medium can turn slightly rosy. Plus, this concealer can crease.

Powder: Chanel's **Loose Powder** *($35)* and **Luxury Pressed Powder** *($35)* tend to go on very chalky in spite of their lovely silky texture. Light and Medium are the best shades, and work for fair-skinned women only. Bronze, designed for women of color, is too orange for most darker skin tones. Mauve, Pink, Peach, and Pink Champagne appear too chalky and have too much color to look natural on the skin. The **Luxury Powder Compact** *($90)* is a stunning gold compact; it would be worth the money if it were a necklace, but it's not. The compact is refillable and the powders are supposed to have "light reflecting properties," but these are still just shiny powders that come in three colors: Dawn, Daylight, and Dusk.

Eyeshadow Colors to Try
All Eyeshadow Colors ($47.50)

The only matte eyeshadow colors in this line are: Black, Les Mats Naturels 4, Les Mats 5, Peach, Chamois, Taupe, Lilac, Buff, and Khaki.

Eyeshadow Colors to Avoid
All Eyeshadow Colors ($47.50)

All of the following colors are too shiny (most are ultra-shiny) to recommend: Escabrilles, Violes, Les Imaginaires, Intensites, Les Fascination, Soleil, Les Coronmandel, Sublime, Les Ochres, Sea Gray/ Petal, Pale/Sable, Mist/Smoke, Brownstone/Fawn, Dusk/Dawn, Earth/Clay, Chestnut/ Crystal, Peach/Sable, Black/White, Purple Smoke, Currant, Golden Leaf, Topaz, Sables 4, and Toffee.

Blush: For the most part Chanel's blushes have a splendid silky texture, but some are too intense for most skin types and most are too shiny. Their blushes also contain cornstarch, an ingredient that can clog pores.

Blush Colors to Try
All Blush Colors ($27.50)

All of these colors are good: Peach Flame (for darker skin tones), Mauve 3 (slightly shiny), Cherry 2 (somewhat shiny), Peach Salon (can be too orange for most skin tones), Tempting Beige (somewhat shiny), Fuchsia 1, and Red Fire (for darker complexions only).

Blush Colors to Avoid
All Blush Colors ($27.50)

All of these colors are intensely shiny, which is a shame because most of them are beautiful: Peony, Pink Satin 2, Natural Pink, and Rose Quartz.

Lipstick: Chanel makes one of the few lip products that actually prevents lipstick from bleeding into the lines around the mouth; it is called **Protective Colour Control** *($18.50)*. Unfortunately, it tends to become caked on the lips as you apply more lipstick over it, and it's expensive. The price may be worth it for those who suffer from feathering, but I did find cheaper drugstore products that worked as well. I also liked Chanel's **Rouge a Levres** *($17)* very much. The texture is somewhat creamy and matte, not greasy feeling like many of the other lipsticks you find on the market today. **Professional Lip Basics** *($35)* is a lip color that goes on in two layers: a wet powder that you let dry and a gloss to apply over it. Interesting option, but it didn't last any longer than most other lipsticks I've tested, and it was really too much trouble to use.

Eye, Brow, and Lip Liners: Chanel's **Crayon Contour Des Levres** *($21.50)* for the lips resembles a dozen other lip pencils on the market that are made in Germany. This one happens to have a lip brush on one end, which I guess is convenient, but it doesn't warrant the steep price tag. The same holds true for Chanel's eye pencils, called **Professional Eye Definers** *($21.50)*; they are standard pencils that are also made in Germany. **Professional Eyeliner** *($38)* isn't all that professional. It is just a powder that can go on dry or wet. This comes in three choices of two colors each. The color combinations are a bit strange and you would be better off buying one deep-colored eyeshadow (not shiny) and lining your eyes with it. **Instant Eyeliner** *($25)* is a black liquid in a pot; it goes on very severe and will remind you of Twiggy lashes (if you're old enough). **Precision Brow Definer** *($24)* goes on rather hard, which means it doesn't look so greasy, but it still tends to make hard lines. **Brow Shaper** *($24)* is a brow gel with a poor color selection: Soft Brown, Taupe, and Clear. There are no shades for brunettes or darker hair shades, but brows definitely stay in place and the gel goes on easily, without smearing, which is very important for this type of product.

Mascara: Chanel's **Luxury Creme Mascara** *($18)* is a good mascara that goes on easily, doesn't smudge, and builds thick lashes.

Charles of the Ritz

Charles of the Ritz is overlooked by many women, perhaps because it is usually found at the lower-end department stores. But take notice: there are some great, reasonably priced products in this line. Charles of the Ritz even has great colors in all of their products for women of color. One point of irritation: many of the product names are silly and childish (a pressed powder called Toast of the Town or Baby Bare; a foundation called The Naked Truth or Tisket-a-Bisquit). You would think a cosmetics company like this expects adults to buy these products, but it is hard to relate to cosmetics that sound like a lame joke.

For the most part Charles of the Ritz is still a low to medium-priced line with an impressive range of products to consider. The display unit is a bit confusing, but the basic concept is a good one. The board is divided into two color groups: Cameo and Rose. Cameo is the yellow and earth tone colors and Rose is the pastel and vibrant blue tone colors. The palette is further divided into smaller groups of blush, eyeshadow, lipstick, lip liner, and nail polish that are all color coordinated. This is helpful, but almost too specific, allowing the consumer little visual room to play with their own color combinations. Still, it can be helpful for those who really need help coordinating all the color elements of a makeup look.

Foundation: Charles of the Ritz makes five different foundations that are really quite good, but the color selection is small and inadequate. They would be better off eliminating one of the lines and adding colors to the others. **Superior Moisture Foundation for Normal to Dry Skin** *($18.50)* provides medium coverage. **Superior Foundation for Normal to Oily Skin** *($18.50)* goes on light and feels great. **Perfect Finish Makeup SPF 6** *($12.50)* comes in a pump bottle (which isn't my favorite because you tend to pump out more than you need and you can't get it back in the bottle), and has a smooth, light, matte finish and a wonderful color selection. However, it does contain alcohol (and smells somewhat—medicinal), so it would only be appropriate for someone with oily skin. **Revenescence** *($30)* is best for dry skin. It has a silky texture, but, unfortunately, a poor color selection. **Powderful Foundation** *($17.50)* is more like a pressed powder than a foundation; it would work as a light matte finish for someone with normal skin only. The color selection is excellent, but be careful: when the product is used by itself, the skin may look dull and powdery.

Foundation Colors to Try
Superior Moisture Foundation ($18.50)
All of these color are very good: Natural Ivory (may turn slightly pink), Soft Beige, New Beige (may turn pink), and Bronzed Beige (great tan shade).
Superior Foundation ($18.50)
All of these color are good choices: Sunlit Beige (may turn pink), Simply Beige, Toffee Beige (good tan color but may turn slightly peach), Warmed-Up Beige (can turn pink), and Toasted Beige
Perfect Finish Makeup SPF 6 ($10)
Ignore the stupid names of these colors; all of them are strongly recommended because they are truly excellent shades: Milkwood, Oh So Bare, The Naked Truth, Sugar Baby Blush, Sunny Disposia, Honey Do, Sandpiper, Tisket-a-Bisquit (could turn rose on some skin types), A Little Cafe (great golden brown), and My Sinnamon.

Revenescence ($30)

All of these colors are very good: Ivory Beige, Warm Beige (good, but could turn peach), Tawny Beige (OK color, but could turn rose), Sienna Beige (great golden brown), and Bronzed Beige (excellent medium to deep color).

Powderful Foundation ($17.50)

All of these colors are good possibilities, even though the names are somewhat childish: First Blush (may be too pink for some skin tones), Beyond Pale (may be too pink for some skin tones), Baby Bare, A French Cafe, Honey Love, and Toast of the Town.

Foundation Colors to Avoid

Superior Moisture Foundation ($18.50)

All of these colors are not recommended: Beige Sand, Deep Beige, Beige Blush, and Tender Beige.

Superior Foundation ($18.50)

These colors are not recommended: Beige Sand, Real Tawny, Beige, and Peach Beige.

Revenescence ($20)

Sand Beige is too rose for most skin tones and Honey Beige is too pink for most skin tones.

Concealer: Hide and Chic Cream Concealer *($10)* is an excellent product that goes on a bit on the dry side, but it stays on great, covers well, and doesn't slip into the lines around the eye. The color selection is small—Light, Medium, and Dark—but they are all quite good.

Powder: Charles of the Ritz has an excellent although small selection of powders. **Powder Glow** *($20)* is a standard talc-and-mineral-oil lightweight powder that comes in four reliable translucent shades. **Translucent Pressed Powder** *($16.50)* is a standard talc-based powder that is also quite sheer and comes in three shades: Light, Medium, and Dark. There is also a **Blemish Control Powder** *($14)* that contains talc and clay. It won't control blemishes, but it is definitely absorbant and comes in three good shades: Light, Medium, and Dark.

Eyeshadow Colors to Try

Singles and Trios ($10/$15)

All of these are soft, lovely colors that have a tiny bit of shine, not enough to stay away from unless you are concerned about crepy skin on the eye. Some of the trio sets are the best color combinations to be found anywhere: Lovey Dovey, Sassy Little Rose, Nutmeg, Brown Bag, Sandbox, Smoky Plum, Thyme Out, Soft Fawn, Moonglow, Dramatic Accents, Woodland Wanderings, Sunset Mauve, Purple Dusk, Neutral Nuance, and Far Horizons/ Windswept.

Eyeshadow Colors to Avoid

Singles and Trios ($10/$15)

All of these colors are either too shiny, too blue, or too green: Blue Mist,

Apricot Cream, Green Gables, Terra Rosa, Blue Moods, and Just Peachy.

Blush: Perfect Finish Powder Blush *($12.50)* comes in a beautiful assortment of colors, with a silky, sheer texture; they are just slightly shiny, but not enough to lose a strong recommendation. Even the vivid colors can go on soft. All of the colors are nice to work with: Tequila Sunrise, Round Robin, Ivory Pink, Rich Rose, Very Sherry, Geranium, Azalea, Rare Wine, Misted Coral, and Desert Peach.

Lipstick: Charles of the Ritz has several types of lipstick to choose from. **Powderful Lipstick** *($10)* contains powder—as the name indicates—and goes on matte and very dry. After a week or two you may find that your lips are getting chapped and dried out. You would be better off using a creamy lipstick with a lip sealer underneath that prevents lipstick from feathering into the lines around the mouth. **Perfect Finish Lip Color** *($10)* has a fairly greasy texture but nice colors. **Revenescence Moist Lip Color** *($15)* has a creamy consistency that is a bit on the greasy side, so it doesn't have much staying powder. The "maximum wear" claim is a fair one; these lip colors have a stain that helps keep them around longer. **Semi Matte Lipstick** *($10)* also contains a stain and has a somewhat soft matte texture.

Eye, Brow, and Lip Liners: Classic Liners for Eyes and Lips *($11)* are fairly standard pencils manufactured in Germany; they have a smooth texture that can be a bit on the greasy side and there aren't many colors to choose from.

Mascara: Charles of the Ritz mascaras are actually quite good. **Perfect Finish Lash** *($11)* is an excellent mascara with great lengthening ability, but it does have a slight tendency to smudge by the end of the day. **High Density Lash Mascara** *($9)* is very good, goes on quickly without clumping, and doesn't smear or flake.

Christian Dior

Dior is a great name when it comes to fashion, but it seems to have lost its footing in the world of makeup. There is nothing particularly outstanding in this line. The eyeshadows are all extremely shiny and the color combinations somewhat difficult. It is one of the few lines with a five-color eyeshadow set, but the colors are almost all too shiny to recommend other than for evening wear. The foundations come in a very limited selection of colors, and although I like some of the textures and coverage very much, the manufacturer charges a fairly hefty sum for makeup that is not particularly special or unique. In spite of the limited foundation choices, the pressed powders come in eight different shades, only a few of which are really worth trying. The lipsticks are fairly creamy, but the fragrance can be a bit overwhelming. The counter displays are nice enough and easily accessible, but the colors aren't organized by color families, which can make finding your color range difficult.

Foundation: Christian Dior has six types of foundation; each has a wonderful smooth silky texture, but limited and somewhat poor color choices. **Teint d'Ete** *($38)* is a very light, sheer foundation that comes in a pump container (not my favorite way to dispense foundation). **Teint Dior** *($38)* is a light foundation designed for normal to dry skin. **Teint Actuel** *($38)* is a thicker, creamier foundation for extremely dry skin that blends better than you would think from the look of it. **Teint Ideal** *($38)* is an oil-free, matte foundation that contains alcohol, which means it can irritate some skin types; the colors are just OK. **Teint Poudre** *($38)* is a pressed powder that is talc- and oil-based, nothing unique or special. This powder is slightly heavier than most and it is meant to be used either as an all-over foundation or as a powder. **Reflet du Teint** *($38)* is a sheer tint that comes in two colors: Soft Light and Golden Light. Both can leave a peach cast on the face.

Foundation Colors to Try

Teint d'Ete ($38)

All of these colors are excellent: Claire d'Ete, Blond d'Ete, and Or d'Ete.

Teint Dior ($38)

Moyen Rose is a good neutral shade that may turn peach on some skin tones; Presque Beige is a good neutral beige tone.

Teint Actuel ($38)

Beige Delicat and Beige Dore are great colors; True Beige is a good medium to tan color, but may turn peachy yellow.

Teint Ideal ($38)

Soft Beige, Golden Beige, and Golden are the only reliable colors for this foundation.

Teint Poudre ($38)

All of these are excellent colors: Champagne, Spice (good tan shade), Dune, Rye, Havana, and Opaline.

Foundation Colors to Avoid

Teint d'Ete ($38)

Both Terre d'Ete and Matin d'Ete are too orange for most skin tones.

Teint Dior ($38)

Moyen Beige may turn orange on some skin tones, Claire Beige may turn pink on some skin tones, and Tres Claire Beige is just too pink.

Teint Actuel ($38)

Rose Tendre is too pink for most skin tones and Rose Beige is too peach for most skin tones.

Teint Ideal ($38)

All of these colors are either too peach or too pink to recommend: Soft Golden, Rose, Medium Beige, Medium Rose, and Medium Gold.

Teint Poudre ($38)

Melon can be too peach for most skin tones.

Concealer: Stick Corrector *($15)* has a good dry texture that tends to crease into the lines around the eyes. **Perfecteur** *($15)* comes in only two colors and both are too peach for most skin tones.

Powder: There are eight **Pressed Powders** *($30)* and **Loose Powders** *($37)* that come in identical shades, though the color selection leaves much to be desired. Pale Mauve is too pink; White Porcelain goes on too white and pasty; Florentine Blonde is too orange for most skin tones; Scandinavian Rose is too pink for all skin tones; Sahara Beige can turn pink on some skin tones; Invisible Plus isn't invisible and it can turn pink. Summer Sun is the only great color in the lineup. The three pressed powders that come in natural skin shades are good: Invisible Plus (has a slight pink tint), Sahara Beige, and Summer Sun (great color for tan skin tones) have a soft consistency and go on sheer. There are also two bronzing colors that are more peach and rust than bronze; Light Tan and Bronze are not recommended.

Eyeshadow: Almost all of Dior's eyeshadows are too intensely shiny to recommend, but they have a new small group of colors called **Powder Eyeshadow and Eyeliner Palette** *($46)*. There are four different sets of totally matte colors with four shades each and one dark powder eyeliner color. This product is actually quite good, with a wonderful silky texture, but the color combinations are a bit strange. The best one is Browns (the shadows) and Blue (the eyeliner, which is really almost black).

Eyeshadow Colors to Avoid
Duo, Quint, and Ombre Express ($26/$46)
> All of these eyeshadow colors are too shiny to recommend or come in sets where more than one color is too shiny: Bouquets, Extreme Blue, Surprise, Images, Caviar/Vodka, Frost/Violet, Terre/Earth, Gold/Brown, Forest/Dune, Havana/Rose, Dawn/Dusk, Champagne/Blue, Ocean/ Mauve, Praline/ Liquorice, Cafe/Creme, Champagne/Blue Champagne, Siam, Sand & Sugar, Scintillating, Discretion, Pearl, Mist, Pansies, and Monochrome.

Blush Colors to Try
Blush Final ($28)
> All of these blushes have a wonderfully silky consistency and texture; these colors are beautiful: Accent (slightly shiny), Soft, Delicat, Attractive, Contour (excellent contour color), Charm, Ardent, Naturel, and Vivacious.

Blush Colors to Avoid
Blush Final ($28)
> Subtle is hardly subtle, and it is too shiny for daytime wear.

Creme-to-Powder Blush ($28)
> All of these colors are too shiny to recommend.

Lipstick: Rouge A Levres *($17)* feels very moist and creamy and there are some great colors to choose from. **Rouge Accent** *($17)* is a small collection of matte lipsticks that have a more vivid, flat appearance. Dior's lipsticks are hard to recommend because their intense fragrance makes them unpleasant unless you really like the perfume. **Rouge Brilliant** *($17)* is a fairly standard lip gloss.

Eye, Brow, and Lip Liners: The lip and eye pencils *($17)* are fairly standard and are manufactured in Germany. The brow pencils *($17)* come in only three shades; each has a rather dry texture and a brush at one end. Even though I don't care to use a pencil on the brow, this one isn't bad, although any pencil with a similar texture and a separate brow brush could function as well.

Mascara: Thickening Lash Mascara *($15)* supposedly has cashmere, which sounds great, but who wants wool in their mascara? Nevertheless, this mascara goes on well, not as thickly as I like, but it does build quickly, lengthens, and stays all day. **Mascara Parfait** *($15)* goes on great, building beautiful thick lashes without clumping; unfortunately, it can smear under the eye by the end of the day. What a shame.

Clarins

Clarins is best known for its imposing procession of skin care products packaged with a French accent and every popular cosmetic ingredient imaginable, specifically botanicals. Over the past few years they've added a relatively small makeup line. I imagine the reasoning goes something like this: If you've captured a woman's attention with your skin care products, why lose her to someone else's makeup products. Despite this effort I think Clarins will lose sales in the makeup arena because these products just aren't that good.

I've heard many cosmetics salespeople say the French have the best neutral-colored foundations. That definitely isn't true for Clarins. The foundation shades are the weakest link in their color line. All the eyeshadows are ultra-shiny; the pressed powders are all fairly peach; the one type of lipstick is fairly greasy and many are iridescent. The counter display is divided into four small but nice color groups— Corals, Rose, Corals Dores, and Les Roses—but it doesn't help the quality of products. If you want to take look at this line, do it from afar and save yourself some major makeup mistakes.

Foundation: Satin Finish Foundation *($28.50)* has a lightweight texture, but it isn't particularly satiny. **Matte Finish Foundation** *($28.50)* isn't exceptionally matte; even though it goes on somewhat light, it feels fairly dry.

Foundation Colors to Try
Satin Finish Foundation ($28.50)
> These colors are OK: Golden Beige (may turn rose), Sunlit Beige (may turn peach), Tender Bisque (may turn peach), Caramel, Cocoa, and Bronze (may turn peach).

Matte Finish Foundation ($28.50)
> These colors are OK: Golden Beige (may turn rose), Soft Beige (may turn rose), Tender Bisque (may turn peach), and Caramel.

Foundation Colors to Avoid

Satin Finish Foundation ($28.50)

All of these colors are either too peach, too pink, or too yellow to recommend: Golden Honey, Peach Beige, Natural Beige, Tawny Beige, and Soft Rose.

Matte Finish Foundation ($28.50)

All of these colors are either too peach, too pink, or too yellow to recommend: Golden Honey, Rose Beige, Soft Rose, Peach Beige, Natural Beige (this isn't remotely natural), Tawny Beige, and Sunny Beige.

Concealer: Clarins' **Concealer** *($13.50)* comes in three shades: Light, which is too pink for most skin tones; Medium, which is more dark than medium but is indeed a good color; and Dark, which isn't really all that dark but is an OK color. The consistency is also OK but not exceptional, and it can crease into the lines around the eyes.

Powder: Clarins' **Pressed Powder** *($22.50)* is a fairly standard powder that comes in four shades, all with strong overtones of peach.

Eyeshadow: All of Clarins' eyeshadows *($21)* are ultra-shiny, and many of them come in a strange combination of colors that are hard to use together. These colors are not recommended: Pink Sorbet/Violet, Tender Mauve/Sky Blue (even the sky isn't this blue), Pearl/Charcoal, Azalea/Ash Brown, Pink Mist/Smoke Sapphire, Seashell/Blueberry, Pink Peony/Stone, Tender Mauve/Raisin, Golden Leaf/Olive, Sunset/Ember, Fresh Apricot/Taupe, and Copper/Rich Plum.

Blush: Just so you don't think I'm Clarins-bashing, I do happen to like their **Cream-to-Powder Blush** *($20)*. The colors and texture are beautiful. All of these colors are recommended: Fawn, Cinnamon, Fuchsia, Heather Pink, Rose Sand, and Rose Petal.

Lipstick: There is only one type of lipstick *($14)* in this line; it is on the greasy side and many of the colors are iridescent.

Eye, Brow, and Lip Liners: A small standard selection of lip and eye pencils *($12.50)* is available; nothing exciting here either.

Clarion

Clarion was one of the first drugstore cosmetics lines to offer a form of sales assistance that didn't require a salesperson. They started using a simple computer system that allowed consumers to punch in specific details about their skin and coloring. After you answer the handful of questions, the computer tells you what products are best for you according to color grouping and skin type. If you want to believe a computer that's a fine way to shop, but it isn't what I would call even vaguely reliable. First of all, the questions are limited and totally dependent on your awareness of your own coloring and skin type, which isn't as easy as it sounds. It also assumes that all of their products are great and you only need to know which ones to use, but that isn't the case either.

Another problem is whether or not you fit or understand their color groupings. Like most drugstore cosmetics lines, all of Clarion's products are arranged into one of four groups representing, to one degree or another, the four color seasons. Color Group 1 has the cool vivid-toned plums (winter); Color Group 2 has cool pastel tones (spring); Color Group 3 has what they call neutral but seems to be yellow earth tones (summer); and Color Group 4 has yellow tones in darker colors (autumn). The groupings are OK but confusing without someone there to help. For example, just because you fall into Color Group 1 doesn't mean you can't wear the eyeshadow colors of Group 3 or 4.

As it turns out, despite these complaints I did like many of Clarion's products, and the prices are great. However, some of the eyeshadows, even though they don't look shiny, are just a little bit, the waterproof mascara runs and smears, and the foundations do not have testers so you can't try one on before you buy it. Not a great idea when it comes to foundation. This line could be a wonderful source of reasonably priced products, but as always you have to be careful what you choose.

Foundation: Clarion makes five types of foundations: **Exceptional Effects Foundation** *($5.95)*, **Visibly Fresh Oil-Free Makeup** *($5.95)*, **Vital Difference Moisturizing Foundation** *($5.95)*, **Perfect Complexion Lightweight Makeup** *($7.50) and* **Protection 15 Makeup** *($5.95)*. These foundations are too pink and orange to recommend, and as I said before, testers were not available in any of the stores I visited. The Visibly Fresh Oil-Free Makeup does happen to contain oil, but that's true for many so-called oil-free foundations. The first ingredient is cyclomethicone, which is a synthetic oil, not terrible but definitely misleading if someone is looking for a truly oil-free product. By the way, the Perfect Complexion Makeup, which comes in a pump container, claims to be a lightweight foundation, but it isn't. It certainly isn't more lightweight than the Protection 15 Makeup. I am glad they made one foundation with such a high SPF. If only they could improve their colors, this would be great foundation.

Concealer: Clarion has two very good concealers that contain sunscreen; one is rated SPF 15 and the other SPF 8, the colors are good, and the price is even better. The only negative is the lack of color choices, with only three colors for each product. **Protection 15 Concealer** *($4.95)* is the one that has an SPF of 15. It comes in a stick and is good for someone with normal to oily skin. I've been using it quite a bit. I even spread it over my nose to protect it from the sun when I'm not wearing a foundation or moisturizer that contains sunscreen. **Line Minimizing Concealer** *($5.25)* doesn't necessarily minimize lines any better than other concealers, but it is nevertheless a very good concealer. It's a liquid and a bit on the sticky side, but it blends easily and lasts.

Powder: Clarion has three fairly standard powders that are worth checking out. **Silk Perfection Pressed Powder** *($7.95)* is talc-free and has a soft consistency; colors are limited to Fair, Light, and Medium. **Natural Finish Pressed Powder** *($6.25)* is talc-based and comes in a small group of colors: Natural Ivory, Gentle Beige, and Medium Beige. **Oil-Free Translucent Powder** *($6.25)* is much like the Natural Finish, only without oil, and comes in three shades: Fair, Light, and Medium.

Eyeshadow: Most of Clarion's eyeshadows are muted and actually quite nice, except many of them have a slight to large amount of shine even though they don't look shiny in the container. Clarion has a new product called **Captive Color Eyeshadow Plus Base** *($4.95)*. It is a combination that looks like it's giving you two products for the price of one, except that the eyeshadow base isn't great, just an extra step that isn't any better than foundation. This also comes in a set of six eyeshadow shades. I don't recommend any of these. Most of them are shiny, and although it looks like you're getting a lot they are not necessarily easy to work with. It is best to only buy eyeshadows one at a time or in sets where every color is worthwhile to use.

Eyeshadow Colors To Try
Eyeshadow Plus Base ($3.72), Silk Palette Singles ($2.22), and Silk Palette Quads ($3.94)

All of these colors are slightly shiny, but not enough to be a significant detraction if your eyelids aren't crepy: India Spice/Mahogany, Sienna Stone, Smoldering Embers, Auburn Spice, Ivory Cameo, Fresh Lilac, Pink Chablis, Rosewood, Pale Shell, Plumstone, Mocha (slightly shiny), Apricotta, Brick Suede, Soft Sable, and Twilight

Eyeshadow Colors to Avoid
Eyeshadow Plus Base ($3.72), Silk Palette Singles ($2.22), and *Silk Palette Quads ($3.94)*

All of these colors are too shiny or too pastel to recommend: Sugar Maple/Ivy Frost, Rose Quartz/Crystal Blue, Copper Glow/Polished Walnut, Heather Grey/Thunder Blue (this one is matte, but it is also exceptionally blue), English Lavender/Claret, Soft Garnet/Plum Smoke, Tea Rose/Wild Iris, Autumn Blaze, Pure Earthtones (great colors but too shiny to recommend), Misty Plums, Azure Skies (too blue for everyone), Moonlit Orchids (can be OK, but the colors are too bright for most skin tones), Emerald Teal (matte but too green), Wedgwood (too blue), and Indigo Blue (speaks for itself).

Blush: I like Clarion's blushes a lot. They go on very smoothly and the colors are lovely. **Exceptional Effects Blush** *($5.75)*, **Luminous Accents** *($4.95)*, which gives you only half the amount of the other blushes, and **Sheer Illusion Creme-Powder Blush** *($7.95)* are excellent options. So is **the Exceptional Effects Contour Blush** *($5.95)*, which has two different colors, one lighter than the other. Both colors are quite good, but only for blush; you should never contour your face with anything other than a brown-toned color.

Blush Colors to Try

These are all excellent colors: Mauve Twilight, Champagne Pinks, Spiced Apples, Amber Sun, Raspberry, Exquisite Orchid, Palest Pink, Pale Sherry, Soft Coral, Plum Sublime, Sweet Peach, Sienna Spice, Hyacinth, Lush Lilac, China Pink, Plum Chiffon, Ginger Spice, Rich Suede, Spring Tulip, Adobe Dawn, Sandalwood, Heather, and Misted Plum.

Lipstick: There are some great lipsticks in this collection, but unfortunately only a few color choices. The best ones to try are the **Lasting Color** *($5.25)*, and **LipSilks** with an SPF of 15 *($5.25)*. The textures are wonderful and they tend not to run, particularly the Creme group. However, you should avoid all of the frost colors in this line.

Eye, Brow, and Lip Liners: For the most part Clarion has standard, very inexpensive pencils in a small array of colors. **Pensilks** *($4.50)* and **Browsilks** *($4.50)* are twist-up pencils that come with their own sharpener. For pencils they are good, but they're a bit on the greasy side and definitely could smear, although they can easily be blended out to a soft smudged look. **Lasting Effects Eye Pencil** *($3.50)* is just a normal pencil, a bit on the greasy side, and can smear.

Mascara: Clarion has some new mascaras that work very well. **Sudden Lash** *($4.95)* goes on thick, doesn't clump, and stays on without smearing. **Infinite Lengths** *($4.95)* is an excellent mascara, one of the best in this line. It is definitely worth a try if you want long lashes without clumping or smearing.

Clinique

In some ways Clinique is a cosmetics junkie's dream. This is a cosmetics line with a lot of product types to play with and enjoy, from blush to eyeshadows and pencils. But you have to be strong and not allow yourself to be carried away by new toys that might be fun but are not practical or worth the time, money, and effort. I have to admit there is a lot of space to poke about at the Clinique counter. If the space a cosmetics company takes up at a department store indicates how well the line is doing, then Clinique is doing quite well—their counter space usually takes up the most area of any cosmetics line.

In the past Clinique was, and to some extent it still is, associated more with the young consumer. The products, particularly those for skin care, are aimed at oily or combination skin types, which is probably why Clinique attracts a young clientele. And the makeup line includes products and colors that are geared toward younger tastes, with items such as color rubs and tints for the cheek, very sheer blushes and eyeshadows, and a clever variety of eye pencils. Unfortunately, many of the pencils, eyeshadows, and color rubs are extremely shiny and not the best for daytime. Clinique does seem to be expanding their potential market somewhat with a new selection of matte shades, exquisite new blush colors, and a new group of matte lipsticks that are less greasy than the rest of the lipsticks in the line.

Many women, regardless of age, are faithful Clinique customers, some because they believe that the products are hypoallergenic and better for their skin (they aren't). The salespeople, dressed in white lab coats, reinforce this belief. There are several counter displays available, but most of the products can be tested only with the help of a salesperson. The line has no color philosophy; the color products are not arranged by skin tone, which leaves you at the mercy of the salespeople. In spite of my hesitation about the counter organization, I am impressed with Clinique's large selection of foundations, lipsticks, and blushes, all of which are quality products that tend to go on softer and more sheer than most. The price range of the products is more affordable than at other counters. You will also get the best service at the Clinique counters; there always seems to be four to six white-jacketed women dashing around behind the counter.

Foundation: Clinique has several foundations designed for different skin types, almost more than I care to count. Their latest addition is **Sensitive Skin Makeup SPF 15** *($18.50)*. This is one of the few foundations available with a nonchemical sunscreen that is high enough to truly protect the skin. It might feel a little heavy for those who want a sheer application, but I would still encourage a test to see if it works for you. The **Stay True Oil-Free** *($14.50)* is one of my favorite oil-free foundations, and the color choices are great. The **Balanced Makeup Base** *($11.50)*, for normal to dry skin, is also quite good, and the colors are excellent. The **Extra Help** *($18.50)* makeup has a nice consistency and would be good for extremely dry skin, except that most of the colors are too pink or too peach. The only foundation I have never recommended is the **Pore Minimizer**, which is now being discontinued, so I can stop complaining about it. It contained alcohol, which is irritating, and provided little to no coverage because it went on too choppy and was hard to apply. The **Double Face Powder Foundation** *($14.50)* is a pressed powder that contains talc and mineral oil; it can be used as an all-over sheer foundation or as a finishing powder, and the colors are so sheer it's really like wearing no makeup at all. **Continuous Coverage Makeup** *($12.50)* is a very thick, heavy, opaque, oil-based foundation intended for those who want to cover scarring. It should not be used as an everyday makeup. The color selection is excellent and it is one of the better foundations of this type for those who need this kind of coverage. It's not a look I recommend, however.

Foundation Colors to Try

Sensitive Skin Makeup SPF 15 ($18.50)
There aren't many colors available, which is disappointing, but all of them are good.

Stay True Oil-Free ($14.50)
All of these colors are great: Stay Beige, Stay Ivory, Stay Porcelain (may be too pink for some skin tones), Stay Sunny, and Stay Golden.

Balanced Makeup Base ($11.50)
All of these colors are very good: Fair, Ivory, Warmer, and Almond Beige.

Extra Help ($18.50)
There's only one really good foundation color and that's Ivory Bisque. The rest are in the "Avoid" category.

Double Face Powder Foundation ($14.50)
All of these colors are excellent: Matte Bisque, Matte Petal, Matte Beige, Matte Honey, and Matte Tawny.

Foundation Colors to Avoid

Balanced Makeup Base ($11.50)
All of these colors are too orange for most skin types: Honeyed Peach, Sun Glow, and Honeyed Beige.

Extra Help ($18.50)
All of these colors are either too pink or too orange for most skin types: Fawn Beige, Golden Almond, Amber Peach, Beige Glow, and Copper Beige.

Double Face Powder Foundation ($14.50)
Matte Ivory can be too peach for most skin types, but it is so sheer that it may not matter.

Concealer: Clinique has an interesting assortment of concealers. **Quick Corrector** *($8.50)* comes in a tube with a wand applicator; there are two shades, Light and Medium, and both are excellent for light or medium skin tones. The texture is smooth without being greasy and it stays on well. **Advanced Concealer** *($10.50)* comes in a squeeze tube and goes on like a liquid but dries to a powder. It comes in two shades, Light and Medium, and again both are excellent colors. Beware: This product works only if the skin under your eye is smooth; any dry or rough skin will look worse when this type of concealer is placed over it. Clinique also has an **Anti-Acne Control Formula Concealer** *($10.50)* that is very thick and heavy and comes in two shades, Light and Medium. The Light is too pink and the Medium is too peach for most skin tones. The anti-acne part of the formula is colloidal sulfur and salicylic acid, ingredients that will not get rid of a blemish and can cause irritation.

Powder: Clinique has a **Loose Powder** *($14.50)* that is talc-based and comes in a good selection of colors. The **Transparent Pressed Powder** *($11)* is also talc-based and comes in one shade that is supposed to be transparent, but it didn't look that way when I applied it over my foundation. It can look chalky on many skin types.

Eyeshadow: Clinique makes several types of eyeshadow. **Soft Pressed Eyeshadow** *($10.50)* goes on very soft and silky, but most of the shades are too shiny to recommend. The matte shades are fine and they do go on soft. **Daily Eye Treat** *($9.50)* is a liquid in a tube. All of the shades are very shiny, and the liquid dries in place, which makes blending tricky. **Lidsticks** *($12.50)* are fat pencils that come in mostly shiny colors and are not recommended. **Beyond Shadow** *($11.50)* is a unique waterproof eyeshadow. The color is squeezed out of a tube and blended over the eye area. It stays surprisingly well (it tends not to crease) and blends thin and soft, almost like skin. Most of the colors have a little shine, but it was not evident when the shadow was applied, so it doesn't affect the smooth look.

Eyeshadow Colors to Try

Soft Pressed Eyeshadow ($10.50)
This is a superb collection of neutral matte eyeshadows: Pink Ginger, Brown Grape, Brandied Plum, Pure Cream, Pure Neutral, Brown Light, Twig, Pure Warmth, and Honey Sun.

Beyond Shadow ($11.50)
All of these colors are soft and beautiful: Natural, Warmth, Smoke, Brown, Bare, Plum, and Fern.

Eyeshadow Colors to Avoid

Soft Pressed Eyeshadow ($10.50)
Many of these colors are beautiful and soft but shiny, which is OK if the skin around your eyes is smooth and has no lines or crepiness. Those who don't meet this standard should avoid all of these: Golden Lynx, Bronze Satin, Tea Leaf, Violet Rain, Sunset Mauve, Teal Haze, Earthling, Starstruck, Twilight Mauve, Starry Rose, Fawn Satin, Star Violet, Olive Bronze, Silver Peony, Periwinkle Blue, Moon Turquoise, Nude Bronze, Rose Warmth, Grapeskin, Jet Stream, Charcoal, Seashell Pink, Extra Violet, Ivory Bisque, and Peach Silk.

Blush: Clinique has several types of blush and cheek products. **Young Face Powder Blush** *($13.50)* goes on very soft and slightly shiny (even the vivid colors go on sheer). **Beyond Blusher** *($15)* also has an exquisite selection of soft blush colors to choose from, with a slightly softer texture than the Young Face Powder Blush. **Color Rub** *($9.50)* pours like a foundation out of a small bottle and spreads over the cheek or face like a very sheer liquid bronzer, but all the colors are too shiny to recommend. **Gel Rouge** *($7.50),* a liquid that comes in a tube, is supposed to be rubbed over the cheek area to stain it with color—not a good idea for dry, oily, or combination skin types, because it may tint open pores and flaky skin. **Creamy Blush** *($9.50)* is applied like a cream but it dries to a powder, very sheer: all the colors are beautiful. **Cheek Base** *($9.50)* is a waterproof cheek color that comes in four very soft colors. It is more like a tint than a blush, and it can stain pores and make the face look dotted. This is best for someone with normal skin. **Bronze Doubles** *($13.50)* have no shine and can be great contour colors. **Transparent Buffer** *($13.50)* isn't very transparent and both colors, Think Bronze and Sun Duster, are too shiny to recommend.

Blush Colors to Try

Young Face Powder Blush ($13.50)

All of these color are beautiful; some of them are slightly shiny, so be cautious: Cheek Bones (slightly shiny), Fig, Honey Blush (slightly shiny), Plum Blush, Extra Clover, Extra Poppy, Rhubarb (slightly shiny), Gold Rust (slightly shiny), Extra Rose, Ginger Apple, New Clover, Powdered Light, and Chestnut (a beautiful contour color).

Beyond Blusher ($15)

All of these colors are wonderful: Honey Bare, Pink Plush, Sweetheart, Full Bloom, and Peaches.

Creamy Blush ($9.50)

All of these colors are beautiful; Bronzed Rose, Warm Glow, Sunny Blush, Basic Blush, Honey Wine, and Satin Mauve (which is very shiny, but may be good for evening wear).

Blush Colors to Avoid

Young Face Powder Blush ($13.50)

All of these colors are too shiny to recommend: First Blush, Extra Violet, Plum Bronze, Baby Rouge, Pink Blush, and Lemon Geranium.

Lipstick: Clinique has four types of lipstick—**Different Lipstick** *($9.50)*, **Semi-Lipstick** *($9.50)*, **Super Lipstick** *(10.50)*, and **Re-Moisturizing Lipstick** *($9.50)*—and all are excellent choices if you prefer sheer, creamy lip colors. The color selection is wonderful and the textures are light but creamy, perhaps even a bit on the greasy side. None of the current selections provide matte or thick coverage. I didn't notice large differences among the four types, although Semi-Lipstick was definitely greasier and more sheer than the others. Clinique has a new matte lipstick coming out this fall. I could not review it before this book went to press, so you'll have to catch the review in my newsletter, *Cosmetics Counter Update.*

Eye, Brow, and Lip Liners: Clinique's **Lip Pencils** *($8.50)* have a soft, smooth texture and come in an excellent array of colors. There are two types of eye pencils available. **Regular Eye Pencils** *($9.50)* come in a good range of colors and go on soft, without a greasy feel; **Quick Eyes** *($13.50)* have an eye pencil at one end of the stick and a powdered eyeshadow section with a sponge-tip applicator at the other. The eyeshadow is released into the sponge tip when you shake it. If the eyeshadow colors weren't so shiny, I would rec-ommend this gimmicky product as a convenient tool for doing a fast eye design.

Mascara: Clinique's **Naturally Glossy Mascara** *($11)* is good but not great. It goes on quickly and builds thickness, but it also tends to spike the lashes, which isn't the best look. Clinique's mascaras also have dates on them so you know when you bought it and can tell when you should get a new one. The salespeople at the counters often recommend a new one every three months. It's hard to get a consensus on that one from dermatologists. I would suggest keeping it no longer than six months or until you're done, which ever comes first.

Color Me Beautiful

Carole Jackson brought the art of color to an entire generation of women. For the past ten years most women have learned or wanted to learn which "season" they are; in other words, what colors work best with a particular skin tone and hair color. Once a woman knew if she was a Spring (blonde hair and pink skin tones; requires pastel colors with a yellow undertone), Summer (blonde hair and sallow skin tones; requires pastel colors with a blue undertone), Autumn (red hair and pink skin tones; requires yellow-based earth tones), or Winter (brunette or black hair and any skin color; requires vivid blue-toned pastels), she could then find colors that enhanced her skin tone instead of draining the color from it. Perhaps even more so than economics, this philosophy has changed the way women shop for clothing and makeup colors. To one degree or another, I (and a horde of other beauty experts) agree with Carole Jackson, and she should be congratulated on her success.

In response to the demand for her color expertise, she created a makeup line with her name and logo attractively headlining each item. Sadly, the line doesn't deliver the color organization you may be looking for. The color trays are divided into the appropriate seasons but many of the colors overlap and not all of the appropriate color swatches are represented. Colors that are in the Winter drawer are also in the Spring drawer, which doesn't make any sense at all given Jackson's beliefs about color. There are also other problems with this line: most of the eyeshadows and some of the blushes are just too shiny, there is only one type of foundation, which is incredibly limiting, and there is only one pressed powder color. I was hoping for better, but this line isn't what I was expecting.

Foundation: Liquid Foundation *($16)* is actually quite good and light, but only for someone with normal to dry skin. The colors are supposedly divided into the four seasons groupings, but because the shades overlap there is really only two color groupings, not four. Although I agree wholeheartedly with the idea of color as a way to enhance skin tone, all foundations should be neutral, with no pink or peach. Dividing the colors of these foundations into color groupings doesn't make sense. Just because a woman has pink tones to her skin doesn't mean she needs a pink foundation: her underlying skin color is still a neutral color, and why would you want to add more pink to an already pink skin color. It would only make the skin color look more pink. There is never a reason to buy a peach-colored foundation. In fact, when I asked the salesperson if they sold much of the peachcolored foundations, they said no. The most popular shades were the neutral ones. There is also pressed powder type foundation called **Perfection Microfine Powder Foundation** *($16)*. It has a great soft texture and the colors are wonderful. This type of foundation is best for someone with normal skin—dry skin can look too powdery and oily skin look caked by midday.

Foundation Colors to Try
Liquid Foundation ($16)
> All of these colors are superior: Neutral Beige, Tawny, Rose Beige, Porcelain, Cool Beige (could turn peach on some skin tones), Bisque, Ivory (could turn peach on some skin tones), Sand (could turn pink on some skin tones), Tender Tan (excellent golden brown shade), and Natural (could turn rose on some skin tones).

Perfection Microfine Powder Foundation ($16)
> All of these colors are excellent: Tabasco Beige, Creamy Beige, Whisper Beige, Sepia Beige, Toasty Beige, Fawn Beige, Cameo Beige, Cocoa Beige, Golden Glow, and Golden Sand.

Foundation Colors to Avoid
Liquid Foundation ($16)
> All of these colors are too intensely peach or pink to recommend: Beige Blush, Peach Blush, Golden Beige, and Warm Beige.

Perfection Microfine Powder Foundation ($16)
> Rose Glow and Pink Sand are too pink to recommend.

Concealer: Cover Stick *($8.50)* comes in two shades: Light, which is too pink, and Medium, which is an OK shade. The texture isn't the best and the color can definitely slip into the lines around the eye.

Powder: There is only one shade of **Pressed Powder** *($10)* in this line. Although it is fairly transparent, it is only suitable for fair skin tones, which leaves out everyone else.

Eyeshadow: Most of these eyeshadow *($8)* colors go on rather heavy and some are very heavy, which makes them tricky to blend. Be careful: most of these colors aren't as soft as they look. Most of them are fairly shiny, so the selection is limited, but the matte colors do have some great choices.

Eyeshadow Colors to Try
> All of these colors are very good: Espresso, Graphite, Cocoa, Claret, Putty, Buff (great neutral), Warm Pink, Honey, Taupe, Smoky Topaz, Tiger's Eye, and Peach.

Eyeshadow Colors to Avoid
> All of these colors are either too shiny or too blue and green or both:

Gray, Evergreen, Smoke, Champagne, Spruce, Violet, Silvered Mauve, Dove Gray, Periwinkle, Steel Blue, Sapphire, Teal Blue, Aegean Blue, Cool Pink, Smoky Turquoise, Wild Orchid, Teal Bright, Cornflower, Soft Aqua, Copper, Coffee, Bronze, Golden Green, Golden Brown, Sage, Mink, Sterling, Emerald, Jardite, and Olive.

Blush Colors to Try

All of these colors go on soft and are good tones to consider: Rosette, Soft Plum, Soft Rose, Clear Pink, Cranberry (for darker skin tones only), Cedar Rose, Desert Coral, Tawny Peach (darker skin tones only), Chestnut (good contour color), Peach Crystal, and Apricot.

Blush Colors to Avoid

All of these colors are too shiny to recommend: Azalea, Soft Rose, Flirtatious Fuchsia, Simply Red, Plum Wine, Warm Pink, Sunset Red, Clear Salmon, Pink Quartz, Carmelon, Ruby, and Peach Crystal, Rose Gold Bronzer, and Copper Sun Bronzer.

Lipstick: There is only one type of lipstick *($9)*; it is very creamy, and even the soft colors have decent staying power.

Eye, Brow, and Lip Liners: Color Me Beautiful has the standard small collection of lip liners *($8)*, brow pencils *($12)*, and eye pencils *($9)*. These go on well and are just like everyone else's, although one end does have a sponge tip for softening or smudging the line. **Brow Fixative** *($9)* is a clear gel meant to keep eyebrows in place. It works well, but no better than hairspray on a toothbrush brushed through the brow.

Mascara: There is only one type of water-soluble mascara, **Sensitive Eyes Mascara** *($9)*, in this line and it goes on fast and thick but clumps lashes together instead of separating them. It does stay on well and doesn't smear, but the brush just isn't the best.

Cover Girl

Cover Girl is probably one of the largest cosmetics lines to be found at the drugstore. In the past, the dense, cloying fragrance that wafted from their products kept me from recommending almost all of them wholeheartedly, but that seems to have changed. I would hardly call the current fragrance annoying; in fact, for most of their products it is about the same as any other cosmetics line. Cover Girl has also upgraded their products in many other categories since I last reviewed them.

As is true with most cosmetics lines, Cover Girl's eyeshadow shades are more shiny than matte. Still, they do offer a number of matte shades, and the ones they have are actually quite good. Cover Girl offers several types of powder blushes in assorted packages, but I found no discernible differences in how these various products went on or how they lasted; most of the colors went on soft and looked fine. Their lipsticks are good, and the mascaras have improved considerably. But the best news of all is the reduced fragrance.

Cover Girl divides almost all of their colors into one of three color families: Warm, Cool, and Neutral. They provide a chart on the back of some of their products, and most drugstores have a small computer-type device that helps you select your category. After you enter your hair color and skin color, it tells you what color family to select. This is a helpful, easy system to use, and their Cool and Warm categories are usually correct. However, they say that their neutral colors work with all skin tones, and I do not agree with that.

Foundation: Unfortunately, testers are still not available for Cover Girl foundations, so I cannot include them in this review. For the most part these foundations are still highly fragranced and would be difficult to recommend even if there were testers. There is one exception to this rule and that is Cover Girl's **Ultimate Finish Liquid Powder Makeup** *($5.49)*. Not only is this foundation fragrance-free (it's about time Cover Girl) but the application is beautiful and the color selection excellent. No shades of peach or pink to be found. There are only six color choices, so these aren't for everyone, but it is worth a try to see if any of them could work for you.

Concealer: Cover Girl has several types of concealer. Their **Clarifying Anti-Acne Concealer** *($3.69)* is basically a tube of foundation that contains salicylic acid. Salicylic acid won't get rid of acne, but it can irritate the skin, and the colors won't work on all skin tones. **Moisturizing Concealer** *($3.89)* comes in four shades that are quite good, and the consistency is creamy without being greasy. **The All Day Perfecting Concealer** *($3.55)* is divided in half. One half is the concealer, the other half (which looks like a lip gloss) is supposed to be a moisturizer. Sounds like a good idea, but it is an unnecessary step. Your moisturizer should take care of any dry skin under the eyes; this "gloss" makes the under-eye area too greasy. **Invisible Concealer** *($3.69)* is an OK light concealer, but it has a tendency to fill in the lines around the eye.

Powder: There are several types of pressed powder in the Cover Girl line that contain almost the same ingredients; they would be great to recommend except that you can't see the color through the packaging. You can flip up the top, but the powder itself is blocked by the powder puff. How strange. And why package a pressed powder with a puff when it should be applied with a brush? At any rate, none of these pressed powders can be recommended because you can't see the color selection.

Eyeshadow: There are a lot of colors here with some good matte shades to try, but there is also an abundance of shine. A cute but useless new product is **Non Stop Eye Color** *($3.57)*, which contains three eyeshadows, one of which is shiny, and an eyeshadow base that matches the color tone of the eyeshadows. Not necessary, and the shiny eyeshadow is a waste of money. **Natural Eyes Breeze-On Shadow** *($3.19)* comes packaged with a large brush, suggesting you can just sweep this color across the eye. You can't without having it look sloppy. The line does have some good colors, but they should be applied with a good professional-size eyeshadow brush.

Eyeshadow Colors to Try

Pro Colors ($1.61)

All of these colors are beautiful: Butter Creme, Fawn, Dewy Pink (can be too white for most skin tones), Marooned, Peach Nectar, Grey Suede (can be too blue for some skin tones), Acorn, Terracotta, Classic Navy, and Amethyst (can be too bright for most skin tones).

Natural Eyes Breeze-On Shadow Single ($3.19)

These colors are lovely and matte: Sunlit Brick, Misty Rose, and Autumn Suede (slightly shiny).

Soft Radiants ($3.70)

All of these are beautiful matte colors: Soft Country Twilight, Soft Desert Blooms, and Soft Forest Glade.

Eyeshadow Colors to Avoid

Pro Colors ($1.61)

All of these colors are extremely shiny and/or too blue or green: Mink, Tapestry Taupe, Rose Mist, Pink Chiffon, Whisper Blue (too blue), South Sea Blue, Magnolia, Snow Blossom (too white for most skin tones), Highland Heather (too blue), Moonlight, Autumn Haze, Ballet Pink, Khaki, Slate Blue (too blue), Silver Mist, Jade (too blue-green), Swiss Chocolate, Glazed Ginger, Milk & Honey, Real Teal, Charcoal Frost, Fern, Wild Iris, Sterling Blue, Forest, and Champagne.

Natural Eyes Breeze-On Shadow Singles ($3.19)

Sienna Peach, Soft Taupe, Brown Sugar, Natural Bronze and Cinnamon Sweep are all too shiny to recommend.

Soft Radiants ($3.70)

Soft Sky Lights is too blue and Soft Misty Morn has one shade that is too blue.

Luminese ($3.25)

The name speaks for itself. All of these colors are too shiny and not recommended.

Blush: Cover Girl has several blush types. I didn't notice much of a difference between the ingredients in any of them or a difference in the way they went on. They are all talc-based with varying amounts of mineral oil and kaolin (clay). Some were too shiny—I don't recommend those and the fragrance was too sickeningly sweet for my taste. But the colors were soft, went on well, and lasted. I particularly liked their new **Ultimate Finish Powder Silk Blush** *($5.39)*. This-cream-to-powder blush went on beautifully and had great staying power.

Blush Colors to Try
Cheekers ($2.85)
All of these colors are great: Rose Silk, Classic Pink, Snow Plum (slightly shiny), Pretty Peach, Crystal Plum, Soft Sable, Sunkissed Pink, Raspberries & Cream, Peaches & Cream, Watermelon Slice, Catalina Coral, Wild Rasberry, Plumberry Glow, Rock 'N' Rose, Peach Sicle, Brick Berry, Cool Berry (too shiny for most skin types), Coral Rose, Pink Flamingo, and Spiced Tea.

Classic Color Brush-On Blush ($4.39)
All of these colors are great: Natural Glow, Sun Warmed Coral, Fresh Peach, Iced Plum, Petal Pink, Cameo Pink, Mocha Mist, and Plum Wine.

Replenishing Blush ($4.25)
All of these colors are great: Precious Plum, Pink Jasmine, Satin Rose, Sandalwood and Rose Petal.

Moisture Wear All Day Blush ($4.50)
All of these colors are great: Empress Rose, Crystal Claret, Tender Peach, Plumberry, Cameo Pink, and Morning Glow.

Continuous Color Moisture Enriched Blush ($4.17)
All of these colors are great: Ruby Wine, Coral Whisper, Morning Glow, Bronze Spice, Satin Rose, Plumberry, and Tender Peach.

Ultimate Finish Powder Silk Blush ($5.39)
All of these colors are excellent: Mauve Mist, Bordeaux, Crushed Cranberry, Pink Camisole, Terracotta, Faded Fuchsia, Pink, and Chestnut.

Blush Colors to Avoid
Cheekers ($2.85)
These colors are too shiny: Iced Ginger and Forever Heather.

Lipstick: Cover Girl makes several types of very impressive lipsticks. **Continuous Color SPF 15** and **Continuous Color (no SPF)** *($3.73)* are both very creamy lipsticks that come in both frosted and cream colors. My strong suggestion is to stay away from the frosted colors. **Soft Radiants** *($3.15)* is a somewhat glossy, sheer lipstick. **Remarkable Lip Color SPF 15** *($4.27)* also has a great texture and a good sunscreen too. All of these lipsticks come in a decent selection of excellent colors. **Lip Advance** *($4.75)* is a half-powder, half-gloss lip color combination that causes many of the same problems that other products of this type do: they tend to cake, they dry out the lips after being used for an extended period of time, and they don't last any longer than regular lipsticks.

Eye, Brow, and Lip Liners: Cover Girl has an absurdly large range of eye-lining products that come in a small selection of colors. **Soft Precision Liner** *($4.37)* is a felt-tip liquid liner that decidedly does not go on soft; **Extremely Gentle Soft Liner** *($3.43)* is a traditional liquid liner that is anything but soft. **Soft Radiants** *($1.79)* is a standard eye pencil that goes on somewhat heavy. **Prolining Self Sharpening Tip** *($3.27)* has a pencil on one end and a sponge tip at the other; most of these colors have a slight shine. **Eye Definer**

($1.75) is a traditional pencil; **Perfect Point Eye Pencil** *($3.15)* is an automatic pencil. The pencils that aren't shiny or blue are fine, but it is hard to tell from the packaging exactly what color you are getting. You are fairly safe with colors like Black and Brown, but that's about it. For those reasons I don't recommend most of the Cover Girl pencils. **Remarkable Lip Definer Lip Pencil** *($3.39)* is a very good twist-type lip pencil that comes in five wonderful colors. The package for the Lip Definer Lip Pencils has the names of the lipstick colors that coordinate with that color—nice touch.

Mascara: Cover Girl has improved the quality of their mascara immensely. There are now several that have great prices and go on great too. **Extension Waterproof Mascara** *($3.43)* is fairly waterproof and goes on well without clumping. **Remarkable Washable Waterproof Mascara** *($3.87)* has a confusing name, but that can be forgiven because it goes on well and doesn't smear. It isn't at all waterproof, but it does wash off with water and a cleanser. **Natural Lash Clear Gel Mascara** *($3.43)* is a clear mascara; for those who want to make stiff lashes without any thickness I guess this is a good enough option. **Long 'n Lush** *($3.87)* is also an excellent mascara. **Professional Mascara** *($3.43)* is not a very professional mascara; it doesn't build thickness very well and it tends to smear

Brushes: Cover Girl has two blush/powder brushes that are just OK. The large blush brush *($4.79)* and the medium blush brush *($4.50)* are both reliable and work well.

Dermablend

Dermablend is a small line of products designed to help women with major skin problems they want covered up. For those women, Dermablend's offer is hard to ignore. The question is how well the products work and whether they are good for the skin. **The Cover Creme Foundation** *($18)*, **Leg & Body Cover** *($15)*, **Quick Fix** (cover stick) *($13)*, **Setting Loose Powder** *($20)*, and **Setting Pressed Powder** *($15)* are supposed to provide complete opaque coverage that hides any kind of scarring or birthmarks (no matter how severe) and spider veins on the legs. These are not lightweight products that magically place a camouflaging film over the face and legs. Not surprisingly, each product has an unusually thick, almost spackle-like quality. This is heavy-duty stuff.

The colors are actually quite good. If you spread an even layer of the foundation, body cover, or cover stick over your face or legs, you can be assured of a good deal of coverage that, depending on the depth of discoloration, will hide it from view. The deeper the discoloration the less likely you will be able to hide it. The question is, Do you really want that much coverage? What you get in place of the discoloration is a thick layer of foundation. Even if you spread it on as thinly as possible it still has a heavy texture. Plus, the thinner you blend it on the less coverage you get. There is no way that these products look natural. Also, the Leg & Body Cover can be a problem to use, because even though it is waterproof and won't come off in the rain, it will rub off, and there's nothing you can do to prevent that from happening. The Setting Powder should not be used at all. It is a white talc powder that looks very pasty on the skin. Almost any neutral pressed or loose powder can be used instead and would work just as well.

This is a difficult product line for me to recommend, yet I know that many women have strong feelings about their facial discolorations. I may think that the heavy look of the foundation is no better than the discoloration itself, but the problem isn't on my face. Emotions are strong when it comes to this issue, so testing the products yourself is probably the only way to make a decision.

Elizabeth Arden

When I first started doing makeup in the 1970s, Elizabeth Arden was the "old ladies' line." The pink-and-white packaging was an age-old mainstay at the cosmetics counters, and indeed the line's clientele was almost exclusively women over 50. All that has changed, and Elizabeth Arden competes well for the baby boomer market.

The counter display is very attractive and easily accessible—always a strong point. The blush and lip colors are divided into four easy-to-understand categories: red tray, coral tray, pink tray, and plum tray. There's enough color variety here to interest women of all skin tones. The eyeshadows are divided into two categories, cool and warm, that are designed to coordinate with the blushes and lipsticks in the four color trays. Cool eyeshadows work with the pink and plum trays, and the warm eyeshadows work with the red and coral trays. Unfortunately, many of the eyeshadows are too shiny and should be avoided. The blush colors are attractive—none are shiny and almost all of them are worth a try.

Foundation: Elizabeth Arden has five types of foundation. **Flawless Finish Sponge-On Cream Makeup** *($20)* is extremely greasy and thick. The color choices are good, but for the most part, it is too heavy for me to recommend to anyone. **Simply Perfect Mousse Makeup** *($17.50)* is a unique foundation; it comes out like a foam and covers the face with a light, somewhat dry texture. The color selection is excellent, but it can take a while to master the application technique. I tend to prefer traditional foundation consistencies and find this one a bit gimmicky. **Flawless Finish Matte Powder Makeup** *($20)* is a talc-based pressed powder that is recommended for use by itself as a foundation. It comes in a good range of colors, but the texture isn't best for use all over the face. It can be used as a regular pressed powder. Arden's two liquid foundations are **Flawless Finish Liquid Makeup, Dewy Finish** *($20)* for normal to dry skin, and **Flawless Finish Liquid Makeup, Matte Finish** *($20)* for normal to oily skin; both have an excellent texture, but limited color choices.

Foundation Colors to Try
Flawless Finish Sponge-on Cream Makeup ($20)
All of these colors are very good: Perfect Beige, Warm Beige, Toasty Beige, and Bronzed Beige.
Simply Perfect Mousse Makeup ($17.50)
All of these colors are excellent (the shades are numbered from lightest to darkest): 4, 5, 6, 7, 8, 9, 10, and 11.
Flawless Finish Matte Powder Makeup ($20)
All of these colors are very good: Honey Beige, Luxury Beige, Natural Tan, and French Bisque.
Flawless Finish Liquid Makeup, Dewy Finish ($20)
All of these are excellent colors: French Bisque, Luxury Beige, Natural Tan, and Warm Bronze.
Flawless Finish Liquid Makeup, Matte Finish ($20)
All of these colors are OK to good color choices: Perfect Ivory (may turn slightly pink), Honey Beige (can turn slightly peach), French Bisque, Subtle Beige, Luxury Beige (can turn slightly rose), Natural Tan (may turn orange), and Warm Bronze (may turn orange on some skin tones).

Foundation Colors to Avoid
Flawless Finish Sponge-on Cream Makeup ($20)
All of these colors are either too peach or too pink to recommend: Porcelain Beige, Gentle Beige, Softly Beige, and Toasty Rose.
Simply Perfect Mousse Makeup ($17.50)
All of these colors can be too pink for most skin tones: 0, 1, 2, and 3.
Flawless Finish Matte Powder Makeup ($20)
Perfect Ivory and Cameo Creme are too peach for most skin tones.
Flawless Finish Liquid Makeup, Dewy Finish ($20)
Cameo Creme, Honey Beige, and Subtle Beige are too peach for most skin tones.
Flawless Finish Liquid Makeup, Matte Finish ($20)
Cameo Creme is too peach for most skin tones.
Concealer: Elizabeth Arden has three types of concealer. **Cream-On Concealer** *($12.50)* comes in a traditional tube and has a good consistency, but is really too pink to use. The **Concealing Cream** *($12.50)* also comes in

poor colors, is greasy, and tends to slip into the lines around the eyes. The sheer **Mousse Concealer** *($11.50)* comes in two shades that are also too pink. The Mousse Concealer is difficult to use until you become accustomed to the squeeze top, and it does not provide the best texture for the job of concealing.

Powder: Elizabeth Arden's **Flawless Finish Pressed Powder** *($18.50)* isn't all that flawless. It is just a standard pressed powder that comes in three shades: Translucent Light, Translucent Medium (fairly peach), and Translucent Dark. All contain talc and cornstarch and are on the dry side, but they do have a sheer texture. There is also a **Bronzing Powder** *($18.50)* that comes in two shades: Golden Bronze, which is too shiny to recommend, and Pale Copper, which is too orange for anyone's skin tone.

Eyeshadow Colors to Try
Singles, Duos, Trios, and Quads *($12.50/$16/$20/$22.50)*
All of these colors are a possible consideration and have a good soft texture: Midnight Mauve/Moonlight Pink, Wild Violet/Lavender, Sophisticated Shadows, Misty Shadows, Horizons (for dramatic looks only), Fresco Shadows, Vintage Shadows, Almond/Slate, and The Classics.

Eyeshadow Colors to Avoid
Singles, Duos, Trios, and Quads *($12.50/$16/$20/$22.50)*
All of these colors are too shiny, too blue, or a difficult combination to use: Wild Grape/Citrus, Haze/Blue Diamond, Art Deco Shadows, Daybreak Shadows, Jade/Pink Lotus, Teakwood/Silver, Aegean Blue/Caribbean Blue, Bittersweet/Heather/Heather Mist, Sunlight/Pink Champagne, Fresh Lilac Shadows, Highland Shadows, Tradewinds, Sandswept (too sheer for most skin tones), Rhythm/Blue, Moonscape Shadows, Gold Lit Shadows, and Sea Glass.

Blush: There are good colors to be found, but many of them are shiny and therefore not for everyone. Look closely before you buy.

Blush Colors to Try
Luxury Cheek Color *($18.50)*
All of these are great colors: Pink 1 (very soft plum), Pink 2, Pink 3 (looks brighter than it goes on—a good pink), Plum 1, Plum 2, Plum 3, Neutral 1, Neutral 2, Neutral 3, Coral 1, Coral 2, Coral 3, and Cocoa 2 (great contour color). Fresh Corals and In The Pink are pretty, but both are too sheer for most skin tones.

Cream Powder Blush *($17.50)*
All of these are great colors: Pink, Mauve, Coral, Mocha, and Cocoa (a great contour color).

Lipstick: Both types of lipstick are easily accessible for testing and are divided into extremely helpful color groupings of plum, pink, coral, and red. **Luxury Lipsticks** *($14)* go on somewhat sheer and moist, and provide light coverage. Elizabeth Arden makes a product called **Lip Fix** *($17.50)* that is supposed to prevent lipstick from feathering into the lines around the mouth. It works well for most but not all lipsticks, and I don't care for the squeeze-tube applicator. Lip Fix goes on like a moisturizer and must dry before you put on your lipstick. For touch-ups during the day, it isn't the best. I prefer anti-feathering products that come in lipstick form.

Eye, Brow and Lip Liners: Elizabeth Arden has a large array of both eye and lip pencil colors called **Slender Liners** *($11)*. Some of the colors are wonderful. If you do consider these pencils, be sure to avoid Peacock and Emerald, both of which are too green for most eyes. There is also a liquid felt-tip eyeliner called **Luxury Eyeliner Pen** *($15)*. It goes on smoothly and evenly, but the color tends to separate when applied. All of the pencils in this line have a good texture, but are nothing unique, just like almost all the other pencils on the market.

Mascara: When it comes to mascara, Elizabeth Arden has its act together. These mascaras are very good. There are three types of mascara available: **Twice as Thick, Twice as Long,** and **Two Brush Mascara** *($13 each)*. They are all great, but it's hard to really tell a difference between them. The only problem with the product is the two brushes. The idea sounds good—one shape does the job of putting the mascara on, the other is supposed to lengthen and separate—but I didn't notice a real difference between the two. I did notice, however, that this mascara dried up faster than others. Two brushes pumping air into the same tube would make any mascara dry faster than usual.

Erno Laszlo

Erno Laszlo's following is just beyond me. I made a bet years ago when the products first came out at the upper-end department stores that this line wouldn't last. I believed there was no way women would pay $14 for a bar of soap or use a foundation that looked powdery and flaky on the skin. I was wrong. It is still here and it still has a following. This curious line is loosely based on the philosophy of its namesake, who was supposedly a medical doctor, although whether or not that's true depends on who you talk to. Mr. Laszlo's thing was skin care: hot water, soap, and a vinegar rinse to reestablish pH. When he died the exclusive use of his name was sold and through various changes is now on the product line you find today.

In general there is nothing worth mentioning about this line. There are only a few token makeup products and they are overpriced and nothing special. This is primarily a skin care line, so there are more foundations than anything else; you won't find any eyeshadows, lipsticks, pencils, or mascara. This line isn't worth it, but I'll review the few products there are anyway.

Foundation: There are three foundations in this line. **Regular Normalizer Shake-It** *($30)* is mostly water, fluid oil, and talc. This is one drying foundation that goes on choppy and thin. **Phelitone Fluid** *($35)* is a light, creamy liquid foundation that has a good color selection. **Oil-Free Normalizing Base** *($30)* won't normalize anything, although it is an OK light-weight matte foundation.

Foundation Colors To Try
Regular Normalizer Shake-It ($30)
> These colors are very good: Honey, Neutral, Light Beige, and Suntan.

Phelitone Fluid ($35)
> These colors are very good: Soft Beige (may turn peach), Beige, Light Beige, Suntan, and Golden Beige.

Oil-Free Normalizing Base ($30)
> All of these colors are very good: Golden Beige, Light Beige, Suntan, and Neutral (may turn peach).

Foundation Colors To Avoid
Regular Normalizer Shake-It ($30)
> All of these colors are too peach or pink too recommend: Beige, Porcelain, and Soft Beige.

Phelitone Fluid ($35)
> Honey Beige is too peach and Porcelain is too pink.

Oil-Free Normalizing Base ($30)
> All of these colors are too peach or pink to recommend: Soft Beige, Beige, Honey Beige, and Porcelain.

Powder: Phelitone Concentrating Pressed Powder *($22)* is a fairly standard powder.

Blush: This line has a small array of **Blushing Powders** *($19)*, all too shiny to recommend. There is also a product called **Phelitone Emollient Duo Phase Concealer** *($28)* that is half blush and half concealer. The concealer comes in only one color choice and it is just OK. The blush half has three color options and is also OK, but the color selection is so small and the concealer so poor that this product is one of the stranger ones on the market.

Estee Lauder

The Estee Lauder Company has set the present-day standard for the world of cosmetics. Their formidable reach is exemplified by the impressive status of Clinique, Origins, and Prescriptives, all part of Lauder family. Of course, Estee Lauder is still the grande dame of make-up lines, with a loyal following and impressive public relations. Ask any of the women who work the counters for this well-respected, veteran cosmetics company and they will tell you the products sell themselves. A few years ago Night Repair and Eyezone were jumping off the shelves. Today the hot product is Fruition, which is supposedly responsible for 5 percent of the line's gross sales (they are hard at work to make it 10 percent). This is a company with dedication to selling and staff sales training. The counter displays are not accessible without the help of a salesperson, so the sales pressure here is fairly intense.

An immense array of Compact Disc shadows was recently added; most these colors are matte, but several are slightly shiny. How disappointing. So close and yet so far. The foundations are still excellent, and there is an excellent selection of colors for women of color. I particularly like the Demi-Matte, Fresh Air, and Lucidity, but you need to be careful about color choice; there are many pink and orange foundations in this collection, and Lucidity doesn't live up to any of the claims the saleswoman carried on about. Most of the blushes are lovely and they too have a good selection for women with darker skin tones. All of the colors are divided into warm and cool, which is an excellent grouping and very helpful. Estee Lauder also offers a set of four **Professional Brushes** for the outrageous sum of $75. These are good brushes but there are better ones on the market for a lot less money.

Foundation: Estee Lauder has eight types of foundation, all of which are quite good. **Demi-Matte** *($20)* is a superior oil-free foundation. **Fresh Air** *($17.50)* is for normal to oily skin and has a lovely finish but exceptionally poor color choices. **Country Mist** *($17.50)* is recommended for normal to dry skin and provides an excellent medium-coverage foundation for dry skin, though I don't recommend it for normal-skin types. **Polished Performance** *($25)* gives a sheer, more natural coverage and is an excellent liquid foundation for normal and dry skin types, although the colors all have a rose tint that is a problem for most skin tones. **Sportswear Tint SPF 12** *($25)* is almost like wearing no makeup, but it does contain a Sun Protection Factor of 12 (15 would be better). **Lucidity Light Diffusing Foundation** *($26.50)* can't diffuse light, although it is a good liquid foundation for someone with normal to dry skin. **Just Perfect Foundation** *($35)* is also supposed to be light-diffusing, but it doesn't change the face or erase wrinkles. It does provide fairly heavy coverage, although it is creamy. **More Than Powder** *($21)* is a pressed powder recommended for use as a foundation. It has a nice consistency but works best on normal skin. All of the Lauder foundations are divided into golden, neutral, and pink shades, and are then rated 1 to 4 for light to fair skin tones. The rating system is helpful, but always avoid foundations with pink or peach tones.

Foundation Colors to Try
Demi-Matte ($20)

All of these colors are very good: Fresh Beige (may turn slightly rose on some skin tones), Champagne Beige, Wheat Beige (may be too yellow), Rose Beige (may turn slightly rose), Natural Ivory, Golden Beige (may be too yellow), Ivory Beige, and Sun Bronze.

Fresh Air ($17.50)

All of these colors are very good: Palm Beige, Linen Beige, Cloud Beige, Nutmeg Brown, and Honey Pecan (may turn orange).

Country Mist ($17.50)

All of these colors are wonderful: Suntan Beige, Golden Beige, Clear Beige, Warm Beige, Misty Tan (may turn slightly rose), Tender Beige, Beige Light, and Vanilla Beige.

Polished Performance ($25)

All of these colors are acceptable, but they all tend to turn rose: Perfect Beige, Outdoor Beige, Cool Beige, Wild Honey, Alabaster Beige, Vanilla Mist, Blushing Beige, Summer Beige, Tender Rose Beige, and Sunlit Beige. Butternut Bronze and Tawny Almond are both great golden colors for darker skin tones.

Sportswear Tint SPF 12 ($25)

All of these are excellent, extremely sheer colors: Light Tint, Bronze Tint, and Golden Tint (can turn peach).

Lucidity Light Diffusing Makeup ($26.50)

All of these colors are very good: Gold Alabaster (excellent pale shade), Ivory Beige (slightly peach), Rich Ginger (may turn peach), Sun Bronze (may turn rose), Gold Caramel, Gold Sand, Bronze Mocha, Medium Beige (slightly rose), Sun Beige, Coffee, and Sable.

Just Perfect Foundation ($35)

All of these colors are very good: Golden Alabaster (may be too yellow for some skin tones), Golden Ivory (may be too peach), Natural Beige, Rich Ginger, Sun Bronze, Hazelnut, Cappuccino, Bronze Mocha, and Golden Caramel.

More Than Powder ($21)

All of these colors are excellent: Ivory, Barely Beige, Warm Honey, Tawny Beige, Tan Bisque, Cinnamon Sun, Toasted Walnut, and Honey Toast.

Foundation Colors to Avoid

Demi-Matte Liquid ($20)

Rose Ivory is too rose for most skin tones.

Fresh Air Makeup ($17.50)

All of these colors are too peach, pink, or ash for most skin tones: Ivory Mist, Meadow Beige, Beige Glow, Newport Beige, Sunrise Beige, and Warm Beige.

Country Mist Liquid ($17.50)

Morning Beige is too peach for most skin tones and Country Beige is too rose for most skin tones.

Lucidity Light Diffusing Makeup ($26.50)

All of these colors are either too peach or too pink for most skin tones: Neutral Beige, Gold Ivory, Cool Beige, Outdoor Beige, and Vanilla Beige.

Just Perfect Foundation ($35)

All of these colors are too peach or too pink for most skin tones: Sienna, Pale Ivory, Cool Beige, and Vanilla Beige.

More Than Powder *($21)*

These colors are too peach or too pink for most skin tones: Sand Beige, Dawn Beige, Radiant Beige, and Blush Beige.

Concealer: Estee Lauder's Creme **Automatic Concealer** *($12.50)* comes in six very impressive shades: Light, Medium, Medium Dark, Warm Medium, Warm Dark, and Dark. The Light is fairly pink, but the other shades are great. The consistency is on the dry side, but it stays on well. Chances are it won't crease, but test it on your own skin first. There are three shades of **Color Primer** *($15)* in this line and they are supposed to do the same thing everyone else's color primer or corrector does: change the skin tone. It doesn't work well at all and adds another unnecessary layer to the makeup. **Shadow Stay Eyelid Foundation** *($12.50)* absolutely didn't work: my eyeshadows creased within a few hours.

Powder: Estee Lauder has three types of powder. **Demi-Matte Oil-Free Loose Powder** *($18.50)* and **Demi-Matte Oil-Free Pressed Powder** *($16)*, for oily skin, are both standard talc-based powders. They have a great texture, but most of the color choices go on too chalky. **Lucidity Translucent Loose Powder** *($25)*, for all skin types, has a great color selection. Lucidity is promoted as a product that can change the way light focuses on your face. It feels good, but it doesn't look any different than dozens of other powders I've tested. **Moisture Balanced Translucent Face Powder** pressed *($18.50)* and loose *($16)*, is just a standard talc-based powder, but it does have a good color selection.

Finishing Powder Colors to Try

Demi-Matte Oil-Free Face Loose Powder *($18.50)*

All of these colors are very good options: Ivory (slightly pink), Champagne Beige (slightly peach), Fresh Beige (slightly peach), Caramel Beige, Cinnamon, and Cocoa.

Lucidity Face Powder *($25)*

All of these colors are wonderful: Light, Medium, Dark, Tan, Copper, and Bronze.

Eyeshadow: Compact Disc Eyeshadows *($10)* are an awesome group of 80 single colors that are almost all matte, but some are definitely shiny, so look carefully. The shadows are numbered 1 through 8 and fall into one of the following categpries: Neutrals, Blues, Teals, Greens, Naturals, Oranges, Browns, Corals, Pinks, and Violets. There are too many colors to list individually, but I would encourage you to concentrate your attentions on the Neutrals (which are wonderful), Naturals, Browns, Corals, and Pinks, for many of these are simply remarkable eyeshadow colors. They also make an **Eye-Coloring Liquid-to-Powder Eyeshadow** *($15)* in an assortment of 12 extremely shiny shades. These are supposed to be waterproof, but you don't want the shine to stick around dry or wet.

Eyeshadow Colors to Try

Singles and Duos *($15/$20)* (not from the Compact Disc collection)

All of these colors are lovely: Arizona, Sand, Cactus, Colorado, Foliage,

Sierra, Clouds, Twilight, Casa Rosa, Granite, Moors, Island, and Aurora.

Eyeshadow Colors to Avoid

Singles and Duos ($20/$25) (not from the Compact Disc collection)
All of these colors are too shiny, come in strange combinations, or, in the case of the quad shadows, are a difficult shape to use: Gala, Trapeze, Rivers, Rainflowers, Oceanic, Bronzewood, and Peach Cream.

Blush: Estee Lauder's new **Just Blush for Eyes and Cheeks** *($25)* has a wonderful selection of soft colors that are meant to work on both the cheek and the eye. It comes packaged with a nice-size retractable brush. **Soft Color Creme Blush** *($20)* goes on like a cream and dries on the skin like a powder. It has a beautiful consistency and is great for normal to oily skin. The **Powder Blush** *($20)* is a standard blush with good color choices for darker skin tones.

Blush Colors to Try

Powder Blush ($20)
Most of these colors are intense and best for darker skin tones, but they are all good color choices: Fresco, Tangelo, Sepia, Terra Rosa, Avant Red, Pastel, Petals, Pot Pourri, Plum, and Fuchsia Silk.

Just Blush for Eyes and Cheeks ($25)
All of these colors are soft, silky, and beautiful: Peach Blush, Ginger Blush, Pink Blush, Just Blush, Rose Tutu, Light Bronze, and Dark Bronze.

Soft Color Creme Blush ($20)
All of these are beautiful colors: Red Silk, Rose Velvet, Sienna Suede, Pink Cashmere, and Peach Chiffon (may be too orange for most skin tones).

Blush Colors to Avoid

Powder Blush ($20)
Most of these colors are too shiny to recommend: Flamingoes, Orchids, Tiger Lilies, and Bronzes.

Lipstick: Estee Lauder has four types of lipstick: **Perfect Lipstick** *($15)*, **All Day Lipstick** *($12.50)*, **Feather Proof** *($12.50)*, and **Polish Performance** *($12.50)*. The Perfect Lipstick, All Day Lipstick, and Polish Performance are wonderful: very creamy and rich. Feather Proof lipstick is one of the few on the market that really doesn't feather. This is a remarkable lipstick and I recommend it strongly if you have this problem. The only disappointment is the small color selection.

Eye, Brow, and Lip Liners: Estee Lauder's **Automatic Pencil Liners for Eyes and Lips** *($22.50)* are wind-up pencils that come in an elegant container. They are among the most expensive pencils on the market, and except for the container they are not unusual or special. These are just like most other pencils on the market. Some of the eye pencils are too shiny and fairly greasy, so be careful. **Liquid Liner** *($22.50)* is a fairly standard liner that draws a wet, serious line across the lid. **Two-in-One Eyeliner and Brow Color** *($22.50)* goes on wet or dry; there is only one color compact available, with two color choices: Brown and Black. Rather limited, especially when you consider that any matte eyeshadow could do the same thing. **Eye Brow Color** *($22.50, $8 refill)* is just a dry, heavy-textured eyeshadow powder that comes in three good shades: Blonde, Soft Brown, and Charcoal. You would be better off and save money if you just used an eyeshadow color that matched your brow color. There is a clear **Brow Gel** *($12)* that works fairly well, but not better than hairspray on a toothbrush.

Mascara: Estee Lauder's **More Than Mascara** *($15)* isn't more than mascara, it's just mascara. Nevertheless, it goes on easily while building nice thick lashes without clumping. **Lash Primer** *($12.50)* is supposed to help make lashes even longer if you apply it before the mascara. It is an unnecessary step; their mascara goes on just fine without help.

Expressions Brushes (Canada only)

Most Canadian drugstores carry these reasonably priced, professional-size brushes *($2.50 to $5)*. All of the brushes are very good and are a great way to affordably invest in the basics necessary for a good makeup application. The only brushes to ignore are the Lip Liner/Eye Liner Brush, which is really too thick for one and too thin for the other; the Fantail Brush, which is pretty but not very practical; and the Eyeshading Brush, which is a little too flimsy to be very useful or long-lasting. The best brushes are the Retractable Lip Brush, the Eyelining Brush, the Fluff Brush, the Blusher Brush, and the Super Powder.

Fashion Fair

Women of color have only two major cosmetics lines dedicated just to them at the cosmetics counters: Fashion Fair and Flori Roberts. My decided preference is Fashion Fair. Flori Roberts just can't compete with the selection of colors and product types Fashion Fair offers. For the widest selection possible, particularly in lipsticks, foundations, blushes, and concealing creams, this line, though not perfect, is nevertheless outstanding. One major drawback needs to be mentioned: almost all of Fashion Fair's eyeshadows are intensely shiny. I don't recommend shiny eyeshadow for women of color any more than I do for women with lighter skin tones. Shiny eyeshadows make eyelids look wrinkly, and they are always inappropriate in daytime. However, Fashion Fair has a line of fragrance-free products that are worth looking at, plus oil-free foundations, blushes, concealer creams, and lipsticks. There is also a selection of products that contain fragrance, and these, too, are of good quality. The display units are all easily accessible, and the saleswomen I met seemed generally well trained and helpful.

Foundation: Fashion Fair has four types of foundation. The fragrance-free **Oil-Free Souffle** *($21)* is applied with a wet sponge and goes on like a pancake foundation. It can be tricky to use, but the color selection and coverage are excellent (although it may look somewhat pasty on normal-to-dry skin). **Oil-Free Liquid** *($17.50)* is an excellent foundation with great color selection for normal-to-oily skin. **Liquid Sheer Foundation** *($12)* works best on dry skin, and there is a superior array of colors. **Perfect Finish Creme Makeup** *($14.75)* is a compact foundation that is fairly greasy, which may cause the foundation color to turn orange. Foundations for women of color, and women with darker skin tones in particular, contain more pigment, and the oil intensifies the pigment.

Foundation Colors to Try
Oil-Free Souffle ($21)
> All of these colors are superior: Beige Glo, Amber Glo, Honey Glo, Tawny Glo, Copper Glo, Tender Glo, Brown Blaze Glo, Bronze Glo, Pure Brown Glo, Ebony Glo, and Pure Pearl Glo (may turn slightly pink on some skin tones).

Oil-Free Liquid ($17.50)
> All of these colors are superior: Beige, Honey Amber, Tender Brown, Copper Blaze, Bare Bronze, Ebony Brown.

Liquid Sheer Foundation ($12)
> All of these colors are beautiful: Alabaster, Beige, Toffee Tone, Honey Amber, Tender Brown, Copper Blaze, Bare Bronze, Ebony Brown.

Perfect Finish Creme Makeup ($14.75)
> All of these colors are worth looking at: Beige Glo (a great color), Tender Glo (a great color, but can be slightly ashy on some skin tones), Brown Blaze Glo (a good color, but may turn orange on some skin tones), Bronze Glo (a good color, but may turn orange on some skin tones), and Ebony Glo (a great color for ebony skin tones).

Foundation Colors to Avoid
Oil-Free Liquid ($17.50)
> All of these colors are poor choices: Toffee Tone (can be too yellow for most skin tones), Tawny (can be too yellow for most skin tones), and Copper Tan (can be too orange for most skin tones).

Liquid Sheer Foundation ($12)
> These colors are not recommended: Tawny (can be too yellow on most skin tones) and Copper Tan (can turn orange on some skin tones).

Perfect Finish Creme Makeup ($14.75)
> All of these colors are not recommended: Pure Pearl Glo (can be too pink

for most skin tones), Amber Glo (can be too yellow for most skin tones), Honey Glo (can be too yellow for most skin tones), Tawny Glo (can be too orange for most skin tones), and Copper Glo (can be too orange for most skin tones).

Concealer: Fashion Fair has three types of concealer. **Cover Tone Concealing Creme** *($12.50)* is for use under the eyes or over blemishes and scars. It has a very dry consistency and provides fairly heavy coverage. It is supposed to be used with a **Setting Powder** *($12)*. The saleswoman told me the powder was waterproof, but all it contains is talc with some preservative. I don't recommend the Concealing Creme or the Setting Powder. The other two concealers are excellent. **Fragrance-Free Coverstick** *($9.50)* has a drier consistency for oily skin; the regular **Coverstick** *($9)* has fragrance and a creamier formula. All of the shades are fabulous and definitely worth a try.

Concealer Colors to Try
Fragrance-Free Coverstick ($9.50)
All of these colors are excellent: Very Light, Light, Medium, and Dark.
Fragrance Coverstick ($9.50)
All of these colors are excellent: Very Light, Light, Medium, and Dark.

Finishing Powder: Fashion Fair has a loose powder *($15.25)* and a pressed powder *($11.50)*; both contain talc and mineral oil. They have good texture and are available in an excellent range of colors.

Eyeshadow: All of the Fashion Fair eyeshadows are extremely shiny. They are not the best option for women of color. The two shades of brown that aren't shiny each come packaged in a set of four colors, and the other three are shiny. I do not recommend any of the Fashion Fair eyeshadows except possibly for evening wear.

Eyeshadow Colors to Avoid
Duos, Trios, Quads, and Quints ($12.50/$13.25/$14.25/$14.75)
All of these colors are extremely shiny: Winter Berry/Golden, Chestnut, Classy Copper/Golden Nectar, Wild Orchid/Caribbean Blue, Frost Rose/Satin Brown, Silver Light, Midnight Blue, Golden Glow, Lavender Beauty, Misty Brick, Black Pearl, Smoky Emerald, Rich Plum, Shades of Mardi Gras I, Shades of Mardi Gras II, Shades of Mardi Gras III, Shades of Fantasy I, Shades of Fantasy II, and Shades of Fantasy III. Shades of Beauty I and Shades of Beauty II both have shiny shadows except for one in each.

Blush: Fashion Fair has a wonderful variety of blush colors, both fragranced and fragrance-free. They go on smooth and include vivid and subtle shades. This is an excellent assortment to consider, although some of the colors have too much shine to be really suitable for daytime.

Blush Colors to Try
Fragrance-Free ($12.50)
All of these colors are worth considering: Rich Ruby (a great color), Terra Rose (too shiny, but may be good for evening wear), Russian Sable (this is a very shiny brown blush, but may be good as an evening-wear con-

tour shade), Metallic Mauve (a beautiful color), Honey Topaz (a great color), and Brandy Mist (a good mauve-brown shade).

Fragranced ($12.50)

All of these colors are beautiful, but fairly shiny: Paradise Pink, Plum Pearl, Fiesta Pink, Rasberry Ice, Crystal Rose, Moonlit Mauve, Chocolate Chip, Quiet Coral, Pearly Paprika, Plum Rose (only slightly), Royal Red, Plum Rich, Wild Plum, Ginger Berry, Crimson, Bronze (an excellent contour color), and Golden Lights (a beautiful bronze highlighter for evening).

Lipstick: Since the range of shades appropriate for women of color is so extensive, it would be nice if Fashion Fair's lipsticks *($10)* were more creamy and less greasy.

Flori Roberts

Given that there are only two major cosmetics lines designed specifically for women of color, I would love to be able to say that I think both of them are wonderful, but that isn't the case. Fashion Fair has its shortcomings, and, unfortunately, Flori Roberts has more. It is by far the weaker of the two in many areas, with an abundance of shiny eyeshadows, poor foundation textures, and dry, grainy blushes. Women of color require stronger colors (which is what grainy textures tend to be), but that doesn't mean the blush textures can't be silky smooth and have stronger pigment at the same time. (Many other lines have accomplished this feat.) And darker skin tones do not automatically require shiny eyeshadows. If the blushes can be matte, surely the eyeshadows can follow suit. It's time to give women of color the products they need. If Prescriptives, Maybelline, Revlon, and M.A.C. can do it, so can this line. There are options to be found in this line, particularly foundations and lipsticks, but choose carefully; many of the other products leave much to be desired.

Foundation: This is where the Flori Roberts line excels. Most of these foundations are excellent and the color choices are great. **Oil-Free Melanin Makeup Base** *($13)* is half glycerin and half makeup color that separates in the container. If it separates in the container it can easily separate on the skin; also, this much glycerin can be irritating to some skin types. **Hydrophillic Foundation for Normal to Dry** *($20)* has a wonderful texture and goes on beautifully, plus the color selection is superior. **Touche Satin Finish** *($15)* is probably too greasy and thick for most skin types, but for those who want more coverage and have dry skin, this just may be an option. The colors are excellent and it does blend well.

Foundation Colors to Try

Oil-Free Melanin Makeup Base ($13)

All of these foundation colors are excellent, although this foundation isn't the best: M-2, M-3, M-3, M-4, M-5, M-7, and M-9.

Hydrophillic Foundation for Normal to Dry ($20)

All of these colors are great and the foundation has a beautiful texture: Chrome A, Chrome B, Chrome C, Chrome D, Chrome E, and Chrome F.

Touche Satin Finish ($15)

All of these colors are excellent choices: Beige, Bronze, Copper, Brown, Topaz, and Ebony.

Foundation Colors to Avoid

Touche Satin Finish ($15)

Caramel is too peach for most skin tones; Honey is too yellow for most skin tones.

Powder: Flori Roberts has two types of pressed powder. **Oil-Free Loose Powder** *($4)* comes in four fantastic colors: Light, Translucent, Medium, and Dark. The texture is fairly dry and grainy, but it would be good for someone with very oily skin. The **Pressed Powder** *($11)* contains oil and the colors aren't as good. Most of them are too peach for most skin tones.

Eyeshadow: Chromatic Eye Compact *($20)* comes in three sets of six shades each. It looks like you're getting a lot, but each shade is barely a drop of color and all of the colors are ultra-shiny. **Signature Eyeshadow Trios** *($14.50)* are all very shiny and the color selection is poor.

Blush: There are two types of blush. **Gold Chromatic Blush** *($15)* has three shades of two colors each, but only two of these have a matte finish. **Radiance Blush** *($12.50)* has some great colors for darker skin tones, but the colors tend to have a grainy dry texture that can look heavy and thick. For the most part these colors would only be good for women with deep mahogany or espresso skin colors. **Enchanted Cheeks** *($16)* is a compact with three very good blush colors: peach, red, and a good brown shade for contouring. If these are your colors, this is a good buy.

Lipstick: Flori Roberts excels in this arena. There are three types of lipstick in this line, some of which are great options. **Lipstick** *($9.50)* has a wide selection of colors (32 shades) and has a good creamy texture almost bordering on greasy. **Matte Lipstick** *($10.)* isn't really all that matte; it's actually more creamy, and is also slightly on the greasy side. **Gold Hydrophillic Lipstick** *($12.50)* has a light, creamy texture, but it also contains a stain, so the color tends to hang around longer than with the other lipsticks. There is also a small but nice selection of tube lip glosses *($10)*, which are nothing special but OK if you want a gloss.

Eye, Brow, and Lip Liners: For the most part the lip and eye pencils *($8)* are fairly standard, but these tend to be a bit drier than most on the market. This makes them a little harder to apply, but they also tend to not smear as fast.

Mascara: This mascara *($10.50)* goes on well and builds thick long lashes, however, it does tend to clump.

Frances Denney

Frances Denney cosmetics have been around for a long time, dating back to 1897. That's quite a history. This is one of the oldest cosmetics lines still on the market today. Along with Estee Lauder, Elizabeth Arden, and Helena Rubinstein, Frances Denney was one of the grande dames who created and established face fashion and skin care for decades. Because of great management, Elizabeth Arden and Estee Lauder flourished, while Frances Denney has had its share of financial woes. Frances Denney has been bought and sold more times than anybody cares to count, which means a lack of stock at the counters and a lack of organization and consistency in management. The color line is weak and dated. Most of the blush and eyeshadow colors are shiny, many of the foundation colors are not the best, and the selection is very small. The strongest and largest area for Frances Denney is skin care, so you may want to look there for some interesting products because you assuredly won't find much to consider in this section.

Foundation: Frances Denney has four types of foundations. **Moisture Silk for Normal to Dry Skin** *($17)* is an OK, smooth foundation with medium coverage. **Moisture Silk for Normal to Oily Skin** *($17)* has an excellent matte consistency. **Incandescent Makeup** *($24)* is for ultra-dry skin. Half of this foundation is a fluid oil, which rides on top, while the color part sits on the bottom. I am not fond of foundation colors that separate because they have a tendency to separate on the skin, but this is indeed emollient and would feel good on very dry skin. **Velvet Fresh Foundation** *($13)* is a rich cream-to-powder foundation that dries quickly and has a soft finish, but it is good for normal skin types only.

Foundation Colors to Try
Moisture Silk for Normal to Dry Skin ($17)
All of these colors are OK possibilities, but they are not the best: Natural Beige (could be too yellow), Ivory (could turn pink), Peach Beige (a very good neutral shade in spite of the name), Light Beige (could turn pink), Medium Beige (OK color but could turn peach), and Tawny Beige (a good light golden brown).
Moisture Silk for Normal to Oily Skin ($17)
All of these colors are OK: Medium Beige (could turn peach), Ivory (could turn peach), Peach Beige (a very good medium shade), Tawny Beige (a good golden brown), and Rose Beige (could turn rosy peach).

Incandescent Makeup ($24)
 All of these colors are surprisingly good: Soft Beige, Natural Beige, and Honey.

Velvet Fresh Foundation ($13)
 All of these colors are quite good: Tan Beige, Soft Beige, Classic Beige (could turn peach), and Peach Beige (which isn't peach at all).

Foundation Colors to Avoid

Moisture Silk for Normal to Dry Skin ($17)
 Rose Beige is too peach for most skin types.

Incandescent Makeup ($24)
 Rose Beige is too peach for most skin types.

Velvet Fresh Foundation ($13)
 Rose Beige is fairly peach and Pink Beige lives up to its name.

 Concealer: Concealer Base Cream *($10)* has a fairly greasy consistency and tends to crease in the lines around the eyes. The colors are also poor; Light is too pink, Medium I is very pink, and Medium II is the only color that might be good for a medium skin tone.

 Eyeshadow: There aren't many colors to recommend here because almost all of them are either too shiny or ultra-shiny. What a waste. The **Moisture Silk Eye Color** *($8)* has only two matte colors available: Honey Dew/Rose Bud, which is a strange combination of pale pink and green; and Violet/Black, which is an OK combination. How strange to have only two matte shades out of more than two dozen colors.

 Blush: Moisture Silk Powder Blush *($11.50)* is a nice enough selection of blush colors, but most are fairly shiny and not my favorite to recommend. However, they do go on well and blend easily. By the way, there is one matte shade: Spiced Neutral. I wonder where this color came from.

 Eye, Brow, and Lip Liners: These are a standard, small array of lip and eye pencils *($7.50)* . Nothing special, just like most thin pencils on the market.

 Lipstick: The lipsticks in this line *($8.50)* are mostly shiny, which I don't recommend, and the color selection is small.

 Mascara: This is not a great mascara *($9.50)*. It doesn't build much length or thickness, and tends to flake.

Guerlain

 If any cosmetic line can be considered sensual and luxurious, this one is it. Without even taking quality into consideration, it is hard to ignore the lavish gold packaging, intricate product design, and awesome price tag that accompanies everything from eyeliner to powder. Imagine, they have a refillable powder compact that sells for $90! Gold and faux jewels bedeck this exquisite little container. Sigh. If it were chic to powder your nose in public, you would be the talk of the party. But that's the problem with overkill packaging: it is essentially a waste because no one but you and your makeup bag see it. All that counts when it comes to your makeup is how it looks on your face. It's not that it isn't nice to have beautiful containers, but if the product is only a blush and the lipstick only a lipstick, there is no real reason to lust after a container.

Looking closer at quality, I do have to say that there are some excellent products in the small but pricey (and I mean pricey) Guerlain line. It would really be an amazing insult to charge these prices and have nothing to offer. The strong point here are the blushes and foundations. The weaknesses are the shiny eyeshadows and pressed powder.

Just a quick aside: I've been asked why I bother to review expensive lines. Why would someone who's looking to save money and find the best buys at the cosmetics counters and drugstores want to know whether or not Guerlain has good products? It's a good question. There are several reasons why I review a diverse range of cosmetics lines, but the main ones are: (1) to stay informed about what is currently available in the world of cosmetics, because I never know where I'm going to find the best products that would then set the standard for my reviews; (2) to reconfirm that expensive rarely means better; and (3) because even women who can afford to spend a lot of money on cosmetics deserve not to get ripped off.

Foundation: Les Voilettes Pressed Powder Foundation *($29)* and **Loose Powder** *($32.50)* are just slightly thick powders that happen to come in eight wonderful shades. **Elysemat Liquid Makeup** *($35)* has a wonderful selection of colors and the texture is great, light and silky. **Halo Line Treatment Foundation** *($35)* won't treat anything, although the brochure carries on for pages about what it can do. The texture is creamy and thick, too thick if you want anything resembling a natural look. Most of the colors are too peach to recommend. **Opalissime Complexion Base** *($30)* is supposed to produce miracles, but it is only a very good foundation with an excellent creamy texture and a small assortment of colors that are not the best. **Terracotta Pearls Hydro Tinting Emulsion** *($35)* is a rather luxurious-looking sheer moisturizing tint that comes in three soft tan color shades. Bronze beads are suspended in an oily liquid. As you rub the color on the beads disappear and impart minimal color. It does go on somewhat oily, which would only be good for someone with very dry skin. This isn't the best bronzing tint on the market, but it is the most interesting.

Foundation Colors to Try
Elysemat Liquid Makeup ($35)
   All of these colors are excellent: 3, 4, 5, 6, 7, and 8.
Halo Line Treatment Foundation ($35)
   All of these colors are great: 15, 20, and 25.
Opalissime Complexion Base ($30)
   All of these colors are good: 4, 7, 8, and 9.

Foundation Colors to Avoid
Elysemat Liquid Makeup ($35)
   The Liquid Makeup has three colors that are called Opalissime. Although they go on quite sheer, they are all shiny.
Halo Line Treatment Foundation ($35)
   All of these colors are too peach to recommend: 30, 35, 40, and 45.
Opalissime Complexion Base ($30)
   Numbers 3 and 6 are too peach to recommend.
   Powder: At these prices you would expect more, but the **Pressed Powder** *($30)* is pretty standard, with a soft, dry texture. The color choice is limited but OK. The loose powders are too highly fragranced to recommend.
   Eyeshadow: Almost all of the eyeshadows *($25)* are either too shiny, too blue, too green, or come in a combination too strange to recommend. Even the texture is poor. All of the following colors are not recommended: Alexandria, Violet (too intense for most skin tones), Vert, Bleu, Roman, Tolede, Casablanca, Balin, Or, Vienne (difficult combination), Miami, Brun/Gris, Mauve/Gris, and Vert/Gris. The only matte shades in the line are: Noir, Lisbonne, Pourpre, and Istanbul.
   Blush: There aren't many, but these shades are beautiful, silky blush colors *($30)*: Blush, Abricot, Mangue, Peche, Pasteque, Fique, and Framboise. Guerlain also has three shades that are meant to be bronzers, but are all shiny to ultra-shiny: Terracotta Mat (which is not at all matte), Terracotta, and Terracotta Dore. Guerlain also has a liquid tint blush called **Star Blush** *($30)*. Like most face tints it is OK if you have normal skin, but if you have open pores it will stain them darker than the skin and look like little dots on the face. Ah, if only the blush in **Rouge a Levres** *($30)* was as fabulous as the container, it would be great. This blush is multicolored and comes in beads and pressed powder that mix together to make one pastel shade that is supposed to react only to your skin. It was OK and kind of interesting, but not worth the price tag.
   Eye, Brow, and Lip Liners: The small, attractive gold containers contain a tiny vial of ordinary **Liquid Liner** *($20)*. It is really too small to apply easily.
   Lipstick: Guerlain has a small but nice array of creamy lipsticks *($18)* that are borderline too greasy.

Joan Simmons Brushes

Imagine a tailor without a sewing machine or a needle and thread, or consider the dilemma a stockbroker would be in without a computer and *The Wall Street Journal.* Every task requires appropriate tools in order to perform the labor properly. It is no different for applying makeup. Using professional-size brushes is the only way to apply makeup successfully, period. The little sponge-tip applicators, tiny blush brushes, and scratchy eyebrow brushes that come packaged with cosmetics are a total waste and are better suited to the garbage than the face. Joan Simmons Brushes *($5 to $13)* are as good an option as you will find for professional-size brushes, and they are reasonably priced. I have found these brushes at major department stores all over the country. Look for them at Nordstrom, Macy's, Saks, or any upper-end department store in your area. These are worth checking out.

There are more than a dozen brushes to choose from. Most are very good, but some are positively a waste of money. The **Foundation Applicator** *($7)* has a big sponge on one end of the handle. Although the idea isn't bad, a hand-held thin round sponge is easier to use and a fraction of the price. **Lash Whirly** *($5)* is just a dry mascara brush meant to separate the lashes if they clump together when you apply mascara. But you could easily take an old mascara brush, wash it, and use it instead for free. The **Blush Blender** *($7)* is a flat-edged, severely shaped brush that can't blend blush well at all. The best it can do is stripe on the color. All of the other brushes are superior and, depending on your makeup needs, worth a closer look. Call (212) 675-3136 to find out if these brushes are distributed in your area.

Lancaster

This upper-end French import has more limitations than assets. There isn't much here to recommend: the eyeshadows are shiny and the foundation colors, while good, are very limited. The blush colors are pretty, but they are all slightly shiny and would be much better if they weren't. The counter displays are very accessible, but it would be nice if they were organized by color so you could more easily match blushes and lipsticks. Still, it is great to have a counter display that you can play with to your heart's (or face's) content.

Foundation: There are some great foundation textures and colors in this line. I loved the way the **Matte Finish Foundation** *($23.50)* went on; unfortunately, all of the colors were opalescent and shiny. A matte foundation with shine seems incredibly contradictory. None of those colors are recommended. **Rich Foundation** *($32)* is very emollient and smooth, but there is only a tiny collection of colors, although they are excellent. Just as this book was going to press I found out that Lancaster is planning to introduce a new foundation. It is being called **Suractif Treatment Makeup** *(price unknown)*. It supposedly will contain an SPF of 15 and retinol (vitamin A). The SPF sounds great and the vitamin A can theoretically reduce some free-radical damage. I'll look forward to reviewing this in my newsletter when it becomes available.

Foundation Colors to Try
Rich Foundation ($23.50)
> All of these colors are quite good: Rivage (slightly ash), Desert, Faience (may turn peach), Fonce (slightly peach), Mordore, and Dune (may turn peach).

Concealer: Concealing Creme *($15)* is a liquid concealer that comes in a tube. It goes on nicely, with minimal slippage into the lines around the eye. The colors, except for the green shade, are worth trying.

Powder: There are two groups of pressed powder *($25/$30)* in this line; both have an interesting array of colors that go on soft and sheer, but they have a fairly dry texture. Both are worth a try.

Eyeshadow: All of the colors available in the **Eyeshadow Trio** *($27.50)* are very shiny, and those in the **Eyeshadow Duo** *($25)* are almost all shiny except for numbers 31, 33, and 90. Number 32 is matte, but it is also very blue.

Blush: All of the blush colors *($27)* are soft and very good, but they do have a slight amount of shine: Hortensia, Pivoine, Coralline, Volcan, Nougatine, and Noisette.

Lipstick: Lancaster offers only one type of lipstick *($16)*, but it is really too greasy to recommend and the color selection is limited. There are also fairly standard tube glosses *($12.50)* that are nothing special or unique.

Eye, Brow, and Lip Liners: There is a nice selection of fairly standard lip and eye pencils *($13.50)*. They also have a good brow powder *($23.50)*, but this is a lot of money for a rather ordinary powder.

Lancome

Lancome remains one of the more popular cosmetics lines for a large group of baby boomers and is one of my personal favorites. Prices are steep but relatively reasonable (I use the term "reasonable" loosely) given Lancome's place at the high end of the cosmetics world. The product line is impressively varied, and many of the items are well liked by the women who responded to my survey. This very French line is extremely low-key and maintains a more casual, although professional, air than the other French lines sold at the department stores.

I like the Lancome display units very much. They are accessible and easy to use, particularly if you want to experiment on your own. I do wish, however, that Lancome would follow the trend of the other makeup lines and divide their blushes, eyeshadows, lipsticks, and lip liners into color groups, but they obviously aren't ready to do that. Their foundations are grouped by color tones, but this organization is confusing and not particularly helpful. A few stores in selected cities now sport "super counters" that take up an entire island. They are really quite impressive.

Foundation: Lancome has quite a large, almost overwhelming, array of foundations to choose from, all of which are excellent. There is even an impressive range of colors for darker skin tones. **Maquivelour** *($28.50)* is for normal to dry skin and has a soft light texture with even coverage. **Maquicontrole SPF 4** *($28.50)* has been reformulated and is no longer the heavy, thick foundation it used to be. It now provides light to medium coverage and feels great on the skin. **Maqui Eclat** *($27)* is a creamy, lightweight foundation that is great for a sheer daytime look. **Maqui Mat** *($27)*, which went on very soft and light but also very matte, was being reformulated as we went to press and will be reviewed in my newsletter, *Cosmetics Counter Update*, when the new colors are available. **Dual Finish Powder** *($25)* is more like a compact powder than a foundation. It comes in an excellent assortment of colors, can be used wet, although I think it tends be too powdery when used by itself, and is an option for someone with normal to slightly oily skin. It also makes a great finishing powder. **Imanance Tinted Creme SPF 8** *($25)* doesn't contain enough sunscreen to provide adequate protection, but it is a very good lightweight, sheer foundation that goes on well. It would work well for someone with normal to slightly dry skin. The color selection is quite limited, so this product definitely isn't for everyone.

Foundation Colors to Try

Maquivelour ($28.50)

All of these are great colors: Porcelain, Porcelain D'Ivoire, Porcelain Delicate, Beige, Beige Camee, Beige Naturel, Beige Sable, Beige Bisque, Rose Clair, Dore Clair, Epice Bronze (can turn peach), Amande Bronze (slightly peach), and Miel Bronze (can turn ash).

Maquicontrole SPF 4 ($28.50)

All of these colors are excellent: Porcelain, Porcelain D'Ivoire, Porcelain Delicate, Beige, Beige Naturel, Beige Camee, Beige Rose, Beige Sable, Clair (slightly peach), Pale Clair, Dore Clair, Epice Bronze (can turn peach), Amande Bronze, and Miel Bronze.

Maqui Eclat ($27)

All of these colors are great: Warm Ivory, Beige, Softly Beige, Buffed Bisque, Shell Beige, Toasted Almond, Truly Bronze, and Beige Sand.

Foundation Colors to Avoid

Maquivelour ($28.50)

Bronze and Cafe Bronze are too ash-green for most skin tones and Clair is too peach.

Maquicontrole SPF 4 ($28.50)

Cafe Bronze is too ash for most skin tones.

Maqui Eclat ($27)

These colors are either too peach or too pink for most skin tones: Pale Peach, Rose Buff, and Blushed Cameo.

Concealer: Lancome makes a waterproof eyeshadow base called **Shadow Base** *($16)*. It is quite waterproof, which means it must be removed with an oil-based cleanser, but because of its color and consistency, it nicely tones down the intense shine of Lancome's iridescent eyeshadows and eyeshadow pencils. However, I never recommend doing two things when you can do one, so it's best to forget the shadow base and instead use foundation on your lid and wear eyeshadows that are matte, not shiny. Besides, I found no difference in how long my eyeshadow lasted when I wore Shadow Base instead of foundation. For covering dark circles under the eye, **Anti-Cernes** *($13.50)* comes in three shades: Light, Medium, and Dark. It is a waterproof cover-up that goes on creamy but dries to a somewhat powdery, matte finish. I'm not fond of this concealer. I have noticed, and several of the Lancome salespeople have too, that the cream fills in the lines around the eye, the colors are a bit too pink or peach for most skin tones, and the tube applicator is hard to control, particularly when the product is almost gone and you have to squeeze a little harder so you can use it all.

Powder: Lancome has four shades of **Poudre Majeur** *($22.50)* pressed powder without talc; they go on smoothly, without a chalky finish. Translucent, Matte Beige, and Matte Bronze are excellent colors, but Matte Peche is too peach for most skin tones. There is also a very good loose powder likewise called **Poudre Majeur** *($25.50)*, which is also made without talc; it contains clay and zinc instead, which can be somewhat heavier than talc. All of the colors are quite good: Ivoire, Sand, Bisque, Rose, Honey, Bronze, and Buff. It also claims to have "micro-bubbles." Whatever that means, it's still only a powder.

Eyeshadow: This used to be the weakest link in an otherwise great product line, but that has truly changed. Although many of the eyeshadow colors are still shiny, a preponderance of them are now matte. In addition, Lancome, like many other lines, has added a large selection of eyeshadow colors from which you can choose two and fill your own eyeshadow compact. **Personal Eyes** *($22.50)* offers a superior selection of matte eyeshadows, so take advantage of this one. It is, a great idea, and one that is way too late in coming to the world of cosmetics.

Eyeshadow Colors to Try

All Eyeshadow Singles, Duets, Trios, Quartettes, and Personal Eyes
($16/$20/$25/$25/$22.50)

All of these colors are exceptional: Country Heather, Cream (this is more white than cream and can be too white for some skin tones), Coleurs au Courant, Les Essentials, Couture de Lancome, Matte Brun, Matte Gris, Matte Beige, Teint Midi, Coleurs du Soleil, Couleurs du Ciel, Peche/Raisin, Abricot, Coquille, Biscotte, Praline, Rose Nuance, Cappucino, Renard, Chocolate Brule, Terre, Le Gris, Fumee, Prune, Aubergine, Ciel du Soir, Violet Moderne, Grappe, Chameau, Parchemin, Le Pinque, and Khaki.

Eyeshadow Colors to Avoid

All Eyeshadow Singles, Duets, Trios, Quartettes, and Personal Eyes
($16/$20/$25/$25/$22.50)

All of these colors are too shiny or too blue to recommend: Silversmoke/Fawn, Golden Leaf, Muscat, French Cream, Bleu Eclipse, Nose Gay (single eyeshadow), Splendeurs D'Automne, Ombres Naturelles, Coleurs Sauvage, Coleurs Impromptues, Coleurs du Moment, Pot Pourri de Lancome, Couleurs Teches, Les Neo Modernes, Ombre de Terre, Les Artistes, Metals Precieux, Effets Dores, Impressions Parisiennes, Silversmoke Fawn/Taupe Vert, Lezard, Raisin, Taupe Vert, Vert Artichoke, Vert Artiste, Sauvage Doree, Peche Cire, Golden Sun, Tiara, Tendre Lumiere, Bleu Cashmere, Bleu Gris, Bleu Fume, and Le Blanc.

Blush: Blush Majeur *($20)* is a cream-to-powder blush with a beautiful consistency. It's worth trying if you want a soft blush look, but only if you can handle the blending. It has a tendency to fade slightly as the day goes by. Most of the **Blush Subtil** *($20)* colors are indeed subtle, and they are all beautiful soft shades.

Blush Colors to Try

Blush Majeur ($20)

All of these colors are beautiful: Petunia, Rose, Berry, Sienna, Hibiscus, Red, Tulip, Sepia, Plum, and Mocha (a great contour color).

Blush Subtil ($20)

All of these colors are excellent: Rouge, Rose Terre, Raspberry, Cappucino, Aplum, Cedar Rose, Rose Ivoire, Peche, Rose Delicate, Rococo, and Naturel.

Lipstick: Lancome's lipsticks are mostly very good and the colors are lovely. **Hydra-Riche** *($15)* is a moist creamy lipstick bordering on a greasy consistency. **Rouge Superb Matte** *($15)* goes on somewhat heavy and is truly matte, but still creamy. **Rouge Superb Sheer** *($15)* is more like a gloss than a lipstick. All are worth checking out, though none of the claims about long-lasting color or reduced feathering were confirmed. **Rouge Absolu** *($15.50)* is a creamy lipstick that has a slight tint so it will stay on longer than the others.

Eye, Brow, and Lip Liners: Lancome sells a standard automatic lip pencil made in Germany called **Le Crayon** *($12.50)* that never needs sharpening. It's convenient to use, though a bit expensive for what you get, since there is no real difference between this and a regular pencil you have to sharpen. **Le Crayon Brow Definer** *($14.50)* is a standard pencil with a comb at the other end so you can brush through the line and soften it. The Taupe color, however, is too shiny for anyone to try, and Brunette can be too red for many skin tones. **Le Crayon Kohl** *($12.50)* is a line of good (though not exceptional) eyelining pencils; they come in a nice range of colors, but they are no better than others I've found on the market for less money. The claim that they don't smudge once they're on is not entirely accurate; smudging is caused by several factors, not just the pencil itself.

Lancome also makes a waterproof pencil called **Le Crayon Waterproof** *($13.50)*. There are more than 15 colors to choose from, but most are shiny, though some of the darker shades, such as Brown and Black, are not. They are fairly waterproof. I find this product difficult to recommend for several reasons: it is hard to get off without using a wipe-off makeup remover, and I never suggest doing that; it is fat and hard to sharpen; and because the darker colors are more waterproof than the lighter colors, and none of them is 100 percent waterproof, they come off unevenly while you are in the water.

There are also two types of liquid liners: **Maquiglace Liquid Liner** *($15)* and **Automatic Eyelining Felt Pen** *($18.50)*. Both make very definite lines that do not blend, although the felt pen goes on softer than the liquid liner. These can be good for some eye designs, but I don't often recommend such an obvious look. If you like it, the felt pen is definitely an interesting way to put on eyeliner. **Le Kohl Poudre** *($12.50)* is a unique pencil that goes on like a powder. It is difficult to sharpen and some of the colors are shiny, but this is actually quite a good option for lining the eyes softly. The **Tinted Brow Groomer** *($14)* comes in only three shades: one each for redheads, brunettes, and ash blondes. Not the best selection, and the applicator isn't reliable. It tends to go on messy.

Mascara: Lancome is known for their great, reliable mascaras that usually don't smudge and are very popular. The best are the **Defincils**, **Immencils**, and **Keracils** *($15)*. Defincils definitely builds the thickest lashes and is by far my favorite, but the others are equally excellent. Keracils is presently being reformulated. **Forticils** *($12.50)* is a clear mascara that is supposed to be a lash conditioner. There is no way to condition or feed lashes to make them grow or be thicker. This product is a waste of time and money.

Lasting Kiss

It isn't worth devoting much space to this review because these products are truly not worth your attention or your money. As you may already be aware, infomercials absolutely drive me crazy due to their conspicuous lack of information in a format that drags on for 15 to 30 minutes at a time. **Lasting Kiss** is no exception to that rule. The setup is the same: an assortment of intensely pleased, very attractive, lesser-known celebrities are sitting around a living room set discussing how their lipstick has never lasted so long as with the **Lasting Kiss** lipsticks. *Not.* Your common sense says you should know better, but it sounds too good, and what if it really does work—after all, why would these women lie? After you are convinced that this lipstick will assuredly last all day, you order the absurdly expensive little package (*$60.78 for three lipsticks with matching nail polishes, a liquid nail polish dryer, a lipstick sealer, a tiny lip conditioner, and a small tube of lip gloss*). What they don't tell you is that these lipsticks are OK, but fairly standard; the lip gloss is ordinary; and the nail polishes are shiny, chip easily, and contain tolulene (an ingredient many cosmetic companies are removing from their nail polishes because it is so caustic). Plus, the lipstick sealer, the *piece de resistance*, is mostly alcohol, and contains hairspray ingredients (acrylates) that are also highly irritating. The leaflet that comes with the products mentions that the sealer burns when you put it on, something left out of the commercial. It will also probably dry out and irritate your lips at the same time. Bottom line: The sealer doesn't help the lipstick stay in place a minute longer than if you didn't use it at all. Send this one back to the manufacturer.

L'Oreal

It is fitting that L'Oreal follows Lancome so closely in my alphabetical listing, because both are owned by the same parent company in France. This is a good drugstore line and I feel confident about recommending many of their products, although the selections are somewhat limited. Because some drugstore lines have an overwhelming array of products, it isn't necessarily a negative that L'Oreal's collection is smaller than most. As is true of most eyeshadows in most lines, their colors are too shiny to recommend. L'Oreal's other products, however, are outstanding. You won't be disappointed with their foundations, blushes, lipsticks, powders, or mascaras. The blush colors, both the regular blush and the cream powder blush, have a beautiful texture and are some of the best around. There are three types of lipsticks in this line, and the colors, wearability, textures, and consistency are all fabulous. L'Oreal's mascaras are some of the best on the market for the money.

Foundation: L'Oreal is one of the few drugstore lines to make foundation tester units available. What a plus! An inexpensive foundation is no bargain if you buy the wrong color. I should also mention that there are some very good to excellent foundations in this line that are worth a closer look to see if they work for you. **Hydra Perfecte Protective Hydrating Makeup, SPF 10 ($7.95)** is a lightweight foundation for normal to dry skin; the SPF isn't the best but it is definitely better than nothing. **Lightnesse Light Natural Makeup ($8.75)** is almost too sheer; it would be good for someone who has normal to dry skin and wants only minimal coverage. **Mattique Illuminating Matte Makeup ($8.75)** has a good, fairly matte texture but has a slightly sticky feel; someone with oily skin might not like the texture. **Visuelle Invisible Coverage Makeup ($8.75)** has a great soft texture and goes on light; it is made for women with normal to dry skin.

Foundation Colors to Try

Hydra Perfecte Protective Hydrating Makeup, SPF 10 ($7.95)
All of these colors are excellent, with a wonderful texture: Pale Ivory (slightly pink cast), Bare Beige, Sand (slightly peach), Almond Beige, and Deep Beige.

Lightnesse Light Natural Makeup ($8.75)
These are excellent colors in a great moisturizing light texture: Ivory, Bare Beige, Ecru Beige, True Beige, Sand Beige, and Warmed Beige.

Mattique Illuminating Matte Makeup ($8.75)
All of these colors are very good: Beige Blush (can turn peach), Nude Beige, Buff Beige, Sand Beige, Honey Beige (may turn orange), and Rich Beige.

Visuelle Invisible Coverage Makeup ($8.75)
All of these colors are great: Ivory, Sand Beige, Honey (can turn peach), and Deep Beige (may turn rose on some skin tones).

Foundation Colors to Avoid

Hydra Perfecte Protective Hydrating Makeup, SPF 10 ($7.95)
Only Shell Pink is too peach to recommend.

Mattique Illuminating Matte Makeup ($8.75)
Soft Ivory is too pink for most skin tones; Golden Beige is too orange for most skin tones.

Visuelle Invisible Coverage Makeup ($8.75)
All of these colors are too peach, too orange, or too pink to recommend: Palest Beige, Pink Beige, and Bisque.

Concealer: L'Oreal's **Mattique Conceal Oil-Control Cover-Up ($6)** is a very good stick concealer that goes on quite sheer and smooth, although it does have a slight tendency to crease into the lines around the eyes.

Powder: Hydra Perfecte Loose Powder ($8.95), Visuelle Pressed Powder ($8.25), and **Mattique Oil-Free Softly Matte Pressed Powder ($8.25)** all come in an attractive assortment of colors and are definitely worth your consideration. The Mattique Oil-Free Softly Matte Pressed Powder has a particularly beautiful texture and color selection. One word of caution: The Visuelle Pressed Powder contains wheat starch, which can be a skin irritant for sensitive skin types.

Eyeshadow Colors to Try
Soft Effects Singles ($4.75)

All of these are excellent matte shades: Sable, Buff, Terra, Blush, and Chocolat.

Eyeshadow Colors to Avoid
Soft Effects Singles and Coleur! Coleur! Trios and Quads ($4.75/$5.50)

All of these colors are too shiny to recommend: Bleu, Plume, Earth, Gris, Rose, Gold Rust, Purple Pink, Desert Stone, Terre Peach, Rose Plum, Fantome (difficult combination), Taupe Peche, Teal, Cafe, Leaf, Soft Perle, Mink, Cornflower (too blue), Grape, Claret, and Violette.

Blush: L'Oreal makes two kinds of blush: a regular blush with an excellent texture called **Visuelle Powder Blush** *($8.25)* and a cream-to-powder blush called **Micro Blush** *($7.25)*. Micro Blush tends to go on dry and somewhat choppy, and the texture isn't as smooth as most, so I no longer recommend this product.

Blush Colors to Try
Visuelle Powder Blush ($8.25)

All of these are gorgeous colors: Plume, Tulipe, Fraiche, Capucine, Rose, Peony Pink, Rouge Russet, and Cameo (an excellent contour color).

Blush Colors to Avoid
Micro Blush ($7.25)

Even though all of the colors are beautiful, the texture is just too choppy and dry to go on smoothly.

Lipstick: L'Oreal makes three types of lipstick: **Colour Supreme** *($6.25)*, **Colour Riche Hydrating Creme Lipcolour** *($6.25)*, and **L'Artiste Enduring Creme Lipstick** *($6.25)*. All are quite creamy, have a wonderful texture, and last slightly longer than average. They rival any lipstick you will find at department store cosmetics counters. I didn't find any significant differences among the three types of lipstick; they all went on, looked, and felt pretty much the same, which is great if you're looking for a good creamy, fairly matte lipstick.

Eye, Brow, and Lip Liners: L'Oreal has a good selection of pencils called **Le Grand Kohl Perfectly Soft Liners** *($5.50)*. Most of these colors are fairly muted, go on smooth without being greasy, and blend easily without streaking. There is also a small selection of standard lip liners called **Lip Precision Self-Sharpening Lip Liners** *($5.50)* that are quite good and last well. **Lineur Intense** *($6.25)* is a traditional liquid liner in a tube; it goes on like the name says—intense.

Mascara: I found most of L'Oreal's mascaras to be exceptional. Their new **Accentuous Precisely Defining Mascara** *($5.75)* went on beautifully and didn't smear like their old standby, **Formula Riche** *($5.75)*. Both separated the lashes nicely without making them look spiked or clumped, and the wand was easy to use. Accentuous is probably one of the best in the group, and that's saying a lot. I also very much liked the **Lash Out Extending Mascara**

($5.75), but I prefer a shorter wand; other than that it is an excellent product. **Voluminous Dramatically Thick Mascara** *($5.75)* was a disappointment; although it went on well, it had a tendency to smear.

M.A.C. (Make-up Art Cosmetics)

This relatively new cosmetics line is gaining a goodly amount of justified attention. Based in Toronto but sold throughout North America, it is found exclusively in upscale department stores. The name is a bit pretentious, but it is nonetheless accurate. M.A.C. claims that it is used by many professional makeup artists, and I wouldn't be surprised if that were true. Most professional makeup artists actually prefer using generic or boutique cosmetics because of the price, but for those who can afford it, this line would be close to perfect. The color line is exceptional. One other important point: M.A.C. doesn't test their products on animals. In fact, the company sells a T-shirt stating "M.A.C. CRUELTY FREE BEAUTY"; the proceeds are donated to research for alternative testing methods.

Please don't get the impression that I'm endorsing a product line, because I'm not—but I truly think many of the foundations, eyeshadows, lipsticks, and blush colors are wonderful and the textures quite good, some of the most reliable and usable tones I've seen anywhere. Full, soft, properly sized makeup brushes are also sold at the M.A.C. counters, and may even be their strongest point. Obnoxious miniature applicators are nowhere in sight. What a pleasure; almost no complaints for any of these color products. (You didn't think it was perfect, did you?) Of course, their skin care line is another review altogether, but for now let's just concentrate on the color part.

Brochures often expound a company's impassioned philosophy and grandiose principles. M.A.C. goes beyond most other companies by ordaining "There must be truth in beauty" and "Ideal colour strikes a perfect balance between art and science." Fairly lofty language for some great neutral foundations and powders. Still, the pompous words don't change what you'll find, which is a wide range of workable colors for most skin tones (although the line is a little weak for women with very dark or black skin color).

One word of warning: The M.A.C. sales presentation for all their products is filled with claims about vitamins, antioxidants, oxygen boosters, prevention of free-radical damage, and pH balance. It's all rather exaggerated and not worth the steep price, but that's to be expected—after all, this is the world of cosmetics.

Foundation: M.A.C. makes several types of foundation that are worth checking out. **Matte Finish** *($17.50)* is for normal to oily skin, **Satin Finish** *($18)* is for normal to dry skin, and **Studio Fix Foundation** *($18)* is a rich powder foundation for normal to oily skin that is really best on normal skin. All of the shades are impressive and provide medium coverage. The colors are divided into cool and neutral, which is a little confusing. The cool colors are sallow in tone and recommended for women with sallow skin. The neutral colors are indeed quite neutral and are for women with pink undertones. The theory is that women with sallow skin should be wearing cool colors of blush and lipstick, although the foundations are supposed to be on the sallow side, and women with pink skin tones should be wearing neutral colors, including the foundation. See: it's confusing. What's important is that most of their colors are pretty neutral and great colors. My strong suggestion for practically everyone is to stay with the color that matches your skin and check it out in daylight.

As far as texture is concerned, the Satin and Matte Finish foundations are actually quite similar; they both go on well and blend easily. The salesperson carried on about the Satin Finish containing vitamins A and E, which is why it would be better for my skin. It turned out that the Matte Finish also contains them. By the way, there are some great foundation colors for women of color.

Foundation Colors to Try
Matte Finish ($17.50)
> All of these colors are great: N1, N3, N4, N5 (can turn peach), N6 (may be too ashy for some skin tones), N9, N10, Summer Dusk (may turn peach), C2, C3, C4, C5 (can turn ashy), C7 (can turn ashy), and Brunette.

Satin Finish ($18)
> All of these colors are great: N1, N2, N3, N4, N5 (may turn peach), N6, N7, N9, C2, C3, C4, C5 (slightly ash), C6 (slightly ash), C7 (slightly ash), and Coppera (may turn peach).

Studio Fix Foundation ($18)
> All of the colors in this group (except for C8, which is too ashy for most skin tones) are excellent.

Foundation Colors to Avoid
Matte Finish ($17.50)
> These colors are too pink, too peach, or too ashy to recommend: N2, N6, C6, and C7.

Concealer: M.A.C.'s **TV Touch** *($10)* goes on rather heavy and thick, but it provides excellent coverage and stays on well without much slippage. The recommendation is to mix the concealer first with the foundation or a little moisturizer and then apply it. All of these colors are great: Natural Beige, Light Beige, Medium Beige, Dark Beige, and Umber. Only Manilla is too yellow for most skin tones.

Powder: M.A.C.'s powders are fairly standard talc-based powders. **Pressed Powder** *($18)* is an ordinary compact powder and the **Loose Powder** comes in a shake-it bottle *($14)* or a traditional tub *($19)*. Both are good, but the shake-it container is one of the most convenient ways to use loose powder. Consider this one a very good buy.

Eyeshadow: The eyeshadows *($10 and $13)* are almost all matte. There is a selection of typically obnoxious shiny eyeshadows, but they are displayed separately, readily identified, and easily avoided. But primarily the color selection is nonshiny and surprisingly neutral. No glaring shades of pink, blue, or green to be found here. Instead, you'll find a large selection of tan shades ranging from pale cream to sable brown, taupe, gray-lavender, and every step in between. If you want to see one of the best neutral color palettes in the business, M.A.C. is the place to look. Warning: Some of the colors can be a bit on the heavy (greasy or grainy) side and go on more intense than they look; nevertheless, they are still worth trying to see how they work for you.

Blush: M.A.C.'s blushes *($10)* are packaged just like the eyeshadows, in round see-through containers. (By the way, the see-through containers are great. You never have to fumble through your makeup bag and wonder if you've picked up the right color.) The shades are just fine, they go on true, and there is a large matte assortment, but basically they are fairly standard colors and not anything exceptional.

Lipstick: There are five types of lipstick *(all priced at $12)* in this line and they are, for the most part, an excellent assortment. That might sound a bit bold, but M.A.C.'s **Matte Lipsticks** don't bleed, and I'm always thrilled when I can find one I don't have to wear over a sealer. I prefer doing one step instead of two. (The only other matte lipstick I've found that doesn't bleed is Estee Lauder's Feather Proof.) The only problem with M.A.C.'s matte lipsticks is they can be very dry and make the lips peel or feel caked by the end of the day. M.A.C. **Satin Lipsticks** are wonderful and nicely creamy without being thick. They're supposed to be semi-matte; I don't see it, but maybe you will. The **Sheer** is more a gloss than a lipstick; it contains a lot of vitamin E, which is a big selling point but not all that essential for the lips. M.A.C also has a unique line of lipsticks called **Liptones**. These are more of a tint that goes on like a gloss, dries, and then becomes sort of a color stain on the mouth. If you can get used to the texture it's an interesting option for lip color that has some amount of staying power. The **Creams** are fairly standard lipsticks that have a great finish. The color selection for all of these lipstick groupings is fairly impressive.

Eye, Brow, and Lip Liners: M.A.C.'s lip and eye pencils *($9)* are the same as almost every other lip and eye pencil on the market. They are made in Germany, where the three major cosmetic pencil manufacturing plants are located. There is also an ultra-dramatic liner that comes in a pot for a very thick matte look. I don't have to tell you to watch out for the Aluminum shade, right?

Brushes: M.A.C. has one of the best selections of brushes you'll find anywhere *(38 different brushes ranging from $6 to $65)*. The big brushes can get a little pricey, but these last forever if you take good care of them, so they are one of the few expensive makeup investments I recommend.

Marcelle (Canada only)

Marcelle is one of the few lines in Canada that sport ingredient lists on most of their products. This reasonably priced drugstore line has some good products that perform well and look great. The packaging is simple and some of the products are fragrance-free. Sad to say, this isn't an exciting line; there are almost no matte eyeshadows and the foundations have an incredibly poor color selection. However, the blushes, one of the mascaras, and the lipsticks are worth investigating. Also, some of the skin care products are very good (see the review in Chapter Eight).

Foundation: Marcelle has four types of foundation; the colors are very limited and some of the textures leave much to be desired. **Oil-Free Makeup** *($8.25)* is half alcohol and half talc and coloring, making it hard to apply. The alcohol is too drying and irritating for most skin types. This product is not recommended. **Moisture Rich Foundation for Dry/Normal Skin** *($8.25)* would be a good foundation to consider if the colors weren't so pink and peach. **Matte Finish Oil-Free Foundation** *($8.25)* also has a poor color selection and is not recommended, and the same is true for **All Day Protection with SPF 8** *($8.75)*.

Concealer: Cover Up *($6.25)* is a lipstick-type concealer with a terrible selection of colors; none of them are recommended. **Concealer Crayon** *($6.25)* is a fat pencil that comes in three OK shades: Light, Beige Cameo, and Dark (which isn't all that dark). I find the texture to be workable, but it tends to crease into the lines around the eye.

Powder: Marcelle's **Pressed Powder** *($8.75)* is an OK powder that comes in a handful of shades of which three are great; the other three match no one's skin tone. Consider trying Suntan, Translucent Medium, and Translucent Dark. Avoid Classic Beige, Rosy Peach, and Translucent.

Eyeshadow Colors to Try
Eyeshadow Singles and Duos ($6.75/$7.75)

All of these are excellent matte neutral shades: Granite, Iris, Caramel, Blush, Chiffon, Soleil d'Or, Moss/Suede (the moss may be too green for most skin tones), Whisper/Nude, and Blue Stone/Pebble Pink (not a great combination, but the blue is grayer than most).

Eyeshadow Colors to Avoid
Eyeshadow Singles and Duos ($6.75/$7.75)

All of these are either too shiny or too blue to recommend: Praline, Smoky Teal, Espresso/Creme Fraiche, Purple Passion/Mango (a strange combination), Algue Marine, Cote D'Azure.

Blush: Moisturizing Blush *($9)* isn't all that moisturizing, but it comes in an excellent group of colors and the price is reasonable.

Lipstick: Marcelle has a good but limited selection of lipsticks *($6.50)* that are worth testing for yourself.

Eye, Brow, and Lip Liners: Marcelle sells a good selection of fairly standard lip *($5.95)* and eye pencils *($6.50)* manufactured in Germany, like so many other pencils on the market. There are two types of pencils; one is waterproof. It does stay on well when wet, but so did the other pencil. Some of these colors are shiny and should be avoided. The lip pencils conveniently twist up so you don't have to worry about sharpening.

Mascara: Superlash Mascara *($8.50)* isn't the best; it takes a long time to build definition. It would be OK if you just wanted a lightweight makeup look. **Ultimate Lash Mascara** *($8.50)* is an exceptional mascara that goes on beautifully and never smeared or clumped. I would definitely buy this one again.

Mary Kay

Mary Kay is one of the original multilevel-marketing home-sales cosmetics companies. The company insists that there is only one level because there are no middle people between you and the company, which is true. However, the person who recruits you to sell makeup does get a percentage of your total sales. It doesn't take away from how much you make, but the incentive is to get more people on the sales team. Since 1963 Mary Kay Ash has built herself (and her sons) quite an empire. There are now more than 300,000 Mary Kay salespeople, and they sold $1.2 billion worth of cosmetics in 1992. Of that total, $840 million was disbursed back to the sales reps. The company also boasts a fleet of 923 pink Cadillacs—the ultimate reward for selling Mary Kay cosmetics—not to mention 4,000 Pontiac Grand Ams. As impressive as this all sounds, and it is impressive, the average salesperson's income is more like $5,000 to $10,000 a year. Obviously, the ability to sell does not come naturally to every member of the sales force.

Since I first reviewed this line I've met several Mary Kay representatives. For the most part these women were exceptionally pleasant and professional, but most of them wore an unattractive, poor makeup application and their skin care information was all product hype—not surprising, but still disappointing. Every sales representative I met was extremely dedicated to Mary Kay and her products; it felt as if they were talking about a religion, not cosmetics. That kind of intensity is not atypical for cosmetics salespeople, but this kind of devotion to the company head doesn't really exist elsewhere. Regardless, their presentations were organized and systematic. Each time I was given new demo-size brushes to use and individual samples of almost every product (including tiny eye and lip pencils), which was wonderful and impressively sanitary.

How do the products hold up two years after I first reviewed this line? There are some good products in the Mary Kay line. The strong points here are great blushes, good foundations, and reasonably priced eye and lip pencils. The colors are also conveniently divided into cool, warm, and neutral tones. There are also lots of pitfalls that you have to watch out for, such as a huge selection of blue eyeshadows, a cream concealer that easily creases into the lines around the eyes, lipsticks that tend toward the greasy side, and a skin care system that forces you to buy all of it or none of it, and that includes the foundation.

Mary Kay does have an amazing training program set up for her representatives. The written materials concerning makeup application are remarkable and for the most part completely credible. The Color Logic book, which organizes the makeup colors according to wardrobe, skin, and hair colors, is one of the best in the business. The drawback is that not every representative has the talent to recreate what she has learned.

Another potential problem arises from the way the products are marketed. Each salesperson buys her products and samples from the company and sells them directly to the consumer, yet because of cash flow not everyone can afford to stock all of the colors. The tendency then is to show the consumer only what the salesperson has in stock, which happened to me almost every time I had a makeup demonstration.

Foundation: Mary Kay has three types of foundations. **Formula 1—Day Radiance Cream** *($10)* is for very dry skin and the coverage tends to be heavy and thick. Be careful with this one; dry skin doesn't mean you have to wear thick, greasy foundation. **Formula 2—Day Radiance Liquid** *($10)* is for normal to dry skin and is an excellent foundation that gives even coverage. **Oil-Free Foundation** *($10)* is for oily skin and provides light coverage. The Oil-Free and Liquid Formula have the best consistencies, go on smoothly, and give an excellent finish. Mary Kay also sells washable sponges to use when applying your foundation. These are great—some of the best I've seen.

Mary Kay's policy is not to sell a foundation to a first-time customer unless she buys the basic skin care products for her skin type, which makes this one very expensive foundation. The rationale for this unusual restriction is that the foundation is considered to be part of the skin care routine. They justify this policy by saying they want to monitor allergic reactions and perfect their assessment of your skin type. This sounds good, but all it really means is that you have to buy products that I would otherwise suggest you avoid. So, I'm caught between a rock and a hard place. If I recommend these foundations, I'm also recommending a handful of other products I think aren't worth it. The list of colors I like is presented for your information, but I can't really encourage you to try them if it means you have to buy $50 worth of other products you may not need or want.

Foundation Colors to Try *(all foundations have the same color names)*
Formula 1—Day Radiance Creme ($10)
All of these colors are good to excellent: Natural Beige, Misty Ivory (slightly pink), Light Beige (slightly orange), Auburn Beige, Creamy Ivory, Bisque Ivory, Sunlit Beige, Honey Beige, Deep Bronze (slightly peach), Burnished Bronze (slightly ash), and Desert Bronze.
Formula 2—Day Radiance Liquid ($10)
These colors range from good to great: Misty Ivory (slightly pink), Creamy Ivory (slightly pink), Bisque Ivory, Natural Beige, Honey Beige, Sunlit Beige, Golden Bronze, Cinnamon Bronze, Chestnut Bronze, and Deep Bronze.
Oil-Free Foundation ($10)
All of these are good colors: Natural Beige, Misty Ivory, Bisque Ivory (slightly pink), Creamy Ivory (slightly pink), Honey Beige, and Golden Bronze.

Foundation Colors to Avoid
Formula 1—Day Radiance Cream ($10)
Rose Beige and Cinnamon Bronze are too peachy orange to recommend.
Formula 2—Day Radiance Liquid ($10)
These colors are too orange to recommend: Light Beige, Rose Beige, Desert Bronze, Auburn Beige, Classic Bronze, and Bronze Sable.
Oil-Free Foundation ($10)
All of these colors are too orange or ashy to recommend: Rose Beige, Classic Bronze, Chestnut Bronze, Cinnamon Bronze, Deep Bronze, and Sunlit Beige.

Concealer: Mary Kay has a **Touch On Concealer** *($7.50)* for covering dark circles under the eye. It is a good product, although the consistency works best on normal to oily skin. Those with dry skin will find it hard to blend unless they use a moisturizer under the eye. All of the colors—Light, Medium, and Dark—are super and definitely worth a try. The **Cream Concealer** *($7.50)* comes in only one shade and it's yellow. This product is greasy, slips into the lines around the eyes, and the yellow color makes you look slightly jaundiced all day long.

Powder: Mary Kay has three shades of talc-based **Translucent Pressed Powder** *($7)*. All have a soft consistency and go on sheer. The shades are Light, which may be too pink for some skin tones, and Medium and Dark, both of which are great colors and definitely worth a try.

Eyeshadow: The eyeshadows are sold in separate tins that can be placed in a refillable compact. You buy the compact separately and then fill it with the colors of your choice. The only negative is that the eyeshadows, although matte, are not offered in the best assortment of neutrals. Just watch out for those blues and greens and you should do fine.

Eyeshadow Colors to Try
Powder Perfect Eye Color ($16 for two shades and compact; $6 per shade, refill only)
> All of these colors are nicely matte and go on softly, perhaps too softly for some skin tones: White Sand, Honey Glaze, Whisper Pink, Taupe, Gray Flannel, Lavender Mist (can look blue on some skin types), Marmalade, Hazelnut, Iris, Truffle, Heather Rose, Smoky Plum, and Blackest Black.

Eyeshadow Colors to Avoid
Powder Perfect Eye Color ($16 for two shades and compact; $6 per shade, refill only)
> All of these colors are either too blue, too green, or too shiny to recommend: Crystalline, Gingerspice, Cranberry Ice, Olive, Misty Pine, Real Teal, Blue Lace, Brilliant Blue, and Midnight Blue.

Blush: The blush colors are sold in separate tins that can be placed in a refillable compact. You buy the compact separately and then fill it with the colors of your choice. Very convenient, you don't have to keep paying for the compact, and most of the colors are great. There are also two shades of **Creamy Cheek Color** *($6)* that are just standard cream blushes. Not the best product for a reliable, long-lasting blush color.

Blush Colors to Try:
Powder Perfect Cheek Color ($15 for compact and one color; $7 for refills)
> All of these colors are great: Wild Rose, Mauve Satin, Very Berry, Lilac, Mulberry, Mango, Coral, Cashmere, Gingersnap, Azalea, Desert Bloom, and True Red.

Lipstick: Mary Kay calls her lipstick **Lasting Color Lipstick** *($9)*, but I didn't find that name to be accurate. The consistency is slightly greasy and the color can feather quickly into the lines around the mouth.

Eye, Brow, and Lip Liners: The **Eye Defining Pencils** *($6.50)* are standard pencils made in Germany. The texture is just fine and the price is reasonable. The **Lip Liner Pencils** *($6.50)* also feature great colors and textures. The **Eyebrow Pencils** *($6.50)* have a slightly slick texture, which can make for a shiny brow.

Mascara: Mary Kay's **Flawless Mascara** *($7.50)* is a decent mascara that goes on OK, but it doesn't build very thick or long lashes in comparison to a lot of other mascaras I've tested. The **Conditioning Mascara** *($7.50)* can smudge, so if you have a problem with mascara smearing by the end of the day, this would not be a good choice.

Max Factor

Max Factor was *the* makeup artist for the rich and famous in the 1920s. He is credited with developing the first mass-produced makeup products that were more than just heavy powders or tints for the cheeks and lips. His task was to find ways to make the men and women in films look exotic, sweet, masterful, wicked, or seductive in a way that was less obvious than on the stage, and this he did with unprecedented flair and creativity. His major creations that have been carried over to the 1990s are Pancake Foundation and Erace, the first foundation and cover stick. I don't recommend that anyone use pancake foundation, but it's nice to recognize the roots of makeup. The Erace stick was the staple of my youthful days; the texture has become somewhat creamier, there are more colors, and it still works well, but the fragrance is too pungent for my taste. I would like to say that I liked this product line but there is a lot lacking here. The only strong points are the lipsticks, one foundation, and two mascaras. Shiny eyeshadows, shiny blushes, concealers that crease, and OK powders are too many weak points to overlook.

Foundation: Max Factor still makes a traditional **PanCake Make-Up** *($5.95)* and a **Pan-Stick Make-Up** *($5.95)*. Both are packaged in a sealed plastic wrap that prevents you from viewing the color selections. For that reason alone these are difficult to recommend, and I happen to find the textures of both the Pancake and the Panstick too heavy and thick. **Satin Splendor Flawless Complexion Makeup** *($7.50)*, however, is a cream-to-powder foundation that comes in a good selection of colors, has a wonderful consistency, provides sheer but adequate coverage for a natural look, and feels great on the skin. Even without testers you can get fairly close in choosing this one by sight. All of the other foundations require testing and samples are not available.

Concealer: Erace Secret Cover-Up *($3.75)* concealer stick is a long-standing Max Factor product. The coverage is good, the consistency is creamy, although slightly greasy, and the color choices are good. It is good for dry skin, but it does have a tendency to crease into the lines under the eye. Unfortunately, it also has an intense fragrance that prevents me from recommending it. There is also an **Erace Plus Cover-Up** *($4.50)* that is heavier and thicker than the Secret Cover-Up. It is almost too thick for most skin types and it also has a tendency to crease into the lines under the eye.

Powder: Creme Puff Pressed Powder *($5.75)* is packaged in such a way that the powder puff blocks the view of the color. Therefore, I can't recommend it.

Eyeshadow Colors to Try
Visual Eyes Eyeshadows ($2.95)
> All of these are excellent colors: Grey Flannel, Cafe au Lait, Sweet Lilac, and Country Pink (a good color for darker skin tones).

Maxi Color-to-Go ($1.50)
> Stormy Weather and Abstract Pink are good matte shades.

Eyeshadow Colors to Avoid
Visual Eyes Eyeshadows ($2.95)
> All of these colors are too shiny: Creme de Menthe (too green) Tapestry Mauve, Perfect Perle, True Blue (no shine, but too blue), Sable, Pink Bouquet, Jade, Champagne, Sky Blue, Blue Lace, Soft Suede, Black Velvet, Brilliant Blue, Soft Teal, Blue Ice, and Karat.

Maxi Colors-to-Go ($1.50)
> All of these colors are too shiny: Goldilocks, Light-as-a-Feather, Medium Rare, Mint Julep, Terrific Teal, Aqua Marine (too blue-green), Blackout, China Sea, Blue Angel (too blue), Paper Moon (can be too white for most skin tones), Blue Lagoon (too blue), and Faded Jeans (too blue).

Shadow Blocks ($3.95)
> All of the colors are too shiny. It's a shame, because the concept of stamping each color with a bold letter that represents where you apply the color is clever; "A" is for accent color, "B" is for base color, and "C" is for contour color.

Blush Colors to Try
Satin Blush ($6.19)
> All of these colors are soft and beautiful: Pinkamelon, Porcelain Peach, Tiger Lily, Mulled Wine, Tender Rouge, Subtle Amber (a good contour color), Pink Velvet, Mauve Rose, and Tea Rose.

Maxi-Glow ($2.75)
> This is a very lightweight cream blush with a beautiful consistency. All of the colors are lovely, but be careful, the color doesn't last very well: Apricoral, Pinkberry, Bittersweet Pink, and Ginger Peach.

Blush Colors to Avoid
Satin Blush ($6.19)
> All of these are too shiny: Sangria, Crystal Sherry, Freshwater Pink, Topaz, Desert Pink, Wild Rose, Shimmering Lilac, and Midnight Rose.

New Definition Perfecting Blush ($6.95)
> The colors are all fine, but the texture of this cream-to-powder blush is somewhat grainy, not something I would recommend.

> **Lipstick:** Except for the intense fragrance, I loved the Max Factor selection of lipsticks: **Moisture Rich Lipstick *($4.75)*, New Definition *($4.95)*, Lasting Color Lipstick *($4.75)*,** and—my favorite—**Maxi's Soft Lustre Long Lasting Lipstick *($4.95)*.** They were all extremely creamy and the color really lasted. **Maxi's Not Quite Lipstick *($5.49)*** is more of a gloss than a lipstick.

Maxi's Soft Lustre Lipstick has to be one of the best lipstick buys on the market. If you can take the somewhat sweet odor that all these lipsticks have, they're great.

Eye, Brow, and Lip Liners: Max Factor has a **Brush & Brow Eyebrow Color** *($5.25)* powder that colors in the eyebrow with a hard brush. The color selection is excellent: Smoky Grey, Soft Black, Natural Brown, Midnight Brown, and Ash Blond. The powder works beautifully, but the firm brush is hard on the brow. It would be better to use these colors with a soft brush. The **Maxi Color Kohl Liner** *($2.10)* has a pencil at one end and a sponge tip at the other for blending. The darker shades, such as Black and Hot Fudge, are good, but stay away from the brighter shades, which are too shiny. Max Factor's **Featherblend Kohliners** *($4.95)* are an excellent assortment of eye pencils; one end is a brush, which blends better than the sponge tips that usually come with these two-in-one-type pencils. **Quick Draw Magic Eyeliner Pen** *($4.95)* is a felt-tip liquid eyeliner that can make the eye look obviously lined. There is also a **Lip Definer** *($4.95)* pencil that is wonderful; one end is a lipstick brush, which can be convenient. **Maxi's Lip Contouring Pencil** *($2.65)* comes in a poor selection of colors and has a fairly greasy texture. Max Factor makes a lip cream called **Lip Renew** *($5)* that comes in a tube and is supposed to prevent lipstick from bleeding. It did not work as well as I would have liked, and I do not prefer this type of anti-feathering product because it makes reapplication difficult.

Mascara: The Max Factor line has an excellent mascara called **2000 Calorie Mascara** *($4.95)* that goes on easily, doesn't smear, and makes lashes thick and long. It tends to flake if you overbuild the lashes. Don't overdo and it should last the whole day. **Super Lash Maker** *($4.95)* is a terrible mascara with a strange tiny brush that is difficult to use and builds no length or thickness. What a waste. **Maxi-Lash** *($2.50)* doesn't work nearly as well as the 2000 Calorie Mascara or many others on the market. Several coats left my lashes short and relatively undefined. The **No Color Mascara** *($4.95)* is simply a clear gel that leaves the lashes pretty much like they were without the product, only slightly more defined. This would do the trick for those who want just a tinge of extra length over already dark eyelashes.

Maybelline

Maybelline has a relatively new line of products called **Shades of You** that is very impressive and very appropriate for women of color, particularly African-American skin tones. It isn't a large selection, but most of the foundation, blush, and lipstick colors are really excellent and worth investigating. There are two types of foundations: **Oil-Free Liquid Water-based Makeup** *($4.25)* and **100% Oil-Free Souffle Water-based Makeup** *($5.50)*. Both have testers available, which is wonderful. There are 12 color choices for each. Both are designed for women with normal to oily skin. The ingredients in both are almost identical, but the texture of the souffle is whipped and feels thicker than the liquid. The souffle goes on somewhat drier than the liquid foundation, providing heavier coverage than I would recommend for daytime. However, if you blend it on carefully with a sponge (not your fingers) it could work well for women with very oily skin who want more coverage, but be very cautious. The liquid makeup is the better choice for a soft daytime look. All of the colors for both of these foundations are surprisingly good, with no overtones of orange or ash, a major problem for darker-colored foundations. Although the selection is small, if your color is there it is worth a try. One overwhelming negative I should point out is that both of the foundations in this line are only for women with normal to oily skin. They have yet to create a foundation for women of color who have dry skin.

There are also wonderful blush colors in the Shades of You collection. The **100% Oil-Free Powder Blush** *($4.10)* colors have a slight shine to them, but only slight and hardly noticeable on the skin. They go on silky and soft without being heavy or greasy. The **Lipstick** *($4.10)* colors are superior, with remarkably appropriate shades for women of color. They have a nice moist feel without being thick or greasy.

Maybelline's primary line has many other products worth checking out and many worth avoiding. There are some impressive colors to consider, particularly for blush and eyeshadows, plus several excellent mascaras. As you already know, the prices are wonderful. With a little caution you can come away with some great bargains and a beautiful look. It isn't the look they show in the ads, but it can be a close facsimile.

Foundation: There are no testers for the foundations in this line, so no recommendations can be made. Maybelline has many types of foundations: **Long-Wearing Liquid Makeup** *($4.35)*, **Sheer Essentials Make-Up** *($4.10)*, **Moisture Whip Liquid Make-Up** *($4.50)*, **Shine-Free Oil-Control Liquid Make-Up** *($3.95)*, **Ultra-Performance Pure Make-Up** *($4.35)*, and their new **Revitalizing Formula** *($4.50)*. Many of the foundations I purchased in each of these categories were too pink or too peach, except for Sheer Essentials, but I still warn against purchasing any foundation that you cannot try on before you buy it.

Concealer: Shine-Free Oil Control Cover Stick *($3.65)* won't control oil, but the two colors—Light and Medium—are both good. However, the product goes on very dry and would only be suitable for someone with very oily skin, plus it has a slight tendency to crease. There is also a basic **Revitalizing Cover Stick** *($4.99)* that comes in three reliable shades, and this too tends to crease. **Revitalizing Concealer with Sunscreen** *($3.65)* has good coverage, but it tends to go on heavy and definitely creases into the lines around the eyes. It has no SPF rating. **Undetectable Creme Concealer** *($3.65)* goes on somewhat dry but stays in place and really covers. I wouldn't exactly call it undetectable, but it does come in three good shades: Light, Medium, and Dark Medium (which isn't all that dark).

Powder: The **Translucent Pressed Powder** *($4)* contains talc and mineral oil, and the **Satin Complexion Pressed Powder** *($4.33)* contains talc and no oil. Both of these are OK and the colors are good, but the powder has a tendency to go on chalky. **Revitalizing Translucent Powder** *($5.69)* is a standard talc-based powder and truly translucent. It comes in three OK shades: Light, Medium, and Dark.

Eyeshadow: Maybelline has several types of eyeshadow combinations that are mostly way too shiny or too brightly colored to recommend. The intensity of their blues and greens are almost without comparison in any other cosmetics line. There are a handful of matte colors that are great, but be careful; don't be swayed by the shine and make a mistake. All of the Shine-Free eyeshadows are iridescent. Did they think we wouldn't notice?

Eyeshadow Colors to Try
Revitalizing Colors Singles, Duos, Trios, and Quads *($1.95 to $4.99)*
> All of these colors are beautiful and matte: Earthy Taupe, Creme de Cocoa, Gray Suede, The Suedes, and Watercolors (which are matte, but may be too bright for most skin types).

Eyeshadow Colors to Avoid
Revitalizing Colors Singles, Duos, Trios, and Quads *($1.95 to $4.99)*
> All of these colors are too shiny, too blue, or too green: Morning Glory, Silver Surf, Sky Blue, Baby Blue, Blue Lagoon, Willow, Misty Mint, Emerald, Empress Jade, Soft Pink, Pink Opal, Snowy Iris, Almondine, Honey Beige, Nutmeg, Spiced Rose, Copper Penny, Woodland Dawn, Crown Jewels, Chocolate Mousse, Sierra Sky, Autumn Mist, and Jamaican Bay.

Blush: Maybelline's **Revitalizing Color Blush** *($5.69)* is an excellent choice, with some great colors and a silky texture.

Blush Colors to Try
Revitalizing Color *($5.69)*
> All of these are excellent colors: Heather, Tea Rose, Desert Sunset, Sandalwood, Roseberry, and Rose Amber.

Lipstick: Maybelline has some really incredible lipsticks that are definitely worth a try. **Moisture Whip** *($4.25)* has a rich creamy texture, as does the **Long Wearing Lipstick** *($4.25)*, which lasts only slightly longer than the Moisture Whip. **Slim Elegance Lipstick** *($5)* is more gloss than lipstick, and many of the shades are frosted. The color selection for all of these is limited, but for a soft creamy look, Long Wearing Lipstick and Moisture Whip Lipstick are both excellent.

Eye, Brow, and Lip Liners: Lineworks *($5.35)* is a felt-tip liquid liner that dries to a somewhat slick finish with a very obvious lined look. **Expert Eyes Liner Pencil** *($3.85)* is an automatic pencil with a sponge tip at one end. On top of the pencil is a device that allows you to sharpen the pencil to an even finer point. **Turning Point Liner** *($4.85)* is an automatic pencil; its point is really too thick to create a thin line, but if you like a wider line this would be just fine. For the lips, Maybelline's **Precision Lip Liner** *($3.77)* is great, but the color selection is limited.

Mascara: Maybelline's ever-popular **Great Lash Mascara** *($4.20)* always gets mixed reviews. I found that it went on well, but it definitely smeared. **No Problem Mascara** *($4.20)* is quite good, one of the better Maybelline mascaras. **Magic Mascara** *($3.95)* has an awkward curved brush that doesn't build much length or thickness. **Perfectly Natural Mascara** *($3.25)* is OK, but it doesn't build up much thickness. For all women, regardless of color, I also want to strongly recommend Maybelline's new **Illegal Lengths Mascara** *($4.55)*. It is excellent without being too thick or clumpy, and it doesn't smear or flake. **Dial-a-Lash** *($5.50)* is a gimmicky mascara that suggests you can turn the base of the tube and adjust how long and thick your lashes will be. This mascara builds wimpy lashes and I saw no difference in the application when I turned the tube. **Fresh Lash Waterproof Mascara** *($4.20)* is one of the better waterproof mascaras on the market because it really stays without flaking or smearing. It doesn't build very long lashes, but it definitely does not come off under water.

Merle Norman

Having never even been into a Merle Norman boutique before, I was astounded by two things: the huge color selection of blushes and eyeshadows (if you can't find a blush or eyeshadow color here it's because you're stubborn), and the slightly worn, outdated feel of the surroundings. There was something antiquated about the two stores I shopped at, and certainly some of the products reinforce that observation. The displays are poorly organized; in fact, they appear almost haphazard. It would be much better if there were some color or style groupings. As it is, the colors have no relation to one another; they seem just strewn all over. While many other cosmetics lines are scaling down their selections of shiny eyeshadows, Merle Norman's is overflowing. There are more than half a dozen types of foundation to choose from, but the colors are exceedingly disappointing, with an overabundance of pink and peach shades. What makes it even more dismaying is that some of these foundations have great textures. The lipsticks are fairly greasy and the concealers crease easily. Regardless of how dismal this all sounds, with a few adjustments this line could really come to life. The matte blushes and eyeshadows are already wonderful, the entire line has an extensive color selection for women of all colors, and the face powders are quite good. A few color improvements and a good reorganization would bring Merle Norman competitively into the '90s.

Foundation: Merle Norman has a startlingly large assortment of foundations. **Luxiva Ultra Powder Foundation** *($22)* is a standard talc-based powder that goes on smooth but can look too powdery on dry skin. **Luxiva Ultra Powder Base** *($12.50)* is a cream-to-powder foundation that is actually more cream than powder. This would only be good for someone with normal to dry skin; it is too greasy for someone with oily skin. **Aqua Base** *($12.50)* is an extremely creamy, extremely waterproof foundation that provides solid medium coverage and has one of the better color selections among these foundations. It can feel too thick if you don't blend it carefully and it can feel like a layer of film when it gets wet or if you perspire. **Remarkable Finish Liquid Makeup** *($15)* is a fairly sheer, matte foundation that goes on very thin with a flat finish. It tends to be very fluid, which makes it hard to control, but it does go on light, which is good for someone with oily or combination skin. **Luxiva Ultra Foundation** *($22)* is very heavy stuff. This is an extremely emollient, almost greasy, foundation that provides rather thick coverage if you're not careful how you blend it on. This would only be for someone with extremely dry skin. **Total Finish Compact** *($15)* is as close to greasepaint as you will find. This foundation is too thick and greasy to recommend. **Oil-Control Makeup** *($15)* won't control oil, but the color selection is great and the foundation quite matte.

Foundation Colors to Try
Luxiva Ultra Powder Foundation ($22)
All of these colors are good: Ivory, Pure Beige (slight rose), Soft Bisque, Creamy Beige, Tan Beige (slightly peach), Soft Honey (slightly peach), Honey Beige, and Tawny Beige.
Luxiva Ultra Powder Base ($12.50)
All of the Ultra Powder Base colors are surprisingly neutral. They are numbered 0 to 12.
Aqua Base ($12.50)
All of these colors are great: Cream Beige, Alabaster Beige, Sandy Beige, Maple Cream, Champagne Beige, Gentle Beige, Fawn Beige, Golden Birch (slightly rose), Spice Beige (slightly peach), Dark, Sunny Tan, Mahogany, and Golden Brown.
Remarkable Finish Liquid Makeup ($15)
All of these colors are good: Ivory, Soft Bisque, Creamy Beige, Cafe Beige (slightly peach), Tan Beige (slightly rose), Sun Beige, Sandy Beige (slightly peach), and Bronzewood (slightly peach).

Total Finish Compact ($15)
   Only Mahogany, Golden Brown, and Amber Beige are good colors to recommend.
Oil-Control Makeup ($15)
   All of the Oil Control Makeup colors are great.

Foundation Colors to Avoid
Luxiva Ultra Powder Foundation ($22)
   All of these colors are too peach, too orange, or too rose to recommend: Soft Honey, Simply Beige, Sandy Beige, Quiet Rose, Alabaster, Blush Beige, and Fragile Beige (ultra peach).
Aqua Base ($12.50)
   All of these colors are too extremely peach, pink, or ash to recommend: Translucent, Midtone, Rose Glo, Blushing Beige, Rose Beige, Bamboo Beige, Caramel Beige, and Latan.
Remarkable Finish Liquid Makeup ($15)
   All of these colors are too peach, too pink, or too rose to recommend: Quiet Rose, Simply Beige, Pure Beige, Alabaster, and Porcelain.
Total Finish Compact ($15)
   All of these colors are too yellow, too pink, too peach or too rose to recommend: Golden Beige, Light Neutral, Alabaster Beige, Medium Neutral, Medium Deep Golden, Delicate Beige, Deep Neutral, Deep Golden, Buff Beige, Toffee, Toasted Almond, Bronze Glow, and Ecru.

   Concealer: Retouch Cover Creme *($9)* has a terrible color selection and easily creased into the lines around the eyes. All of the colors were either too peach, too pink, too yellow, or ashy. Not one of the six colors came close to a neutral flesh tone. **Oil-Free Concealing Creme** *($9)* goes on drier than the Retouch and has a slightly better range of colors, but it still tends to crease into the lines around the eyes.

   Powder: There is a wide range of powders in this line. They are all standard talc-based powders that go on rather translucent. **Remarkable Finish Loose Powder** *($16.50)* and **Remarkable Finish Pressed Powder** *($14.50)* both have six good color selections that range from Translucent to Deep. **Remarkable Finish Oil Control Loose Powder** *($16.50)* and **Remarkable Finish Oil Control Pressed Powder** *($14.50)* won't control oil, but they are oil-free powders that go on soft and have six good color selections that range from Translucent to Deep.

Eyeshadow Colors to Try
Powder Rich Eyeshadows Singles, Duos, and Trios ($11/$14/$15)
   All of these colors are very matte and blend on smoothly: Cloud Pink, Pink Mauve, Soft Lavender, Deep Plum, Eggplant, Rose Taupe, Cashmere, True Navy (more gray than navy), Yellow Gold, Kohl (good black), Taupe, Taupe Suede, Cinnamon Spice, Sienna, Harvest, Warm Naturals, Cool Naturals, Rich Brown, Peach Blossom, Sable, Wisteria, Soft Umber, and Wheat.

Eyeshadow Colors to Avoid
Powder Rich Eyeshadows Singles, Duos, and Trios ($11/$14/$15)

All of these colors are too ultra-shiny, too blue, or too green to recommend: Pink Shimmer, Rosewood, Country Rose, Powder Frost, Mauve Dust, Violet Haze, Lavender, Blue Haze, Blue Suede, Gold Dust, Honey, Pearl Grey, Soft Grey, Smoke Grey, Butternut, Yellow, Sepia, Rococo, Coffee Mist, Pink Innocence, Tender Rose, Mist, Mystique (strange combination), Sunwashed, Twilight Beige, Delicate Pastels, Blue Lagoon, Mystic Teal, Rosewood/Deep Plum, Imperial Blue, Pure White, Elite, Rosegold, Spirited Sun, Rosy Brown, Maroon, Topaz, Burnished Bronze, Rose Petal, Teal, Black Pearl, Turquoise Teal, and Smoke Grey/Soft Grey.

Blush: There is a vast selection of blush colors here for a wide range of skin tones. The textures vary a bit, but for the most part they are soft and blend on easily. Merle Norman also has a **One Powder Eyes & Blush** *($12.50)* that is meant to be safe for use around the eyes, and the color is also compatible as a blush shade. It comes in only four colors, but they are very nice.

Blush Colors to Try
Blushing Powder ($12.50)

All of these colors are great and have a soft, silky texture: Soft Peach (not soft but bright), Coral Blush, Spirited Fuchsia, Cinnabar, Umber (good contour), Nutmeg (good contour), Woodland Rose, Caramel, Barely Blush, New Copper, Matte Red, Woodland Peach, Apricot, Blushing Red, Cayenne, Candied Rose, Matte Rose, Matte Pink, Mauve Blush, Cafe Rose, Claret, and Raspberry.

Blush Colors to Avoid
Blushing Powder ($12.50)

Only Opalescent is too shiny to recommend.

Lipstick: Moist Lip Color *($9)* was a very greasy, almost gloss-like lipstick that didn't have much staying power. The regular lipsticks *($10.50)* were creamy, but still on the greasy side.

Eye, Brow, and Lip Liners: Trimline Lip Pencils *($11)* are standard pencils made in Germany that come in a small but good color selection. **Lip Pencil Plus** *($9.50)* is a fat pencil with a lip liner on one end and a lipstick on the other. This would be a great idea except the lip liner and lipstick combinations are too contrasting. A more subtle, complementary color match for lipstick and lip pencil is required. The **Trimline Eye Pencils** *($9.50)* have a poor texture and many of them are shiny.

Mascara: Creamy Flo-Matic Mascara *($10)* is an OK mascara. It doesn't clump, but it also doesn't build very thick lashes.

Brushes: The Merle Norman boutique I went to sold two different sets of brushes; one was good and the other was poor quality. The only way to distinguish between the two were their handles. The black handle brushes were more dense but stiff. The red handle brushes were less dense but softer. My preference was the red handle brushes; prices range from $5 to $23.50.

Monteil of Paris

How is it that I've overlooked this line for so many years? It could just be my reluctance to review another high-end French line. There are so many of them, and the prices are always so unreasonable and the products so often lackluster. Yet, I am always pleased to find a cosmetics line that has a respectable number of good products, colors, and textures, which Monteil just happens to have. I've learned my lesson: never judge before you look. In many ways this is just another fancy overpriced cosmetics line and the prices are beyond the upper limits of tolerable, but if price isn't a consideration, there are some interesting items to check out.

By the way, don't be all that impressed by the French-sounding name of this cosmetics line. (You may remember that Monteil of Paris used to be Germaine Monteil, but the first name is now gone.) For a long time it was owned by Revlon, which loses some prestige in the translation. Revlon went crazy in the 1980s, buying up a large number of cosmetics lines, and ended up mired in management hell. Much-needed financing to improve these lines just wasn't there. Monteil was recently bought by the Lancaster group (which is French), so there might be some needed improvements in the works. One of the things Monteil can use is good organization of their color line and better tester units. The colors are just there, in no workable or cohesive order. It is always helpful to the consumer to have colors grouped by color families such as roses, corals, reds, and neutrals. Perhaps Lancaster will do what it takes to help a line that already has some strong points, such as blushes, foundations, eyeshadows, and lipsticks.

Foundation: One of the better foundations I've tested for this book is Monteil's **Habitat Natural Foundation with Chemical-Free SPF 4** *($30)*. It has light to medium coverage and goes on silky smooth; the SPF 4 isn't great (it should be at least 12), but it is chemical-free. Regrettably, the rest of Monteil's foundations are disappointing, with poor color selections and merely OK textures. **Soft Cover Liquid Makeup** *($25)* has a terrible selection of colors that are all either too pink or too orange. **Supplegen Lasting Makeup** *($30)* has only four shades, which are all very pink or orange and also cannot be recommended. **Soft Cover Creme Makeup** *($25)* has only three neutral colors to recommend—Ivory, Sheer Beige, and Natural Beige—but even they can turn slightly peach; all of the other colors are just too peach, too pink, or too rose to recommend.

Foundation Colors to Try
Habitat Natural Foundation with Chemical-Free SPF 4 ($30)

All of these colors are excellent: Buff (may turn slightly pink), Beige, Nude, Sand, Toast, and Shell (may turn slightly pink).

Concealer: Who would have thought that my favorite concealer ever would be hiding in Monteil's cosmetics line! **Hides Anything Moisturizing Concealer** *($17.50)* won't hide everything and it is not at all moisturizing—in fact, someone with dry skin might not like the texture at all—but it is an excellent under-eye concealer and rarely creases into the lines around the eye. It comes in three colors; Light and Medium are both great, but Deep can turn peach on most skin tones.

Powder: The **Moisturizing Pressed Powder** *($18)* is talc-based and comes in a small but impressive assortment of colors. Sheer 1, Sheer 2, Sheer 3, Sheer Natural, and Tan (a bronzer color without shine) are all quite good.

Eyeshadow Colors to Try
Rich Powder Eyeshadow Singles and Duos ($15/$17)

What a great selection of primarily matte attractive eyeshadow colors: Chambord, Sande, Mellowed Sienna, Coquille, Gris Classique, Limoges, Volcane, Limonette, Bisque, Dijon, Cafe/Creme, Eden Roc/Gris Pale, Terra Rose/Terra Wood, Aubergette/Rochelle (one of the colors is ultra-pink and may be difficult to use), Souffle de Peche/ Vermeil, Brun/Chamois, Twilight Blush/Twilight Oyster, Warm Khaki/Mellowed Ochre, L'Aire/Barque, and Woodsmoke/Flax.

Eyeshadow Colors to Avoid
Rich Powder Eyeshadow Singles and Duos ($15/$17)

All of these colors are either too shiny, too blue, or too green to recommend: Anis Pale, Teal Charbon, Mahogany/Rose Blush, Shelle/Rocque, Rose/Bleu de Nuit (a strange combination), Duske/Inkling, Silver/Si Bleu, Ashe/Gazelle, Patina/Pumpkin, and Mahogany/Rose Blush.

Blush Colors to Try
Silk Powder Blush ($18)

The colors aren't really all that silky—actually, they are rather dry in texture—but the shades are beautiful and blend on easily: Apricote, Peche-En-Fleur, Rose Valmont, Berrie D'Ambroise, Rose-En-Fleur, Fleur de Mai, Fountain Glow, Peche Naive (slightly shiny), Rose de Luxe, Petalique, Naturelle-En-Fleur, and Rose Avril.

Creme Blush ($13)

This is a traditional, greasy cream blush with only four colors. It is hard to find this type of blush anymore in any cosmetics line because powder blush is easier and doesn't dissipate like cream blush. If cream blush is what you are looking for it is OK, but using cream blush is not the best.

Blush Colors to Avoid
Silk Powder Blush ($18)

Cordovan, Brique, and Shimmer are too shiny to recommend.

Lipstick: The lipsticks *($12.50)* are creamy and feel great, but they are not unique or anything special.

Eye, Brow, and Lip Liners: The lip and eye pencils *($11)* are fairly standard; like so many other pencils on the market, these are manufactured in Germany.

Mascara: Ideal Mascara *($12.50)* is hardly ideal. It builds poorly and can smear.

New Essentials

New Essentials is a relatively new cosmetics line sold at department stores such as J.C. Penney. It's a fairly small line, but there are a handful of interesting products and color choices, and the prices are reasonable. The testers are fairly accessible and there was little pressure from the salespeople I encountered. Colors are grouped into three categories: Pastel (soft colors), Neutral (more earth tones), and Brights (vivid strong colors). This arrangement is a little confusing because yellow and blue tones are tossed together. Apparently no one at New Essentials felt that color tone is the most essential aspect to choosing shades of blush, eyeshadow, and lipstick. If you're wearing a vivid coral blush, it wouldn't be best to wear a bright pink lipstick; the contrast would be similar to wearing a pink blouse with a coral skirt. You can get away with it, but you have to be careful. Color divisions that divide yellow tones from blue tones are usually the most helpful.

Foundation: Surprisingly, the two foundation types in this line are excellent and definitely worth trying. Both come in pump containers, which I don't recommend because they tend to waste product. When you pump out too much, how do you get the excess back inside? **Skin Balancing Foundation Moisturizing SPF 8** *($12.50)* won't balance anyone's skin, but it does have excellent colors and a light, smooth texture. **Skin Balancing Foundation 100% Oil-Free** *($18.50)* isn't 100-percent oil-free, but it is fairly matte and has a wonderful texture.

Foundation Colors to Try
Skin Balancing Foundation Moisturizing SPF 8 ($12.50)
> All of these colors are quite good: Bisque (may turn pink on some skin tones), Ecru (may turn pink on some skin tones), Buff, Sand, Cream, and Sienna.

Skin Balancing Foundation 100% Oil-Free ($18.50)
> All of these are excellent colors: Bisque (may turn rose), Ecru, Buff, Cream, Sand, and Sienna.

Concealer: New Essentials **Concealer with SPF 8** *($8.50)* isn't bad, but it isn't great. It comes in three colors: Ivory, Nude, and Beige, which are all pretty good. On some skin types it can have a slight tendency to crease into the lines around the eye.

Powder: This line has a **Loose Powder** *($15)* and a **Pressed Powder** *($15)* that both come in one shade called Transparent. It is fairly transparent, but it still has some color and won't work on medium to darker skin tones.

Eyeshadow Colors to Avoid
Eyecolor Duos ($14)

All of these colors are fairly shiny and come in strange color combinations that are hard to use: Violet/Chrome, Apricot/Empire Blue, Slate/Royal Pink, Beige/Smoky Blue (Beige is matte, but the Smoky Blue is shiny and very blue), Organdy/Copper, Forest/Moonrose (Forest is too green, but Moonrose is a great matte), Soft Pink/Silver, Lavender/Pale Yellow, Celadon/Salmon (blue and coral, who could wear this?), and Cream/Sand (both are matte, but Cream is too white for most skin tones).

Blush Colors to Try
Cheek Color ($12.50)

All of these are great soft colors that have a slight amount of shine, but not enough to make them a problem: Pale Pink, Cedar Rose, Peach Blossom, Apricot, Cinnabar, Sienna Pink, Fiesta Rose, Tender Peach, and Mulberry Wine.

Lipstick: The lipstick *($9)* comes in some great colors; unfortunately, they are fairly greasy and the color just won't last very long.

Eye, Brow, and Lip Liners: There is a very small selection of standard eye and lip pencils *($8)*.

Origins

Estee Lauder started off the 1990s with a new cosmetics line called Origins, and what a concept it is. A quote from one of the brochures sums it up quite nicely: "Origins marries the forces of nature with the vigor of modern science to make provocative differences in the way you experience cosmetics." To put it in my own words: "Origins utilizes all of the current fads on the market to create one of the most distinct makeup and skin care collections around." The brochures, like most of the packaging, are made of recycled paper. The ad copy is loaded with names of exotic-sounding botanicals, herbs, and oils. References to Egyptian and Roman know-how are frequent. When it comes to the allure of "natural" products, nothing else comes as close as Origins to living up to that claim. Modern science plays a part in the technical-sounding promotions that describe theories about skin care and makeup application. It's going to be hard to ignore this line in the '90s. They even sell sensory therapy oils and gels that are "thousands of years old." Of course, the oils and gels aren't that old, but the idea is to convince you that whoever was around thousands of years ago used these concoctions, and that they must still be good.

I was very impressed with the color presentation at the Origins counter. The lipsticks, eyeshadows, blushes, and lip pencils are all divided into three color groupings: Peach to Rust, Beige to Tan, and Ivory to Pink. All of the colors have minimal or no shine and most are soft and muted and therefore extremely easy to use. The textures are wonderful and the application is almost flawless. Although I like the eyeshadows, be aware that a few have some shine present; many of the salespeople I talked to insisted that the colors were all matte and they are not. There is also a problem with the amount of flower extract used in many of the Origins products. If you have any hay-fever-type allergies, these are going to cause you problems. "Natural" ingredients are not automatically the best for all skin types.

Foundation: As this book was going to press there were only two foundation types available in this line and they are both being discontinued. **Moisture Makeup** *($16)* came in an extremely poor assortment of colors and contained talc and kaolin, which are terrible for dry skin. The **Matte Makeup** *($16)* provided medium coverage, was nicely matte, and had several good colors. Origins is planning to introduce three kinds of foundation in different consistencies: some coverage, more coverage, and most coverage. There will be 18 shades for each type of foundation, which is a promising range of colors. I'll look forward to reviewing these in my newsletter when they become available.

Foundation Colors to Try
Moisture Makeup ($16)
> Birch is an excellent color but the only one. Sugar Cane, Pecan, Clove, and Freesia are acceptable but could turn peach on some skin tones.

Matte Makeup ($16)
> All of these colors are excellent: Linen, Paperwhite, Chestnut, Shell, Allspice (slightly ash), Wheat, Flax, Warmspice, and Hazelnut (slightly peach).

Foundation Colors to Avoid
Moisture Makeup ($16)
> All of these colors are either too orange or too pink to recommend: Ginger, Biscuit, Vanilla, Coffee, Cocoa (too ash-green), Honey, and Sand (very orange).

Matte Makeup ($16)
> Lily and Maple are too peach for most skin tones.

Powder: Origins' **Translucent Powder** *($17.50)* is mica- and talc-based. It is soft and sheer, although it's hard to imagine who would use some of these colors. Nature's Cream, Nature's Almond, and Nature's Copper are good colors; Nature's Peach is too peach, Nature's Rose is too pink, and Alabaster is pure white.

Concealer: Origins' concealer *($10)* comes in two shades. Light is an excellent shade, but Medium can be too peach for most skin tones. This is a fine concealer if the Light shade happens to be your color.

Eyeshadow: Origins has a superb array of matte eyeshadows *($12.50)*. Although I dislike almost all shades of bright blue and green eyeshadows, I feel that almost all of the eyeshadow colors in this line are worth a try. Even the blues are some of the nicest blues on the market. Warning: Not all these colors are matte; a very few do have a small amount of shine.

Eyeshadow Colors to Try
Singles ($12.50)

All of these colors are splendid: Quince, Seashell, Cayenne, Cinnamon, Primrose, Cabernet, Daphne, Sherry, Rosebud, Driftwood, Raisin, Winter Bloom, Umber, Snow (may be too white for most skin tones), Mocha, Blue Sage (may be too blue for most skin tones), Tourmaline (may be too blue for most skin tones), Malachite (may be too green for most skin tones), Olive, Kiwi (may be too green for most skin tones), Maize, Pineapple, Lapis, Wisteria, Iris, Heather, Amethyst, Fog (superb shade of gray), Slate, and Onyx.

Blush Colors to Try

All of the blush *($15)* colors are superb and unquestionably worth a try: Nutmeg, Persimmon, Nectar, Orchid, Laurel, Hyacinth, Claret, Tulip, Brick, and Dusk.

Lipstick: Origins' lipsticks *($10)* are very glossy and the color won't survive to the midmorning break. If you have a problem with lipstick bleeding into the lines around your mouth, you'll feel this lipstick traveling the second you put it on.

Eye, Brow, and Lip Liners: The eye and lip pencils *($9)* come in great colors, though the selection is limited. The brow pencil *($9)*, like all brow pencils, has a slightly slick texture and is not recommended unless you are a wizard at penciling brows that don't look fake.

Mascara: Origins makes a gimmicky mascara product called **Underwear for Lashes** *($10)*. It is an undercoating for the lashes that you apply before the mascara. The claim is that it helps the lashes grab more mascara. A good mascara should suffice, so this is an unnecessary layer on fragile lashes. Origins' **Fringe Benefits Mascara** *($10)* is a good mascara that builds evenly and doesn't smear.

Payot

Payot is a French line that has a very elegant appearance. It is usually found in department stores like J.C. Penney, which makes it one of the more expensive lines there. Although I wouldn't even begin to call this line exceptional, the blushes and powders do come in silky textures, the displays are easily accessible, and some of the colors are good. On the other hand, most of the eyeshadows are shiny, the foundation colors are poor, and the lipsticks, although quite good, have an unusually small selection.

Foundation: Payot's foundations actually have wonderful textures and I would love to be able to recommend them, but the color selection is so small as to be practically nonexistent and the colors are almost all too peach or pink. What a waste.

Foundation Colors to Try
Fluide Mat Hydrant ($21)
There is only one good neutral color, called Naturel.
Teint Creme Traitant ($37)
Teint Lumineux and Teint Hale are good neutral tones for medium to deep skin tones.
Creme to Powder Foundation ($35)
Although the texture of this foundation is exceptional, the only color recommended is Naturel.

Foundation Colors to Avoid
Fluide Mat Hydrant ($21)
None of these colors are recommended: Fluide Dore (too ashy), Fluide Clair (too pink), and Fluide Invisible (which is hardly invisible because it is vividly peach).
Teint Creme Traitant ($37)
Teint Porcelaine and Teint Opaline are both too pink for most skin tones.
Creme to Powder Foundation ($35)
Beige is too pink, Dune is too peach, and Epice is practically orange.
Concealer: Payot's **Concealer** *($15)* comes in only one color, Naturel, that is actually quite good, but it has a fairly greasy texture and can crease into the lines around the eyes.
Powder: The **Pressed Powder** *($23)* comes in two types; both have a very silky texture and appearance, but the Voile colors are more sheer than the others. Most of the shades are actually quite good, although some miss the mark; try Ambre (a great neutral), Premier Soleil (a great deep brown), Voile Ambre, Voile Rose (fairly rose), Voile Naturel (this is indeed natural), and Bronzant (an excellent deep golden brown). Avoid Rose (too pink).

Eyeshadow Colors to Try
Eyeshadow Singles and Duos *($19/$23)*

All of these colors are good and very matte: Rose Santal (great pale peach), Vison Ecru, Lilas Naturel, and Duo Prune Cendree.

Eyeshadow Colors to Avoid
Eyeshadow Singles and Duos *($19/$23)*

All of these colors are either too shiny or too blue or too green: Eclat Rose, Eclat Naturel, Eclat Dore (too peach for most skin tones), Petale Rose, Pacifique (more blue than the Pacific), Nacre, Gris Volcanique, Bronze, Aigue Marine, Soleil Levant/Terre Brulee, Brique Rose/Blue Lilas, Rose Aurore/Blue Orage, Sable Bloue/Vert Ocean, Blue Hemisphere (this one's matte, but the blue is too much), Violet Sauvage (one side is matte and the other is ultra-shiny), Duo Vert Givre (one side is matte and the other is ultra-shiny), and Duo Pain Rose.

Blush: All of the blush *($23)* colors are excellent and the texture very silky and soft.

Lipstick: There is a small selection of lipsticks *($15)*, but the colors are soft and lovely and the texture is wonderfully creamy and velvety.

Eye, Brow, and Lip Liners: Payot has an **Eyeliner Compact** *($23)* that you can use either wet or dry. It comes in two sets of two colors each: Nuit Bleu (black and navy) and Terre Indigo (brown and navy.) Any eyeshadow can serve the same purpose.

Mascara: This is an excellent mascara *($17)* that makes the lashes thick and lush without clumping or smearing.

Physicians Formula

There are some great products in this line, but before I review the wonderful blushes, eyeshadows, and lipsticks I have to tell you how much I dislike the name Physicians Formula. It is deceptive. You would logically assume by the name that all of the Physicians Formula products are formulated by physicians. Wrong. According to David Lozano, Vice President of Marketing and Research, the chemists at Physicians Formula are neither doctors nor dermatologists. These chemists are chemists just like the ones working for every other cosmetics line. They study ingredients that have been researched in universities and reviewed in various investigative journals, and based upon their experience and knowledge they choose "reliable" supplies of ingredients. This process is no different from that used by hundreds of other cosmetics companies. So why the name Physicians Formula, besides the fact that it sounds very professional and official to the consumer?

In 1937, Dr. Frank Crandell, an allergist, created Physicians Formula's first product, called Le Velvet, for his wife, who had photo-sensitive skin. Thus the name Physicians Formula. (An allergist *is* a physician, after all.) Does today's Le Velvet even remotely resemble the original product that Dr. Crandell invented 56 years ago? Well, Physicians Formula today claims to emulate Dr. Crandell, striving to create hypoallergenic, noncomedogenic ingredients and products. But given the new cosmetic ingredients on the market, I would be shocked if the original formula was still in use.

According to David Lozano, you can be sure that Physicians Formula's products are hypoallergenic because they are tested on ani-mals in outside laboratories and were reported to cause zero allergic reactions. This is hard to believe, but we weren't given the test results. Products are also supposedly tested on in-house employees, but again we were not provided with any results. I was told by David Lozano that product quality is further ensured by a medical committee, which evaluates each and every product before it is put on the market. Naturally, you would expect a *medical* committee to be comprised of doctors, particularly given the name of the company. Wrong again. This committee is headed by one dermatologist, Dr. Stuart Martel, who became a board-certified dermatologist in 1955. Surprisingly (or maybe not surprisingly), he is the only certified doctor on the committee. The rest of the medical committee is made up of sales, marketing, and con-sumer representatives. Physicians Formula is a misleading name, but it is not the only cosmetics company with a less than meaningful name. It is only the most obvious.

Having said all this, I want to report that Physicians Formula does have some products that are worth recommending, so ignore the name and look closer at the products. There are some great buys here.

Foundation: Physicians Formula has three types of foundation that I was hoping would go on much better than they actually did. **Le Velvet** *($7.25)* is a compact foundation that goes on surprisingly light and creamy, plus it con-tains a good titanium dioxide-based sunscreen with an SPF of 15. Unfortunately, it leaves a whitish film on the face, making it look chalky and pale regardless of the color. **Sun Shield Liquid Makeup SPF 15** *($5.25)* is a good option, but there are no testers available. **Oil Control Matte Makeup** *($5.25)* won't control oil; it does go on well, but the color selection isn't the best. There are no testers available for any of these foundations, so you could easily go home with the wrong color. One more recommendation: Physicians Formula sells **Refill Sponges** *($2.50)* for the Le Velvet foundation that work well with any foundation. I prefer the round thin shape to the thick wedge sponges you normally find at cosmetics counters and drugstores.

Concealer: Gentle Cover Concealer Stick *($4.35)* comes in four shades: Green, Ice Blue, Light, and Medium. The texture is too heavy and tends to crease into the lines around the eyes. I also never recommend using green or blue concealers. Physicians Formula also has a **Color Corrective Primer** *($3.75)* that comes in Mauve, Yellow, and Green. The texture is very heavy and thick and can feel tacky under foundation.

Eyeshadow: This is a wonderful collection of matte eyeshadows. They go on beautifully and blend easily.

Eyeshadow Colors to Try
Matte Collection Singles and Duos ($2.95/$4.25)
All of these colors are excellent: Taupe, Cinnamon, Peaches 'N'Creme, French Vanilla, Smoke, Perfect Pink, Jade (may be too green for most skin types), Rosewood, Plum Smoke, Praline, Chocolate Fudge, Khaki, Dusty Mauve, Autumn Dusk, and Vanilla Marble.

Eyeshadow Colors to Avoid
Matte Collection Singles and Duos ($2.95/$4.25)
Midnight Blue, Misty Blue, Stormy Skies, and Sky Blue/Pink are all too blue, Teal is too green, and Flamingo is a difficult color combination of peach and green.

Blush: The package says "silky smooth" and this is almost right. I wouldn't call these blushes silky, but they do go on smooth and are totally matte. **Matte Blush** *($5.75)* is a great find. Only one word of warning: Most of these colors are very muted, bordering on dull. Check them out only if you are looking for a very natural tawny blush color. Natural Shadow Blush is one of the best contour colors to be found anywhere.

Lipstick: Total Perfection Lipstick *($4.50)* is a good creamy lipstick. Unfortunately, the only way to select a color is via color swatches that don't really match (or sometimes even come close to) the color of the lipstick. It would be nice if you could see the lipstick color itself.

Eye, Brow, and Lip Liners: Gentlewear Eye Pencils *($3.95)* may be gentle but the pencils are fat, which makes them hard to sharpen and hard to control, plus most of them are shiny.

Mascara: Length Plus Mascara *($4.50)* and **Full Lash Mascara** *($4.50)* are just OK but not recommended. These mascaras weren't great. They didn't build much length or thickness and they tended to smear.

Prescriptives

Prescriptives prides itself on having a wide range of colors that are appropriate for almost every woman's skin color. For this they win high marks. More so than any other line, Prescriptives has an outstanding selection of eyeshadows, blushes, foundations, and lip colors for every skin tone you can think of. More so than any other line at the cosmetics counters, Prescriptives acknowledges that Caucasian women are not the only women in the world. And they do so beautifully. Congratulations, Prescriptives, I only hope the other cosmetics lines follow your lead.

Prescriptives is an extension, or cousin, of Estee Lauder, but that is about all they have in common. Many of the reservations I have about the makeup products in the Estee Lauder line do not apply to most of Prescriptives' products. Almost all of their colors—blushes, eyeshadows, lipsticks, pencils, and powders—are matte with no shine whatsoever. Now that's a find! The major problem is that selecting a product is somewhat complicated, at least from a consumer's point of view. The counter personnel I interviewed had a wide variety of training, and this line requires training—you're better off talking to someone who has been with the line for a while. Actually, that's true of almost all lines, but especially for this one.

The counter displays are incredibly well organized and the color selections, for the most part, are terrific. All of the shades are divided into four color groups: Yellow-Orange, Red, Red-Orange, and Blue-Red. It is the job of the salesperson to color-type your skin and to indicate what foundations and principal color group you should be wearing. The hitch is that once you know what your principal color group is, you are told that you can wear certain colors in all the other groups for a more natural, dramatic, or intensified look. Not a concept that everyone would agree with, particularly me, but great for selling more products. No matter how the woman tried to convince me that I would look great in Yellow/Orange colors for my natural look, there is no way I felt comfortable in those shades. In spite of this sales tenet, I like their color selections and find many of their products to be quite good. And almost all of Prescriptives products are fragrance-free.

Foundation: Prescriptives has seven types of foundation made for a variety of skin types—more than 125 shades altogether. Although this large selection is impressive, many of colors are too peach or too rose. Be sure to follow my suggestions carefully. **Makeup 1** *($28.50)* is an excellent light foundation designed for normal to dry skin; **Makeup 2** *($28.50)* is for dry skin and has a somewhat heavier coverage than Makeup 1. **100% Oil-Free Liquid Makeup SPF 15** *($28.50)* is a very good oil-free foundation designed for oily to combination skin that provides a sheer light coverage and is a superior sun block at the same time. **Oil-Free Foundation** *($28.50)* looks strange in the bottle. Half of it is glycerin and water, which floats at the top of the jar, while the other half is the makeup color, mostly talc, which sits on the bottom until you shake it (and you have to shake it vigorously to mix it thoroughly). This is a tricky product to use and I don't recommend it, because if it can separate in the bottle it can separate on the face. Furthermore, in concentrated amounts, glycerin can cause allergic reactions. **Custom Blend** *($50)* is prepared for you personally and assumes that the salesperson can match your skin tone better by mixing and matching than by selling you the ready-made shades they have. I did not review the Custom Blend foundation. It sounds like a good idea, but it relies too much on the expertise of the individual salesperson, which is, at best, undependable. **Soft Matte Foundation** *($28.50)* provides medium coverage and isn't all that matte, although it feels great on the skin. This foundation has the weakest color choices. However, all the foundation types have excellent foundation colors for women of color. **Quick Cover Compact Makeup** *($28.50)* is a soft powder foundation that is slightly heavier than regular pressed powder. There are 12 colors to choose from that are surprisingly neutral and sheer. These compact powder foundations are good for normal skin types, but can look too powdery on dry skin and tend to streak on oily skin.

Prescriptives' foundations are grouped in the same color categories used for the entire line. A specific foundation shade is chosen for you from the existing foundation colors by a process they call "color printing." Four of the potential foundation color groups are drawn in a line on your cheek with the Makeup 1 foundation and then allowed to dry. One will seem to disappear into your skin and that is considered the foundation color group that is best for you. Within the color group chosen for you, there is a range of shades from light to dark. I found this to be one of the more reliable ways to test foundation, except that the final selection can vary from salesperson to salesperson. Some of the foundation colors that are "accepted" by your skin may still look too pink or orange in the sunlight, and there is still the question of proper intensity. Regardless of how scientific color printing sounds, be sure to check the foundation in the daylight to assure true compatibility.

Foundation Colors to Try
Makeup 1 ($28.50)
> All of these colors are great: Verona Beige, Fresh Peach (nothing peach about this color), Pale Gold, Bisque, Ivory Silk, Pale Cream, Fresh Cream, Burnished Gold, Rosewood, Victorian Porcelain, Cyprus Umber, Mosaic Gold (can turn orange), Amber Beige (can turn peach), and Warm Peach (nothing peach about this color).

Makeup 2 ($28.50)
> All of these colors are very good: Sunny Peach (can turn peach), Amber (may turn peach), Tan, Perfect Bisque, Rich Cream, Creamy Gold, Soft Ivory, Fresh Camellia (may turn pink) and English Porcelain (slightly pink).

100% Oil-Free Liquid Makeup SPF 15 ($28.50)
> All of these colors are beautiful: Suntan, Tuscan Beige, Rich Gold, True Bisque, Fresh Ivory (slightly pink), Pure Porcelain (slightly pink), Rose Silk (slightly pink), Copper Beige, and Quiet Beige.

Soft Matte Foundation ($28.50)

All of these colors are very good: Mocha (may turn pink on some skin tones), Desert Rose (may turn pink), Deep Tan, Truffle, Sun Beige, Espresso (great black foundation color), Sienna, Soft Gold (may turn peach), Taupe (may turn pink), Sun Bronze, Sepia, Light Cream (may turn pink), Soft Ivory (may turn peach), Macassar, and Cappuccino.

Foundation Colors to Avoid

Makeup 1 ($28.50)

All of these shades are too peachy-pink: Blue-Red Porcelain, Blue-Red Alabaster, Blue-Red Camellia, Blue-Red Rose Porcelain, Red Pale Blush, and Red Warm Blush.

Makeup 2 ($28.50)

All of these colors are too peach or too pink to recommend: Classic Beige, Pure Peach (the name is accurate), Almond, Rose Cameo, Cool Alabaster, and Blush.

100% Oil-Free Liquid Makeup SPF 15 ($28.50)

All of these colors are too peach or too pink for most skin tones: Soft Gold, Rose Earth, Tea Rose, Pale Alabaster, Pure Gold, Roman Peach, and Natural Peach.

Soft Matte Foundation ($28.50)

All of these colors are too peach, too pink, or too rose to recommend: Blush, Deep Blush, Petal, China Rose, Honey Beige, Roman Beige, Tawny Peach, Pale Peach, Patina Gold, and Pure Beige.

Concealer: Prescriptives has 11 shades of concealer called **Camouflage Cream** *($13.50)*. Most of the colors are for those with medium skin tones; there are only one or two colors for fair to medium skin tones, but these colors are great. There are particularly good choices for women of color. The consistency is somewhat creamy when it goes on and slightly dry when blended, but it can crease into the lines around the eye. If you have any lines around your eye, this isn't the concealer for you. These colors are very good: Yellow-Orange Light, Yellow-Orange Medium, Yellow-Orange Dark, Red-Orange Light, Red-Orange Medium, Red-Orange Dark, Blue-Red Light, and Red-Orange Extra Dark. All of these colors are either too pink or too peach to recommend: Red Light, Blue-Red Medium, and Blue-Red Dark.

Powder: The **Better Pressed Powder** *($22.50)* is talc-based and contains mineral oil. It is available in a great selection of colors. The loose powder comes in two types: **Oil Control** *($17.50)* contains talc, zinc, and clay; **Moisture Rich** *($22.50)* contains talc, mineral oil, and lanolin oil. All have a silky soft texture. **All Skins Pressed Powder** *($22.50)* has an impressive array of colors for a wide range of skin tones. The texture is light and slightly on the dry side, which is great for most skin types. The **Suncolors** *($18.50)* are meant as an all-over dusting of tan color, but they are shiny and not recommended.

Eyeshadow: There are some great matte colors to be found in this line. The **Quad Eyeshadow** *($10)* compact colors have three matte shades and one shade that's shiny. The strips of color are so thin and tiny that it's hard to get a brush through the color evenly. Prescriptives has introduced **Pick 2** *(color tins $10 each; compact $2.50)*, an eyeshadow compact that lets you pick your own two colors to insert. Great idea, and many of the colors (and there are a lot of colors) are matte and excellent color choices.

Eyeshadow Colors to Try
Singles and Pick 2 ($16/$22.50)

A superior collection of beautiful matte colors: Cameo, Biscuit, Mocha, Pink Sand, Swiss Chocolate, Cocoa, Navy, Stone Mist, Rose Powder, Mushroom, Heather, Rose Smoke, Suede Storm, Midnight Brown, Twilight, Eggplant, Honey, Grey Smoke, Pongee, Toast, Pumpkin, Adobe, Walnut, Tea Leaves, Coal, Peach Dust, Chamois, Clay, Red Earth, Clove, Moss, Seal, Pale Taupe, and Dove.

Eyeshadow Colors to Avoid
Singles and Pick 2 ($16/$22.50)

All of these colors are too shiny, too blue, or too green to recommend: Sandalwood, Garnet, Hot Pink, Jade, Mulberry, Violetta, Iris, Bambi, Blue Angel, Henna, Gold, Ink, Canary, Opal, and Hazel

Blush: Most of the blush colors *($18.50)* are worth trying. These are beautiful shades and most have no visible shine, although some of the colors tend to go on quite sheer. The browner tones—Sandalwood, Cherrywood, Tulipwood, and Rosewood—are superb contour colors. They also have a two-in-one blush container called **All Skins Face Colors Refillable** *(blush tins $12.50 each; compact $5; total cost $30)*. What a great concept. You can pick a contour and a blush color, or two different blush colors, or a blush and a pressed powder of your choice. One caution: Most of the colors have a slight amount of shine, although not enough to be a problem. However, a handful of these shades are intensely shiny and should be avoided: Peach, Mocha, Bronze, Rose, Rosewood, Cocoa, and Orchid.

Lipstick: Prescriptives has a beautiful array of **Classic** *($12.50)*, **Demi-Matte** *(12.50)*, and **Matte** *($14)* lipsticks. The Classic is by far the preferred choice, with its nice array of colors and good consistency. The Demi-Matte has a nice range of muted colors, but the texture can be a bit on the dry side and they have a tendency to bleed. **The Hots** is an intriguing color selection of red lipsticks. The line also offers a lipgloss *($15)*, but there is no reason to spend this much money on a gloss.

Eye, Brow, and Lip Liners: Prescriptives has a huge selection of lip and eye pencil *($12)* colors. They have a great texture but are not unusual as far as pencils go. The eye pencils come in good colors, but they are crayon-like and go on too greasy.

Mascara: Prescriptives' new **Gentle Mascara** *($12.50)* may be gentle, but it doesn't build much length or thickness and tends to smear.

Revlon

Revlon's **ColorStyle** for women of color is a remarkable collection of products and colors. The color selection is decidedly superior. Much like Maybelline's *Shades of You* line, the ColorStyle products avoid orange, red, or gray overtones in almost all of the foundations, blushes, lipsticks, and powders. An added enhancement is the availability of testers for every shade of blush, foundation, and powder. (There are no testers for lipsticks.) The tester unit can be a bit awkward to use; the lid covering the testers kept falling on my hand. After a few tries I was able to work it out, but it was definitely worth the effort. This is one of the most complete tester units I have ever seen in a drugstore.

There are two foundations available in the ColorStyle line: **Natural Color Oil-Free Makeup** *($8.25)* and **Natural Color Creme-Powder Makeup** *($7.50)*, which is also oil-free. Both have an excellent variety of colors and the textures are good. The oil-free liquid makeup is very good for someone with oily skin, but it can prove too drying and heavy for someone with normal to dry skin. Great colors combined with a good blending technique can make this a foundation to consider. The Creme-powder Makeup can go on a bit choppy, and the color can flake. Blending this one on evenly can be tricky, but if you have normal to slightly oily skin it can be great and there are 16 shades to choose from, an impressive assortment. (The only color to avoid is Teak, which can turn orange.) Much like Maybelline's Shades of You foundations, an overwhelming negative is that both of the foundations in this line are only for women with normal to oily skin. They also have yet to create a foundation for women of color who have dry skin.

Another strong point for Revlon is their outstanding selection of concealers and pressed powders. **ColorStyle Natural Blend Concealer** *($5.75)* comes in five shades that are very good; they go on well, with only a slight tendency to crease into the lines around the eyes. **Color Balancing Pressed Powder** *($8.25)* comes in six different colors. The texture is lightweight and soft, and the powder goes on evenly. These are all excellent.

Soft Color Powder Blush *($7.50)* offers an interesting choice of colors, the texture is good without being greasy, and the color goes on evenly. Most of the colors are matte, except for Coral Sands, Ginger, and Gold, which are extremely shiny and should be used only for an evening look.

The ColorStyle Color-Enriched Lipstick *($5.75)* comes in a small but attractive selection of matte colors with only a few shiny choices that you should avoid for daytime use. The texture is slightly on the dry side, but that helps the staying power. (A previous problem with lipsticks designed for women of color is that they were terribly greasy, so this group is a welcome change of pace.) A good variety of colors is available, with many appropriate for lighter-skinned women of color.

The rest of the Revlon line has several interesting strong points. Consider checking out the matte eyeshadows, the Eye Shapers set, a couple of the mascaras, the blushes, and, most of all, the lipsticks. You won't be disappointed.

Foundation: Revlon has several types of foundation in its drugstore line: **New Complexion Makeup for Normal to Dry** *($8.25)*, **New Complexion Makeup for Normal to Oily** *($8.25)*, and **Touch & Glow Moist Makeup** *($6.30)*. Almost every shade is either too pink, too orange, too peach, or too rose. I can't recommend any of them. Revlon's **Powdercreme Makeup Base** *($7.50)* is a good product with a smooth texture and easy application. **Springwater Oil-Free Makeup** *($8.25)* is a lightweight foundation in mostly neutral shades of beige or tan. **DoublePlay** *($9.49)* is a lightweight cream-to-powder foundation in stick form. This is actually an impressive foundation with a handful of good colors and there are even testers available in most stores. If you have normal to combination skin, this one is definitely worth a try.

Foundation Colors to Try
DoublePlay Stick Makeup ($9.49)

All of these colors are good: Bare Buff, Creamy Natural, and Rich Beige. All of these colors are OK but may turn peach: Porcelain Rose, Sandrift, Fresh Beige, Warm Honey, and Bronzing Stick. Ivory may be too pink for most skin tones.

Concealer: Revlon's **New Complexion Concealer** *($6.75)* comes in three shades: Light, Medium, and Deep. This lightweight concealer leaves a sheer residue that covers beautifully. It is one of the better concealers I tested, and definitely worth looking into. The **Springwater Oil-Free Concealer** *($5.50)* goes on very light yet covers well. Unfortunately, it does have a slight tendency to crease.

Powder: Revlon has a good selection of pressed powders. They are all talc-based and go on soft. The problem is the color selection; many of these shades are a bit too peach or too pink for most skin tones. The **Love Pat Pressed Powder** *($6.75)* colors are too pink or too peach for most skin tones. **Springwater Pressed Powder Oil-Free** *($8.25)* has three good color choices: Light, Medium, and Dark. **Touch & Glow Pressed Powder** *($7.50)* is almost identical to Love Pat Pressed Powder and the color selection is also poor. **New Complexion Powder** *($8.25)* is a talc-based powder with a poor color selection. Most of the colors are peach.

Eyeshadow: Revlon has a superior selection of matte eyeshadows that I feel comfortable recommending to anyone who wants a soft, natural-looking eye design. Be careful—not all of the colors are matte, and many have quite a bit of shine. The only ones I am recommending are the matte shades. Revlon also offers a **Day into Night Shadow Stick** *($4.95)* that has a creamy texture when it first goes on and then dries like a powder. This one is tricky to use. It can go on somewhat choppy and is difficult to blend, but once it's on it does stay put. An interesting new addition with just a handful of colors is the **Eye Shapers Shadow and Liner Set** *($4.47)*. The shadows go on nicely; the black eyeliner powder is excellent and can be used as a shadow or liner. This would be a great option, except one of the eyeshadows is shiny. What a shame.

Eyeshadow Colors to Try
Singles and Duos ($3.10)
All of these are excellent colors: Beaches, Dawn, Twilight (for fair skin tones), Desert, Slated Grey, Granite, Cedar, Rose Briar (for darker skin tones only), Currantine (for darker skin tones), Bluestone (if you have to wear blue, this will do), Not Quite White, Bali Brown (a good liner or accent color), Ranch Mink (a good liner or accent color), Peach Whisper, Slightly Pink (may be too white for some skin tones), and Lilac Lucense (intense lilac color, for darker skin tones).
Overtime Eye Shadows ($5.15)
All of these colors are beautiful: Nudes, Mauvestones, Lilacs, and Naturals.

Eyeshadow Colors to Avoid
Singles and Duos ($3.10)
All of these colors are too shiny: Dusty Pink Frost, Cameo Blush, Superfrost Pink, Mauve Gold, Baby Blue, China Blue Frost (speaks for itself), Silverlace, Mint Julep, Superfrost Beige, Peach Blast, Burnished Khaki, Ipanema Gold, Taupestar, Sheer Sky, Clear Seas (too blue), Gauze Grey (too blue), and Aquarium (no shine, but too blue). Paradise Matte, Lilac Matte, and Smokies Matte have no shine, but each set contains two or more blues, and who needs more blue eyeshadows?
Overtime Shadows ($5.15)
All of these colors are too shiny: Smokies (too blue), Foliage, Paradise (too blue), and Aquatines (too green).

Blush: Revlon has an interesting assortment of blushes that range from ultra-frost, which is too intense for daytime, to soft, exceptional colors that are great anytime. My favorite is the **Powdercreme Blush** *($7.35)*, a superb product with a silky texture that glides on smoothly and evenly. It would be hard to make your cheeks look overdone with this blusher.

Blush Colors to Try
Powdercreme Blush ($7.35)
All of these colors are great: Amberfrost, Pink, Mauvefrost, Primrose, and Plum.

Naturally Glamorous Blush-On ($7.35)
All of these colors are excellent: Revlon Red, Mauve, Wine, Sandalwood Beige, Neutral Umber, Neutral Tan, and Bronzetta.

In the Pink Cheek Color ($4.50)
All of the shades in this group are soft and beautiful, a great but small assortment of blue-toned blushes.

Sheer Face Color ($7.25)
All of these colors are excellent: Sheer Tawny (a great contour color), Sheer Rose, Sheer Peach, and Sheer Pink.

Springwater Blush ($7.35)
All of these colors are matte and go on dry. They would be good only for someone with oily skin.

Blush Colors to Avoid

Pure Radiance ($8.50)
Original Sun Glow is supposed to be used as a bronzer. It is not a great idea to change the color of the skin; no matter how good the color is, you always end up with color at the jaw or on your collar.

Soft Lustre Blush-On ($7.35)
All of these colors are too shiny: Fresh Peach, Sunrise Pink, Rose Lustre, Irrepressible Rose, and Honey Brown Lustre.

Lipstick: Revlon has a large and wonderful selection of lipstick colors with great textures and staying power. Most of the **Moon Drops Moisture Creme ($5.75), Super Lustrous Creme ($5.75),** and **Velvet Touch ($6.25)** lipsticks are excellent. All are wonderfully creamy, go on evenly with good coverage, and have good staying potential (Velvet Touch has a good matte finish). Avoid **Moon Drops Moisture Frost** and **Super Lustrous Frost**; all of these are too shiny. I am extremely impressed with Revlon's **Outrageous Creme Lipcolor ($5.99).** It has an unusually creamy, moist texture with surprising staying potential, and it feels great. The choice of colors for all of these products is extensive, and even the **Outrageous Lipcolor Luminesque,** which is too shiny for my taste, is a good option if you like a soft, pearlized look on your lips. There is a specialty lip product called **Triple Action Lip Defense ($5.75).** The lipstick tube is striped with a line of blue, pink, and white. It does have an SPF of 19, which is great for the lips, and it is quite emollient, but all the other claims on the package are overstated and contrived. **Color Lock Anti-Feathering Lip Base ($5.75)** really does keep lipstick from bleeding. What a find.

Eye, Brow, and Lip Liners: Revlon has a nice selection of standard lip and eye pencils in a nice variety of colors. There is an assortment of other pencils, but these are the best. **Micropure Slimliner ($5.50),** in spite of its fancy packaging, is just a pencil, but a rather good one. **Fabuliner ($5.75)** is a standard liquid liner. **Precision Eyelining Pen ($4.75)** is a felt-tip pen applicator. Because of the packaging, there is no way for you to see the color of any of these products. The same is true for the pencils, so it's difficult to recommend any of them. The **Waterproof Eyeshaper** *($4.49)* is basically an acceptable liner, but it tends toward the greasy side and would be better if it weren't waterproof. Because of the greasy texture you would not want to use this on your eyebrows, and if you are concerned at all about eyeliner smearing this is not a great option. **Jetliner Intense** *($5.50)* is a liquid eyeliner pen with a hard tip that actually scratches the eye and hurts when you apply it. Revlon also has an eyeshadow stick called **Softstroke Powderliner** *($4.95)* that is waterproof as well. It comes in a good selection of colors, but I find it difficult to recommend because it can smear too easily, although it can aid in creating an eye design in a hurry and without mess. For the brows there is **Natural Brows Color & Style System** *($4.95)*, a powder that comes in four excellent shades: True Blonde, Rich Brown, Soft Black, and Light Brown. The brush it comes with is terrible, but it is a rare cosmetic that comes packaged with a good applicator. A professional angled brush would work just fine.

Mascara: Two of Revlon's latest mascaras—**Impulse Long Distance Mascara** *($3.95)* and **Impulse Quick Thick Mascara** *($3.95)* —are both excellent: no smudging, easy, quick application, and they make lashes thick and long. They also make a waterproof version called **Impulse Water Tight Mascara** *($3.95)*, which is water-tight up to a point. Once you rub or wipe your eyes the mascara peels right off. **Lengthwise Mascara** *($3.99)* is excellent and I strongly recommend it. **Lashfull Mascara** *($5.35)* is another very good mascara that goes on well and really makes it through the entire day. **Fabulash Big Brush Mascara** *($5.15)* is a good mascara, but it can't really compete with the Lengthwise Mascara.

Brushes: Revlon has several brushes in good shapes and sizes, but the blush brush *($6.50)* and eyeshadow brush *($4.25)* have oversized handles that are cumbersome and hard to carry in a makeup bag for touchups during the day. Also, the bristles are too soft to apply the color evenly.

Shiseido

I was surprised to find that very little of Shiseido's products and color line had changed since I last reviewed this line three years ago. It is still the only Japanese name-brand cosmetics line sold in U.S. department stores. I'm sure part of its sales appeal is its uniqueness and the reputation the Japanese have for creating excellent, reliable products. Shiseido is a rather limited makeup line, however, some of their products are excellent. I particularly like their lipsticks, which are very creamy. Some of their foundations are also excellent, and the blush colors are quite nice and have a beautiful silky texture. Like many cosmetics lines, Shiseido has a large array of shiny eyeshadows that make the skin look wrinkly and too made-up for daytime, but they have also added some excellent matte shades that are worth checking out. The counter displays are attractive but inaccessible.

Foundation: Shiseido makes five types of foundation. **Stick Foundation** *($30)*, for dry skin only, goes on fairly greasy; after blending it can be surprisingly sheer and it does feel great on dry skin. **Fluid Foundation** *($27)* has a great consistency, but a poor selection of colors. **Creme Powder Compact Foundation** *($30)* looks like a cream but dries to a silky and light finish; it can look powdery and choppy by the end of the day for some skin types. It can be used either wet or dry. **Dual Compact Powder** *($27)* is basically a talc and mineral oil pressed powder that can be used wet or dry and comes in an excellent assortment of sheer colors. **Oil Control Treatment Compact** *($17.50)* is a confusing cream-to-powder foundation. It isn't oil-free because it contains shark oil, and although the salesperson told me it's medicated, it isn't. This product won't control oil, but it is a good foundation with a great light texture and a small but excellent color selection.

Foundation Colors to Try
Stick Foundation ($30)
All of these colors are excellent: I2, I4, B2, B4, B6, and G1.
Fluid Foundation ($27)
All of these colors are excellent: Natural Light Ivory, Natural Fair Ivory, Natural Light Beige, Natural Fair Beige, Natural Fair Pink (almost too pink to be in this section), Natural Warm Beige, Natural Deep Beige, and Warm Bronze.
Creme Powder Compact Foundation ($30)
All of these colors are excellent: Natural Light Beige, Natural Fair Beige, Natural Deep Beige, Natural Light Pink, Natural Fair Pink, Natural Deep Pink, Warm Bronze, Natural Light Ivory, and Natural Fair Ivory.
Dual Compact Powder ($29)
All of the colors for this powder foundation are excellent.
Oil Control Treatment Compact ($17.50)
All of these colors are good neutral shades: 01, 02, 03, 04, and 05.

Foundation Colors to Avoid
Stick Foundation ($30)
All of these colors are either too orange or too pink for most skin tones: P2, P4, P6, and C1 (this is a green primer color for the skin, something I never recommend).
Fluid Foundation ($27)
Natural Light Pink (no one is this pink) and Natural Deep Pink are not recommended.
Concealer: There are only two shades of *concealer ($15)* in this line. Both are poor color choices; 01 is too peach for most skin tones and 02 is too gold for most skin tones. I wish the colors were better because the texture of this product is smooth and blends well.
Powder: Shiseido has a large selection of compact powders *($26)* that go on very sheer and contain talc, clay, and mineral oil. Nothing special for a fairly steep price tag, and the colors are only just OK.

Eyeshadow Colors to Try
Single, Duos, and Trios ($18.50/$21/$23)
   All of these colors are excellent: Brown Red Trio, Brown Beige Trio, Black Variations, Brown Variations, Blue Variations, Black/Dark Brown, Light Brown/Chestnut, Underwood/Almond, Beige Plum Dream, Grey Saffron Dream, Moss, Roseate, Desert Hues, Taupes, and Tres Tres Peach.

Eyeshadow Colors to Avoid
Single, Duos, and Trios ($18.50/$21/$23)
   All of these colors are extremely shiny or too blue or too green: Copper Shell, Shell Pink, Hot Gold, Mauve Pink, White Gold, Celadon, Pure Gold, Crystal Lavender, Shiny Shell, Steely Blue, Pink Quartz Nuance, Golden Green Nuance, Azure Nuance, the Anthracites, the Jades, the Indigos, Bronze/Copper, Violet/Rust, Bronze/Copper, the Tortoise Shells, the Purple Quartz, Golden Coral/Rose Coral, Clove/Violet, Brick Tones, Soft Petals, Rose Opal, and Pearls & Onyx.

Blush Colors to Try
Singles, Duos, and Tri Effect ($22.50/$28)
   All of these colors are beautiful: Coral Brown (a good contour color), Rose Ochre, Brown Beige, Hot Brown (a good contour color), Grape (preferably for darker skin tones), and Soft Pink.
   Lipstick: Shiseido's lipstick *($14)* has a wonderful creamy texture, with a matte finish that is really beautiful. I like these lipsticks a lot. They also have a small selection of traditional lip glosses *($14)* that come in lipstick form and are nothing special.
   Eye, Brow, and Lip Liners: The lip liners *($11.50)* have an excellent dry texture and come in a lovely array of colors. The eye pencils *($13)* have a wonderful texture and come in soft muted colors. The brow pencils go on heavier than most and need to be blended carefully. They also make a **Moisture Mist Liquid Eyeliner** *($17.50)* that creates a definite liquid line across the eye. The **Eyebrow Shapeliner** *($20)* is a clear brow gel that goes on just fine, but hairspray on a toothbrush works just as well.
   Mascara: Shiseido makes two kinds of mascara *($18)*, one with fiber and one without. Both are just OK but not great, and the fiber mascara can flake and get in the eye. There are better mascaras at both the drugstore and the other cosmetics counters.

Ultima II

   The Ultima II line has definitely grown since I last reviewed it three years ago. A wide variety of products is offered and the quality of most is impressive. The display units are attractive, though you need to ask the salesperson for assistance in order to use most of them. I found the

Ultima II sales staff less aggressive than most wherever I went, which made shopping at their counters less discouraging.

From lipsticks to eyeshadows, the color range, which includes superior colors and textures for women of color, is nothing less than astounding and sometimes a bit bizarre. I often wonder who would ever consider buying some of them, some of the eyeshadow colors are that strange. They have a wide range of lipstick shades that vary from natural to full, bold colors. Ultima II has the most confusing product divisions and display units. There are two product lines within this one cosmetics line: **The Colors** and **The Nakeds**. I've lumped them all together because their division is arbitrary and illogical. Also, The Nakeds are no longer all that naked; in fact, there are some rather strange vivid colors in this category, not to mention ultra-shiny ones. Ignore the divisions, concentrate on color choice, and be careful: there are some weird shades in this line.

Foundation: Ultima II has seven foundation types, more than any one line should carry. **Smooth Cover Makeup** *($20)* is a glycerin- and oil-based foundation that separates in the bottle and can also separate on the skin, but the color selection is nice, the application sheer, and the texture can be good for some dry skin types. **ProCollagen Foundation SPF 6** *($28.50)* is supposed to firm the skin with collagen; it can't. It would be an OK foundation for dry skin if the color choices were better, but they're not. **CHR Foundation** *($33)* has medium coverage and is best for someone with very dry skin. **Ultimate Coverage** *($18.50)* is an accurate self-description; use it only if you really want a heavy makeup to cover a skin discoloration. **The Foundation Moisturizing Formula SPF 6** *($24)* is a lightweight, soft foundation with great colors. **The Foundation Oil-Control Formula SPF 6** *($24)* is also lightweight and soft, but matte, and has great colors. Many of these foundations are divided into yellow-, pink-, and neutral-based tones, but you should never wear a pink-toned foundation just because your skin has pink undertones. The cream-to-powder foundation, called **Brush-On Foundation** *($20)*, goes on very sheer and comes in a beautiful array of colors. This product applies better with a sponge than it does with the brush that comes in the compact.

Foundation Colors to Try
Smooth Cover Makeup ($20)
   All of these colors are very good: 2N, 4Y, 5N, 6P, 8N, 10Y, 11N, 13Y, 14Y, and 15Y.
ProCollagen Foundation SPF 6 ($28.50)
   All of these are good color choices: Chamois Y, Blushing Beige P, Wheat N, Oat N (may turn pink), and Cameo Beige Y (may turn pink).
Ultimate Coverage ($18.50)
   All of these are excellent colors, but this foundation is too heavy to rec-

ommend for most skin types or problems: 9Y, 11N, 14Y, 13Y, 10P (may turn peach on some skin tones), 12Y, 15Y, Manila, and Tuscan Beige (may turn rose).

CHR Foundation ($33)

There are only a couple of good reliable neutral colors to consider: Almond, Toffee, Shell, and Fresh Tawny (may turn peach).

The Foundation Moisturizing Formula SPF 6 ($24)

All of these are excellent colors: F1Y, F2P, F3P (may turn pink), F5N, F8Y/N, F9Y, F10N, F11P, F12Y/N (may turn peach), and F13Y/N. F14Y/N and F15Y/N are both excellent color choices for darker skin tones.

The Foundation Oil-Control Formula SPF 6 ($24)

All of these are excellent colors: F1Y, F2P, F5N, F7Y/N, F9Y (may turn yellow), F10N, F12N, and F13Y/N. F14Y/N and F15Y/N are both excellent colors for darker skin tones.

Brush-On Foundation ($20)

All of these are beautiful colors: 2Y, 3Y, 1N, 2N, 3N, 1P, 2P, and 3P.

Foundation Colors to Avoid

Smooth Cover Makeup ($20)

These colors are too peach or too pink to recommend: 3P, 7Y, and 9Y.

ProCollagen Foundation SPF 6 ($28.50)

All of these are either too peach or too pink and are not recommended: Light Beige, Ivory Silk, Linen, Medium Beige, Cool Beige, Deep Beige.

Ultimate Coverage ($18.50)

All of these are either too rose, too pink, or too peach for most skin tones: Bronze Umber, Cashew, Natural Beige, Ivory Bisque, and Desert Peach.

CHR Foundation ($33)

All of these colors are too peach to recommend: Light Ivory, Light Beige, Light Peach, Medium Beige, and Deep Beige.

The Foundation Moisturizing Formula SPF 6 ($24)

These colors are too peach on most skin tones: F4Y, F6P, and F7.

The Foundation Oil-Control Formula SPF 6 ($24)

All of these colors are either too peach, too pink, too orange, or too yellow for most skin tones: F3P, F4Y, F5, F6P, F8P/N, and F11P.

Concealer: Ultima II's **The Concealer ($11.50)** has a good selection of colors. The consistency is smooth without being too dry or too greasy, and there's only a small chance it will slip into the lines around the eye. I recommend this one. One problem is that there is a huge color difference between C1 and C2, and C1 isn't a great color, so there isn't anything for light to fair skin tones.

Concealer Colors to Try

The Concealer ($11.50)

All of these colors are excellent: C2, C3, C4 (a great color for dark skin tones only), C5, and C6 (a great tan color).

Concealer Colors to Avoid
The Concealer ($11.50)

C1 is too pink for most skin tones.

Powder: Ultima II The Nakeds has a **Loose Powder** *($19.50)* and a **Pressed Powder** *($15.50)*. Both have almost identical talc-based formulas, though the loose powder does have a slight shine added to it. They go on quite sheer and have a nice silky texture, but they are fairly expensive for what you get. The superior colors are numbered 1 to 6 and range from almost white to bronze.

Eyeshadow Colors to Try
Singles, Duos, The Colors, and The Nakeds ($12/$15.50)

All of these are excellent matte shades, but be careful—some colors are very hard to use: Mango, Bikini, Neat-O, Push-Up Pink, Big Pink, Earth, Deep Purple, Girls Night Out, Matte PC, Tatoo, Call Me, Thorn, 1, 2, 3, 5, 6, 7, 8, 14, 22, 29, 47, 48, 49, 50, Matte Chip, Matte Data, Matte Wow, Matte Topline, Bikini, and Almond Cocoa.

Eyeshadow Colors to Avoid
Singles, Duos, Trios, The Colors, and The Nakeds ($12/$15.50)

All of these colors are either too shiny or too strange to recommend: Peach Sorbet, Tropic Moondust, Fairy Dust, Candlelight, In-the-Pink, Prairie Mauve, Va-Va-Va Violet, Moonlit Orchid, Midnight Mauve, Sheer Silver, Cool Blue, Lagoon, Blue Smoke, Aquamarine, Black Emerald, Big Teal, Spunsilver Beige, Ochre, Spungold Wine, Plumstone, Wine Mist, Dusty Pink, Taupe, Bombshell Bronze, Clear Opal, RSV Pink (it's matte, but too white for most skin tones), Pink Fluff/Pink Buff, and Bronze/In the Buff.

Blush: Unfortunately, most of the Ultima II blushes have some amount of shine—not a lot, but enough to make oily skin look shinier than it already is, and they also tend to make dry skin look more dry. A few colors are ultra-shiny. **The Nakeds Blushing Cream** *($13)* is a traditional cream blush that is not all that easy to use and only works well on normal skin types. There are only four colors to choose from and they are all fairly deep, muted colors.

Blush Colors to Try
The Colors Powder Blush and The Nakeds Powder Blush ($15/$16.50)

All of these colors are quite good: Coral Lite, Cheeky Pink, Coral Reef, Ready or Not, Sweet Bordeaux, Pink Vermeil, 4, 5, 6, Valentine, and Tickled Pink.

Blush Colors to Avoid
The Colors Powder Blush and The Nakeds Powder Blush ($15/$16.50)

All of these colors are too shiny to recommend: Rose Feather, Sahara Rose, Burnished Bordeaux, Rose Amethyst, Glazed Heather Plum, Frosted Honey Umber, Bronze Bordeaux, Chestnut Frost, Ginger Plum Frost, Grenadine Fizz, Bronzing Glow, and Bronzing Tan.

Lipstick: Ultima II has several types of lipstick with a wide range of color choices. **Mattes** *($13)*, **Lip Chrome** *($11)*, and **Super Luscious** *($13)* mostly have excellent textures and go on in a variety of consistencies, from creamy to extremely dry. **Lip Sexxxxy** *($11)* is a new group of lip colors with a very interesting dry but light texture. It goes on almost wet and then dries in place. It doesn't feel like a powder, but it definitely doesn't feel like a lipstick, nor is it all that sexy. It's hard to explain. The texture isn't for everyone, but it is an ultra-matte look.

Eye, Brow, and Lip Liners: All of the pencils are fairly standard and, just like many others, they are manufactured in Germany. The eye pencils have a sponge tip at one end to help soften lines after application. **Styleliner** *($9.50)* is a standard liquid liner in a tube that comes in three colors: Grey Blue, Black, and Brown. The **Super Luscious Lipliner** *($9.50)* comes in a nice variety of colors, has a smooth texture, but is not anything outstanding.

Mascara: Extra Full Mascara for Sensitive Eyes *($12)* is not a great mascara; it goes on OK but doesn't rinse well and it can smear. Plus there is nothing about this that is particularly good for sensitive eyes. **Big Finish Mascara** *($12)* is an excellent mascara. It goes on well, doesn't clump, creates long lashes, and doesn't smear.

Victoria Jackson

Did you know that only two out of ten television infomercials actually make a profit? That is an amazing statistic, specifically in light of the fact that there are so many of them trying to get you to pick up the phone and dial in your order for everything from motivation tapes to diets to less real estate courses to, of course, cosmetics. What makes Victoria Jackson Cosmetics so intriguing is that it has one of the most successful infomercials on television. I find that statistic both shocking and disheartening at the same time. I'm shocked because I know that women are not buying this line because the products are in any way superior or unique (they aren't and they have some real drawbacks). Rather, it is because the slick half-hour television sales presentation comes off as sincere and convincing. As many of you already know, I am strongly opposed to buying makeup that you can neither try on nor see before you buy it. When television sales techniques are the only thing you can base your decision on, that's dangerous. We all need more information, not advertising rhetoric, to make decisions on anything we buy.

When you call the 1-800 number for almost all of the infomercials you are connected to a clearinghouse of operators, used for many "call-in-now" products. I was asked a couple of questions—my skin tone (light, medium, tan, or dark) and what colors I prefer (red, peach, or pink). I answered medium and red. After being given two payment options, I was told my products would be delivered in four to six weeks. Two weeks later my package arrived.

Almost everything you would need to do a complete makeup application and cleansing routine was sent in the **Introductory Kit** *($119.85)*. The makeup items included a brush set (no sponge tips), four eyeshadows, two shades of foundation in one compact, a retractable lip pencil, three retractable eye or brow pencils, four shades of lip color that come in a compact, two blushers, pressed translucent powder, mascara and lash conditioner, a packet of instruction cards, an instructional video tape, and reorder forms. Quite a kit. Each item in the kit was marked at a higher price than what I actually paid. For example, the foundation was marked at $24.95, although I received the "special" price of $12.95 that was listed on the order form. All of the Victoria Jackson products have two price categories. If you order a certain amount of products, you can get the cheaper price every time. This is a cosmetics line that likes making deals. But what about the products? The makeup items I received, for the most part, were fine, although nothing special, and a few of the products didn't work well at all.

Once you order you also start getting their product catalogue. One of the "money-saving" offers (of course, not my definition of money-saving) in here is a group of eyeshadows, eye pencils, blushes, and lipsticks divided into Morning, Noon, and Night *($99)*. These are three different intensities of makeup in a similar color family of Red, Peach, or Pink. Morning is the softest, Noon is a little deeper, and Night is the darkest. The package is arranged so that you get these three sets of products, a total of 15 products. That's more makeup than anyone needs, plus it assumes that you need drastically different makeup for morning versus afternoon and night. There are easier ways to change morning makeup into night than buying entire new sets of makeup. Also, are you supposed to wash your face at lunch and start over again? Regardless, the eyeshadows are shiny and the lip colors greasy. The blush and pencils are nice enough, but fairly pricey when purchased individually.

One other product offered in the catalogue is the **Ultimate Space-Saving Makeup Kit** *($49.95)*. It looks great in the picture, all your makeup packaged in a neat little box that unfolds in an organized, orderly fashion to reveal the colors. It is indeed small and looks convenient, but the containers are not refillable, so once one runs out the prospects are expensive to refill it.

The makeup demonstration video tape that came with the introductory kit was very interesting. I didn't always agree with Victoria's application techniques. For example, she recommends applying eyeliner and brow color before the eyeshadows, which would undo or mess up the eyebrow you created and the liner you applied. Those are minor points; basically this is a good, understandable makeup video. The problem I had with the tape is that 50 percent of it made me feel as if I was sitting through another television ad, listening to Victoria and a guest celebrity talk about how great the products are. I had already bought the products; now I wanted to learn more about how to use them. I suppose that sometimes it's hard to stop selling when you have to pay for expensive television time.

Foundation: Victoria Jackson has one type of foundation (*$24.95/$13.95*) that comes in a single compact with two shades for each of four categories of skin tones: Light, Medium, Tan, and Dark. The colors are good, though the Medium shades are a tad on the ashy-green side, the Light is a bit pink, and there is only one color for darker skin tones. In order to create the right color for you, you are supposed to mix the two colors together, which is fine if you know how to mix the right proportions. If you don't, you're likely to have trouble. I found the foundation to be quite thick, and I would not call the application sheer as the commercial claims. The foundation is petrolatum-based and therefore somewhat greasy. Oily or combination skins would not be happy with this one.

Concealer: There is no individually packed concealer in the Victoria Jackson line. The suggestion is to use the lightest shade of foundation in the dual foundation compact for the under-eye area. This would be a great idea if the foundation weren't so greasy. It easily slips into the lines under the eye and any liner you then place around the eye will probably smear.

Powder: The pressed powder compacts (*$16.95/$10.95*) come in four shades Light, Medium, Tan, and Dark and are talc-based. The colors are all fine and the textures sheer and light.

Eyeshadow: The eyeshadow sets (*$19.95/$10.95*) come in a single compact of four different colors. The color combinations are excellent; unfortunately, almost all are slightly shiny.

Blush: Each color family kit (Peach, Red, and Pink) comes with a blush compact (*$19.95/$10.95*) that contains two colors. One of the colors is always a pale shade of peachy-pink and the other is a more vivid color. The textures and colors are very good. The Red kit's blush color is a nice shade of coral (which is not red, by the way); the Pink kit's blush is a soft shade of pink; and the Peach kit's blush is a brown-peach shade that is probably too brown for most skin tones.

Lipstick: Victoria Jackson includes a lipstick compact (*$17.94/$10.95*) in each color kit that contains three shades of lip creams and a lip color powder.

The colors are fine, but the lip creams are very greasy; if you have any problem with bleeding lipstick, these are not for you. The lip powder is a problem because it tends to cake on the lips and dry them out when used alone or over an extended period of time. Lipsticks that come in tubes are listed on the order sheet, but there are no color swatches provided to assist in making a decision.

Lip, Eye, and Brow Liners: All of the pencils *($9.95/$6)* in the introductory kit are retractable and have a great texture. There are three eye or brow pencils in each kit—Black, Chocolate Brown, and Taupe—and a lip pencil that matches the color categories of Peach, Pink, and Red. They are all great, and at the $6 price, an excellent buy.

Mascara: Every introductory kit comes packaged with a dual black mascara *($13.95/$8.50)*: one end is a clear conditioner; the other a black mascara. The mascara is good but the conditioner is mostly a plastic-like substance and glycerin. It won't do much for the lashes and I didn't notice a difference whether I used it or not. Victoria Jackson's traditional black mascara *($13.95/$8.50)* is great just by itself.

Brushes: Victoria Jackson includes a set of brushes in the introductory kit that are adequate but not great. A retractable brush set *($40/$24.95)* that includes a retractable blush brush and a retractable lip brush is overpriced at either cost. A professional brush set *($18.95/$9.50)* includes a lip brush, an eyebrow brush/comb, a two-sided eyeshadow brush, and a blush brush. The brushes have sparse hair and are not firm enough to hold the color well. These brushes are useful, but there are better ones on the market.

Yves St. Laurent

Many of the upper-end (meaning expensive) cosmetics lines have an air of snobbery about them. The salespeople seem to sniff at you in disdain if you don't have the appearance they deem worthy of their time and assistance. If I look like I have don't money to spend, ask pointed questions, or act in any way startled by the prices, it is obvious that I am wasting their precious time. Yves St. Laurent fits into this category, which is a shame, because some of their products are actually quite lovely. I found this snobbish attitude not only at the cosmetics counters but at their customer service department as well. My recommendation to management, not that they care what I have to say, is drop the attitude, it will only help you sell more product.

Foundation: Most of these foundations have wonderful textures and good colors. **Line Smoothing Foundation** *($44)* doesn't smooth lines, but it does have a lovely texture. It goes on easily and blends well with the skin, providing medium to slightly heavy coverage. The sales pitch is that it has light-reflecting properties. One salesperson said that meant it would light up the dark areas in my wrinkles. Please, it simply can't do that. **Teint Libre Moisturizing Foundation** *($32.50)* has only four shades, but the colors are OK and the texture is very smooth. **Teint Poudre Foundation** *($36.50)* is a cream-to-powder foundation. It isn't really all that creamy (it has more of a dry texture), the color choice is poor, and some of the colors are shiny. **Teint Spontane** *($31)* is an ultra-sheer face color/moisturizer, but it still rubs color over the face. I generally don't recommend these products, but if you like face tints this is a good one.

Foundation Colors to Try
Line Smoothing Foundation ($44)
   All of these colors are great: 1 (slightly peach), 3 (slightly peach), 7, 8, 9, and 10.
Teint Libre Moisturizing Foundation ($32.50)
   All of these colors are great: 2, 3 (can turn peach), and 4.

Foundation Colors to Avoid
Line Smoothing Foundation ($44)
   All of these colors are either too pink or too peach to recommend: 2, 4, 5, and 6.
Teint Libre Moisturizing Foundation ($32.50)
   1 is too pink for most skin tones.
Teint Poudre Powder Foundation ($36.50)
   All of these colors are too pink, too peach, or too shiny to recommend; 1, 2, 3, 4, and 5.

   Concealer: Radiant Touch *($27.50)* is an impressive concealer that is marketed as a way to touch up makeup at the end of the day and equal to "plastic surgery in less than a minute." The concealer is automatically fed into the brush tip like a pen; it is a very sheer cream, lightweight and moist, and doesn't crease into the lines around the eye. It really does look great to apply this under the eye or on top of the cheekbone at the end of the day for a lift. If you've ever tried to put under-eye concealer on a second time to touch up your makeup, you know how thick that can feel. This eliminates that problem. About the plastic surgery comment; forget it, it doesn't work that well.

   Powder: Sunny Complexion Powder *($35)* has a great silky texture, but is too shiny to recommend. **Silk Finish Pressed Powder** *($33)* has a wonderful silky texture and some of the colors are quite good. The best colors are 3 and 6; the others are too pink or too peach to recommend.

   Eyeshadow: All of the eyeshadow colors are ultra-shiny and are not recommended. What a shame, because the texture is quite nice. **Variation Solo** *($21)* is a quad set of colors, but two of the shades are shiny. **Eyeshadow Powder Duo** *($31)* has only ultra-shiny colors. Number 3 is the only good combination of matte colors in this entire line. Where this one came from is anyone's guess.

   Blush: Variation Blush *($31)* and **Blushing Powder** *($30)* are way too shiny to recommend, even though the textures are quite silky.

Lipstick: Yves St. Laurent has two types of lipstick. **Rouge Intense** *($21.50)* is a matte lipstick with a vivid array of colors; it has a tint, which means the color stays on the lips somewhat longer. **Sheer Conditioning Lipstick** *($20)* has a soft, creamy, beautiful texture and feels great. If you can swallow the cost, this is a good lipstick.

Eye, Lip, and Brow Liners: The small selection of standard lip *($16)* and eye pencils *($16.50)* are manufactured in Germany. The **Automatic Pencil** *($33/$10 refills)* comes in five shades and is convenient to use, but absurdly expensive. The **Eyebrow Pencils** *($15)* have a dry mascara wand on one end to stroke through the brow after you apply the pencil to soften the line. Good idea, but a less expensive pencil and an old clean mascara brush can do the same thing for a fraction of the price.

Mascara: Conditioning Mascara *($20.50)* is a good mascara, but for this price it should be great.

"God, I love makeup—I just wish it stayed on permanently."

Overheard at a Makeup Counter

Evaluation of Skin Care Products

THE PHILOSOPHY

If one thing has remained the same in the world of cosmetics since I first wrote *Don't Go To The Cosmetics Counter Without Me*, it is the absurd, almost ludicrous claims made about the products sold to clean, tone (whatever that word means), exfoliate, clear up, and moisturize the skin. My head reels from the elaborate language and preposterous explanations of why you should buy one company's products over another. The reason you've picked up this book (and probably flipped to this section first) is because somehow you and your skin know that the $25 cleanser, the $45 moisturizer, and the $50 eye cream may just not be worth it. Well, you're right: they're not. But that blanket statement probably isn't enough for you. (It wouldn't be for me either.) You still want to know if Estee Lauder's Fruition, Elizabeth Arden's Ceramide, or Avon's Anew really works, and why. Those with access to a maximum cosmetics budget will want to know if Guerlain's Serennissme Issima at $170 for 1 ounce is anything more than a way to take advantage of someone who can afford to waste money.

But even if you can afford to spend the money, should you be wasting money, at any income bracket? For some people a $15 product is a stretch, for another person the limit may be $75, but both are probably wasting their money. And just because you can afford to stretch, in any price category, should you? Should you be so susceptible to the cosmetics industry's marketing and sales pressure?

This search for better, more expensive products exists because the never-ending question of whether a $15 moisturizer is better than a $5 one, or whether a $65 moisturizer is better than a $30 one, is just that: never ending. Never ending because what I (and most dermatologists, at least those who don't sell or work for a cosmetics company) will tell you isn't going to agree with what the companies who make the more expensive stuff tell you, so it just depends on who you want to believe. Can I end this dilemma? Although I'll try to give you some answers in the next several pages, the truth is that you must base your opinion on facts and information. I know that's not as easy as it sounds. If you assume that the cosmetics industry isn't trying to put one over on you, the proverbial pulling the wool over your eyes, then no matter what facts I present to you, regardless of what the ingredient lists divulge, or how I demonstrate that the words on the label are vague, ambiguous jargon, the bottom line remains the same: the final purchase is yours alone, and your decision will be fraught with emotion.

Women spend a little to a lot more than they need to in all price categories in the hope that it will make a difference on their skin. Nutraderm or L'Oreal? Lancome or Borghese? Yves St. Laurent or La Prairie? One recurring theme rang in the background as I shopped the cosmetics counters: women explaining to their friends or the cosmetics salesperson that they were purchasing such and such a cream because it couldn't hurt, they had to do something, or they needed to feel good about the way they took care of themselves. One woman in particular seemed to epitomize the position most women find themselves in when they decide to spend money on skin care. With great earnestness and frustration she declared, "I don't know if it works, but it's better than nothing, isn't it?" Confusion mixed with hope and a touch of desperation makes for a very vulnerable consumer. Those of you who want to escape the confusion have to first change your belief system.

It isn't that there aren't good skin care products available from the cosmetics counters, home sales companies, health food stores, infomercials, and drugstores, but they are just not as spectacularly wonderful as they sound. Also (you can see this one coming), spending more money doesn't automatically mean you are getting more for your money and spending less doesn't always mean you are getting a bargain. Yes, there are decent products out there. There are cleansers that clean the face without leaving the skin greasy or dry, toners that exfoliate the skin without irritation (although they never "tone" anything), and moisturizers that alleviate dry skin (but can't in any way, shape, or form get rid of wrinkles). It's just that the hoopla, hyperbole, and expense are impossible for me to hear without groaning in exasperation and anger.

You will notice a generous amount of sarcasm mixed in with my evaluations of each product, but I just couldn't help myself. I feel that I come by my jaded perspective honestly. After all, if I weren't skeptical I wouldn't make a very good consumer reporter, and I challenge anyone to listen to lengthy explanations of why spleen extract, or a special grade of yeast, or an exotic plant from Africa is going to rejuvenate the skin without becoming jaded themselves.

Just to set the record straight: Anything you can buy at the department store cosmetics counters can be bought for much less from a much less expensive line, and the cheaper product will not be less effective. In fact, it is often just as effective, and many products are actually considerably better than their expensive counterparts. It's easier to believe this basic cosmetic fact once you realize that many of the drugstore products contain many of the same ingredients as similar items carried in the higher-priced lines.

I want you to look past the marketing language and the sales tactics and begin to understand how products work and what they can do for your skin. While I want to emphasize the extent and depth of the misleading and illusive portrayal of cosmetics by the media and the cosmetics industry, I also want to underscore what great products do exist for all skin types. However, it is difficult for me to describe my elation or enthusiasm about any product without always being careful to let you know what can really be expected. Erring on the side of skepticism is safer when you are talking about the possibility of wasting, and I mean wasting, $35. A product that costs that much should not only be exceedingly good, it should be remarkable. If it is only good (which is almost always all it is), it isn't worth the extra money if you can get "good" for $5 or $10. My reviews will always reflect that philosophy.

DUCKING SALES TECHNIQUES

If women were better prepared to handle the persuasive language they run into when they are buying cosmetics, saving money would be easy. There are many ways to accomplish this, but the best is to know what you need, what you don't, what is optional if you want to splurge, and what you need to ignore when the product is being described.

The sales pressure and advertising promises at the cosmetics counters and any other place where you can buy makeup haven't changed since I wrote the first edition of this book. If anything they have gotten worse and are likely to carry on in that direction. Step up to any counter or talk to any cosmetics salesperson anywhere and you are likely to hear the saga of cleansers that deep clean, creams that diminish wrinkles, masks that close pores, lotions that feed the skin, and scrubs that rejuvenate the skin. Perhaps I would be more forgiving of the foolishness that takes place during most cosmetic purchases if I felt that women were purchasing products that were really worth the money, but that is rarely the case. If I could only get women to realize that there is no reason to spend more than $15 on any cosmetic (and I think even that's high). Their skin and their pocketbooks would both be happy.

Aside from the sheer waste, regardless of the expense, I am also unhappy that in so many cases women are being sold the wrong products. Women with dry skin are told to use toners that contain alcohol or cleansers that dry the skin; women with oily skin are sold moisturizers or oil-free moisturizers, even though their skin isn't dry; women with normal skin end up with an armload of products in hopes of warding off the inevitable disasters of age, sun, and environment.

One of the ways to better equip yourself when shopping for makeup or skin care products is to be aware of what you need and what you don't need. That isn't as difficult as it sounds, and I will remind you of it throughout the entire skin care evaluation. Although everyone's skin is different, some basics are universal. For example, everyone has to clean their face and protect their skin from the sun, however, not everyone needs a moisturizer. A toner may feel good on the skin, but it is not an essential step that will change your skin. Once you understand the essentials, you will be more able to resist the endless array of extras that are, to say the least, unnecessary and can actually cause skin problems such as irritation and cosmetic acne. The following list outlines what products are necessary, unnecessary, and optional for most skin types.

Necessary: Cleanser, irritant-free toner, a sunscreen of SPF 15 in either your foundation or your moisturizer (but not both), an exfoliant (including AHA products), and, for breakouts, a topical disinfectant.

Unnecessary: Eye makeup remover, wipe-off cleanser, a nighttime moisturizer if you have oily skin, two or more products that contain a sunscreen, facial masks, eye creams, throat creams, cellulite creams, emergency skin treatments that are supposed to "repair" your skin in a week or two, and pre-moisturizers that are supposed to be worn under a moisturizer.

Optional: Bath gels, foot creams (only ones that contain salicylic acid or AHA because these ingredients can peel calluses; other foot creams are just moisturizers and not worth an extra product), Retin-A (not a cosmetic), cuticle creams, facial masks (only those that do not contain irritants).

Follow this list closely and you can duck most sales techniques because you will know ahead of time when you should simply say no, I don't need that. If all this seems to be glaringly simple, it is meant to be just that: simple. The cosmetics industry makes things too complicated and involved, and it doesn't have to be that way. I can tell you that using an eye cream or an expensive moisturizer isn't the least bit necessary, but when the attractively dressed sales representative is telling you that it can smooth, refine, restore elasticity, protect, reduce stress, soothe, plump, revive, improve cell turnover, increase moisture, reduce visible signs of aging, firm, repair, hydrate, diminish wrinkles, and is dermatologist- and ophthalmologist-tested, designed by makeup artists, designed by dermatologists, designed by pharmacists, and won't cause breakouts, it isn't so easy to remember my warnings anymore. And these are only some of the buzzwords a woman is bombarded with when she goes shopping for makeup; the list goes on and on. These terms get bandied about as if they were truth itself. If a woman can deflect these come-ons by ignoring them or realizing that they have little meaning, she will be way ahead of the game.

Besides, what it really boils down to is that every product label and every cosmetics salesperson at every the cosmetics company in the world says the same thing: that their line is the indisputable, consummately beautiful best. Now here's the tricky question. How can you tell which of the 300-plus cosmetic lines is telling the truth? Which one really does have a wrinkle cream that smooths, refines, plumps, and diminishes wrinkles? Can it be that 299 of these lines are deceitful and only one is telling the truth? It gets even more absurd when I inform you that if you wanted to go out today and buy a moisturizer for normal to dry skin, you could choose from among well over 5,000 products. Astounding. I can help narrow the field, but you have to be the one to keep the cosmetics industry in perspective. Remember the following caveats when you consider your next cosmetic purchase.

Beware of hyperbole. Regardless of the product, practically every salesperson earnestly declares that each and every item in their line is the best available and that it can vastly improve your skin if you use it. The formulations, regardless of the line, are all described as superior—nothing less than phenomenal. There are no phenomenal skin care products. There are good products. I have yet to see a woman use a skin care product and no longer have acne or lose a wrinkle (and I've been in this field for almost 14 years).

Beware of the authority claim. Every product is promoted as having been tested and certified by the proper scientific authorities, including dermatologists, pharmacists, and ophthalmologists. Physicians do not formulate cosmetics. That is not what they are trained to do. When we called many of the lines that make these kind of claims, such as Clinique and Physicians Formula, there were no doctors to be found. There were cosmetic chemists, but no physicians. Actually, I am much more comfortable knowing cosmetic chemists are formulating cosmetics.

Beware of universal approval. The salesperson assures you that all of the people who shop the line, including themselves, use the product/products and can't live without it/them. Recently a dignified saleswoman at the Estee Lauder counter told me, "You would be making a big mistake if you don't try Fruition. It's 5 percent of our total line sales. It is the biggest thing to ever come out of Estee Lauder. Everyone loves it. It is perfect for everyone's skin, really." Very convincing. I can understand how easy it must be for consumers to believe what is told them when it comes to the products they need to take care of their skin. Fruition ($45) is an OK product, but it does not alter the skin or do anything that isn't done equally well by less expensive drugstore products such as Alpha Hydrox ($6).

Beware of special ingredients. A product can contain one or even several novel or unusual ingredients and still not take care of your skin care needs. If you are dead set on finding a product that contains vitamins A, E, and C because they are good antioxidants, you might forget to also look for a high SPF number in your daytime moisturizer or good emollients such as oils and water binding agents in your nighttime moisturizer. One ingredient does not make a product.

Vitamin A (retinol, retinyl palmitate) the other vitamins, thymus extract, yeast, placental extract, herbs, proteins, and amino acids are the least important ingredients, yet the ones that attract the most attention. If you disagree with me on this point, that's fine, but please notice that often these "exclusive" ingredients are listed at the end of the ingredient list or after the fragrance and preservatives, which means you are getting a negligible amount of the so-called good stuff. If you really want these ingredients don't get sold short. They should be in the first half of the ingredient list.

THE CRAZY THINGS COSMETICS SALESPEOPLE SAY

They say the most amazing, inconceivable, preposterous things. Cosmetics salespeople will tell you that a moisturizer can make your cells produce better cells; that a firming cream containing elastin and collagen can reinforce the structure of the elastin and collagen in your skin, firming up sagging skin; or that the amino acids in a toner can merge into the deepest layers of your skin where it will fuse to your own DNA, building new layers of stronger cells that will make your face look younger in only two weeks. I've even heard cosmetics salespeople describe a freshener as a liberating liquid that can purify the toxins from your skin and improve circulation, helping the skin to regenerate younger skin, because old skin is caused by poor circulation to the face. Wow! I'll take ten of those.

I've heard facial masks, standard clay masks with some herbs or oils thrown in, described as nothing less than answers to prayers. One of the spiels I heard recently claimed that the mask in question pulls the water and garbage (garbage?) right out of your skin and automatically reduces puffiness and blemishes; that the botanicals and essential oils in it reduce the stress and tension that build up in the face and cause wrinkles (sounds like Valium for the face); and that (this is the best one) it combats pollution by feeding the skin nutrients and vitamins that the environment has depleted, and once your skin is fed properly it can generate new, youthful skin that can't be harmed by pollution again, as long as you use the mask once a week, that is.

I recently overheard a woman questioning a cosmetics line representative about the effects of a specific eye gel. I know you'll appreciate her reply. The saleswoman told her that "we can't even tell you everything it [the gel] can do for your skin because then it would be a drug and it would cost them [the company] too much money to keep it on the market." The epitome of cosmetics insanity is this sincere sales pitch I listened to involving a new moisturizer: "This night cream penetrates down to the birth area of the skin, where cells are produced, and then feeds it oxygen so that the cells have the ability to make healthy new cells. Of course, oxygen is essential to making new cells, and because of pollution there's so little oxygen left in the air that it destroys the skin and you can't have good skin without oxygen." Incredible!

The most popular ruses at the cosmetics counter these days are the distortions about alpha hydroxy acid products and products containing vitamins A, E, and C. It isn't surprising that AHA products are getting so much ballyhoo. This interesting cosmetic ingredient can temporarily smooth the skin, but in no way can it change, alter, restructure, or permanently improve the skin; it is just a very good moisturizing ingredient that can exfoliate the skin at the same time. Nevertheless, at the cosmetics counters you will be told that it can "rearrange the fibers of the skin to make them firmer and more elastic," or that it "works in harmony with the skin's own natural balance, returning it to a younger state." And the hype concerning vitamins in skin care products is nearly as bad: "There are conclusive studies that show free-radical damage is tearing down our skin, causing wrinkles, and that the only way to stop the damage is using products that contain vitamins." There are no conclusive studies on this subject anywhere; there are some theories, but no conclusive evidence.

And then there's the assertion that one line's ingredients are better than the next guy's, regardless of what they are—AHA, protein, sea salts, collagen, herbs, or oils. As if every cosmetics manufacturer didn't have access to the same distributors of these trendy little gems or only one distributor is selling the good stuff and the rest are selling inferior ingredients.

Are any of those enticing promises true, or even remotely possible? Bottom line: No, none of them are achievable from a cosmetic. If they were true, the products would indeed be drugs and scrutinized in a very different manner by the FDA. As wonderful as these sales pitches, and millions of other sales pitches, sound, they all lead you to believe what isn't true: that a cosmetic can change the inherent nature of your skin. It cannot. That a cosmetic can feed the skin from the outside in. It cannot. That a cosmetic can in any way, shape, or form alter the wrinkles on your face. It cannot.

How do the salespeople get away with it? Because the FDA is simply unable to monitor the thousands of people selling cosmetics, and is barely staffed to monitor the ads and product labels.

You may be wondering which products received those excessive descriptions. I didn't include names for two reasons: first, I didn't want you misunderstanding that these explanations were anything but false and have you accidently running out and buying it for yourself; second, many cosmetics salespeople, regardless of the product line, say crazy things that are either blatantly false, like all of the descriptions above, or so misleading as to be essentially false. Why pick on one line when all are guilty of the same offense?

A LITTLE LESS DESPERATION WOULD HELP

Almost everyone reaches *a certain age* and begins to worry that this certain age is the point of no return and they had better start doing something about it immediately to somehow shore up the impending breakdown. What is the certain age? Consensus indicates it is a highly relative number. Some women reach it when they turn 30, others 35, still others 40. Some women even wait until they become 50 to commence worrying. Then there is that rare specimen of woman who never reaches a certain age and never worries about it. This uncommon group is divided into two personality types. A woman who feels the same at 50 as she did at 30 is either the type of woman who simply cruises through life celebrating every moment to its fullest or she is someone for whom every age is the same: dull and boring. Hopefully we can all learn to celebrate.

I am always espousing a balance in life. I don't want to be a woman who doesn't recognize her age, but I also don't want to be constrained or frightened of it. I don't want to be so fearful of the media's interpretation of my eventual life that I run out and cover every line I see with either a new product or a cosmetic surgeon's skill. Besides, I see no special benefit in looking 25. I was once 25. All it got me was no respect and a lot of irresponsibility. I much prefer it here in my 40s, where the world is clearer and I feel stronger. Every age should be celebrated, but that takes self-esteem and self-confidence, and you won't find them in a cosmetics bottle or jar. Believe that one; it will save you time and money.

Facing life with a sense of goals and accomplishment, separate from how we look, can save a lot of bruised egos and money thrown away on products that won't change a thing. Women approach cosmetics with an attitude of near faith. "Sell me anything that will stop or slow down what is going to happen to my face." "Keep me beautiful so men don't start ignoring me." There is so much more than wrinkles involved in that kind of thinking. Giving the cosmetics industry so much credit and power is a huge mistake. This is where women turn the flashy hype into hopeful self-delusion.

MAKING THE FINAL DECISION

Which moisturizer, foundation, toner, or whatever should I buy? Which cosmetics line do you like the best? These are the two questions I am asked most frequently. The second question is the easiest to answer; as many of you already know, there is no one line I like the best. All cosmetics lines in all price categories have products I like and dislike. No one line has only good products or bad products. I sometimes wish that weren't true. Of course, then I would be out of this job because I would just say buy such and such a line and they would hire me as a spokesperson. But that isn't the case, because the perfect, or even close to perfect, cosmetics line doesn't exist.

The first question is more tricky. The truth is that many of the thousands of moisturizers, foundations, toners, and whatevers you can buy out there are pretty good. It's not that there aren't grades of good, but most products, particularly moisturizers, do their job fairly well. How well any product works depends more on your skin's needs and your personal preferences than on what the product contains. Do not expect me to tell you that one cosmetic ingredient or a series of ingredients are the only ones you can use or are the absolute best on the market. There are many bests and many possible combinations. Actually, the combinations of possible formulations are limitless, which explains the plethora of cosmetics. I am not ignoring the heartfelt request of so many consumers when I say that there isn't one best moisturizer, cleanser, or toner. There are products that don't work well and many that can irritate the skin, but of the ones that work, there isn't a best, there is just the one that works best on your skin.

In Chapter Nine, I list a series of bests and best buys, but I can't point to any one of those and say it is the ultimate best. That step is up to you, to discover what works best for your skin. In that regard, you are the one who determines what to buy. After all, out of 5,000 moisturizers on the market, do you really believe there can be only one best?

THE INGREDIENTS

It is important for you to understand how I went about making decisions about the skin care products I reviewed. Fortunately, the cosmetics companies have provided all of us with the very tool we need to implement an objective evaluation—the ingredient list. Every skin care item (and makeup item for that matter) lists the exact contents, in descending order, on the box or container. This ingredient list can be your best friend, because it can't mislead you. All of the information in that one small spot (often covered up by the price tag) has to be accurate, by law. Every skin care product I reviewed was evaluated on the basis of what it contained. You will have to test for yourself how it feels on your skin. My mission was simply to compare the promises made about a particular product with the ingredients listed on the label. Whatever the claim, the ingredients are the basis for whether or not a claim can be verified. For every product I explain what the ingredients are and then what the product can and can't do based on that published fact.

You will notice in the product reviews that I frequently use the terms *thickener(s), emulsifier(s), standard water binding agent(s),* and *slip agent(s).* Many ingredients perform one or more of these functions. There is a large group of universal cosmetic ingredients used in every cosmetic product to create texture, appearance, and help bind other ingredients together. Look at any ingredient list and you will see names such as cetyl or stearyl alcohol, myristyl myristate, glyceryl stearate, cetyl esters, peg-8, peg-100 stearate, caprylic-capric triglyceride, sorbitan stearate, cetyl acetate, polysorbate 80, acetylated lanolin alcohol, tea stearate, myristyl lactate, cetearyl alcohol, and ceteareth-20. All of these and hundreds more are standard, wax-like ingredients that I clump together as thickeners and emulsifiers.

Slip agents and "standard" water binding ingredients are those ingredients that allow the cosmetic to glide over your face and help bring water into and on the skin, keeping it moist and smooth. Again, there are dozens of these that show up in cosmetic after cosmetic, regardless of their price; propylene glycol, butylene glycol, hexylene glycol, lecithin, glycerin, dimethicone, and cyclomethicone are the most common standard water binding/slip agents. Then there are the more current, but not necessarily more effective, water binding ingredients that I usually refer to simply as water binding agents. These include hyaluronic acid, mucopolysaccharides, sodium PCA, NaPCA, collagen, elastin, and protein. They all work equally well but should not be considered the perfect moisturizing ingredients because they are not. They are what they are: good water binding ingredients.

On the occasion where an ingredient is used primarily for sudsing or degreasing ability I use the term *detergent cleanser.* Ingredients in this category include sodium lauryl sulphate, sodium laureth sulphate, tea-lauryl sulphate, cocamide DEA, ammonium laureth sulphate, and ammonium lauryl sulphate. When preservatives, fragrances, or coloring agents were listed I have indicated so; if a specific preservative was a problem I mentioned it within the review.

Many products list an assortment of exclusive-sounding adjectives for just plain water: deionized, purified, triple-purified, demineralized. You will also find phrases such as "infusions of" or "aqueous extracts of" and then the name of a plant or plants. That means you're getting plant tea or plant juice and water. They are almost 95 percent water, but they sound pure and natural, which we automatically think means our skin will do better (it won't). Water is water in a cosmetic, regardless of the type. What kind of water is used does not affect the skin or the product. After the water is combined with other ingredients its original status is unimportant.

Many of these ingredients, despite their complicated names, do have natural origins. In fact, some companies list the plant source next to the complicated-sounding ingredient. Keep in mind that the source of the ingredient doesn't have anything to do with the process the plant went through, which is often anything but natural and pure. An ingredient's natural origin has nothing to do with the eventual cosmetic ingredient you end up with, nor does it have anything to do with its effectiveness.

The questions I asked myself as I examined each item were simple: Can this product do what it says it can do? (If a product says it gently cleans the face and it leaves the face feeling tight and dry, I wouldn't call it gentle.) Is this product substantially different from similar products out on the market? (If all eye makeup removers have essentially the same ingredients, does it make sense to buy one that costs $17 versus one that costs $5? If a $50 wrinkle cream is essentially the same as a $10 wrinkle cream, does it make sense to spend the $50?) To establish these points, I've listed each product's specific, key ingredients so that you can begin to familiarize yourself with the repetitive nature of cosmetic formulations.

What I was not able to do is explain or refute all of the claims every product made regarding its efficacy or miraculous ability to improve and transform your skin. That alone would make this tome something of an epic, impossible to read, and, even worse, a problem to take to the cosmetics counters. Every product is summarized according to what the product contained and what those ingredients could and couldn't do. Skin care products are nothing more than a combination of ingredients. If a toner is supposed to be soothing or designed for sensitive skin but it contains irritating ingredients, the answer is simple: someone with sensitive skin or someone who is worried about a negative skin reaction shouldn't be using it.

UNDERSTANDING THE INGREDIENTS

Below is a list of typical cosmetic ingredients you will see on most product labels in all price ranges. Each ingredient is examined briefly as to what it is and what it can or cannot do for the skin. Although there are a lot of skin care formulations that don't make sense and many that you could easily do without, a number of them are beneficial to the skin. The information included here is truly the nuts and bolts of the cosmetics industry. Understanding the ingredient list may not change the way you buy skin care products altogether, but it will definitely make you more aware of what you're buying.

Acetone: This is used in some astringents and toners for its ability to remove oil from the skin. It is extremely drying and can cause severe irritation.

Alcohol, SD Alcohol 10-40: Alcohol is found in many different types of skin care products, but most frequently in astringents, toners, and fresheners. It can severely dry out the skin, and the resulting dryness can irritate the skin.

Algae Extract: Derived from seaweed and any water where green stuff grows. The claim is that it can do something special for wrinkles; it can't.

Allantoin, Panthenol, Aloe Vera: These cosmetic ingredients are well known, legitimately, for their ability to soothe the skin.

Amino Acids (Proteins and Animal Protein): Amino acids constitute the protein in human skin. Twenty-two of these extremely complex substances are used in cosmetics. Proteins provide a smooth covering on the skin and are considered beneficial in helping the skin absorb water. They provide no other benefit such as building or supplementing the protein in your own skin.

Ammonium Glycerhizinate: This strange-sounding ingredient is a very good anti-inflamatory agent. It helps to soothe skin and reduce irritation.

Amniotic Fluid: This ingredient is derived from the liquid surrounding the embryo in animals. In cosmetics the claim is that this fluid can rejuvenate the skin. There are no independent studies that support this claim.

Animal Extracts: Animal extracts include the following: spleen, matrix, neural lipid, epidermal lipid, thymus, animal tissue. These are dead fat or skin tissues from the thymus, testes, ovaries, udder, placenta, or other parts of a cow, pig, or sheep. The cosmetics industry would like you to believe that they have some rejuvenating effect on the skin. There is no evidence that these extracts can do anything for the skin, much less make it look younger, or even keep water in the skin for that matter.

2-Bromo-2-Nitropane-1, 3 Diol: When this ingredient and the compound triethanolamine are used together in a cosmetic they can combine to form a potentially carcinogenic material. By itself it is a potent skin irritant.

Camphor: This can cause irritation upon contact with the skin.

Caprylic/Capric/Lauric Triglycerides: This is an oily substance derived from coconut oil, and it helps keep water in the skin.

Cholesterol, Triglycerides, Phospholipids, Lecithin: These elements are all found in human tissue. In cosmetics, they very nicely help bind water to the skin and keep it there. Nothing special, but very good for dry skin.

Collagen and Elastin: These two well-known ingredients keep water in the skin. The distorted belief that somehow collagen and elastin rubbed on the skin would help rebuild the collagen and elastin in your own skin is hopefully a thing of the past. The collagen and elastin found in cosmetics, because of their structure, cannot even penetrate the skin.

Fatty Acids: Stearic acid is the most popular fatty acid used in cosmetics. It is a substance found in skin tissue. Used in a cosmetic, it helps keep water in the skin.

Glycerin: This is a fairly standard skin care ingredient that helps attract water to the skin and keeps it moist.

Hyaluronic Acid: You will be hearing quite a bit about hyaluronic acid over the next several years. It will be one of the buzzwords of the 1990s, just as collagen and elastin were in the 1980s. Hyaluronic acid is a mucopolysaccharide (another ingredient you will find in skin care products), which is a basic element found in skin tissue. When used in creams and lotions it helps water penetrate the skin. There is no evidence that hyaluronic acid can aid the skin besides keeping the surface soft.

Isopropyl Myristate: This chemical has a reputation for causing blackheads and other skin irritations when used in concentrations of 10 percent or greater. Most cosmetics don't use that much, but you don't want to find this in the first few ingredients in a cosmetic you are thinking of using.

Kaolin, Bentonite: Both are clays that are used in cosmetics to aid in the absorption of excess oil. They can be slightly irritating.

Lanolin: The only negative thing you can say about lanolin is that it is a potential skin sensitizer. Other than that, it is very effective at keeping the skin moist and supple. You will see several types of lanolin on skin care product labels: hydroxylated lanolin, lanolin alcohols, lanolin oil, and acetylated lanolin. All of these work as well as or better than pure lanolin in helping to keep moisture in the skin.

Liposomes (Ceramide): This is an interesting, unique chemical compound. You will see it used more and more in skin care products because of the way it helps keep water and oil in the skin for longer periods of time than other skin care ingredients can.

Mineral Oil: For some reason, this widely used cosmetic ingredient has gained a bad reputation in the past. In spite of the occasional bad press, mineral oil is considered one of the most nonirritating cosmetic ingredients available and is superior at keeping water in the skin.

Minerals: Minerals such as salt (sodium chloride), iodine, magnesium, chloride, and potassium are potential skin irritants when found in the first part of a cosmetic's ingredient list.

Mucopolysaccharides, Glycosamnioglycans: Along with collagen and elastin, these substances are found in the lower layers of human skin. In skin care products they offer exactly the same benefit to the skin as collagen and elastin.

Oil: Oils keep water in the skin. Lots of kinds of oils are used in skin care products, everything from jojoba oil to egg oil, rice bran oil, castor oil, and shark oil (squalene), and the list goes on and on. If you have dry skin you would not want to buy a moisturizer that didn't use a combination of oils as the primary ingredients.

Petrolatum: Petrolatum is one of the more effective moisturizing ingredients around. Study after study indicates it performs as well as or better than any other skin care ingredient for keeping water in the skin and does not clog pores.

Plant Extracts: There are an endless array of plant ingredients that range from algae to chamomile. They offer little benefit other than to boost the appeal (and price) of a product. They won't enhance cell production, youthful appearance, or anything else when it comes to your skin.

Propylene Glycol, Butylene Glycol, and Polyethylene Glycol (PEG): These skin care basics are present in almost every cleanser, toner, lotion, cream, or specialty product you will ever buy. These ingredients help attract moisture to the skin and help the product spread evenly over the skin.

Salicylic Acid: This ingredient can be very irritating to the skin. It is used frequently in acne preparations for its ability to exfoliate the skin.

Serum Albumin, Serum Protein: These elements are derived from the blood of cows or pigs and are used as moisturizing ingredients. Neither provide any benefit for the skin in spite of sounding like a blood transfusion.

Sodium Lauryl Sulfate, Zinc Lauryl Sulfate, Ammonium Lauryl Sulfate, and Magnesium Lauryl Sulfate: These compounds are all cleansing agents found mostly in shampoos and skin cleansers. These are considered to be somewhat drying when used as the primary ingredient in a skin cleanser.

Sodium Laureth Sulfate, Magnesium Laureth Sulfate: Both of these, and a dozen or so similar-sounding ingredients, are considered to be more gentle detergent cleansing agents than the ones listed above. They are found most often in shampoos and water-soluble cleansers. They can be gentle, but they can also be somewhat drying on the skin.

Sodium PCA: This ingredient is a component of human skin that is used in cosmetics for its ability to hold water to the skin.

Tocopherol: This is the chemical name for vitamin E. It is used in cosmetics as an antioxidant, which means it helps keep the air off the face, and that helps prevent dehydration and possible free-radical damage. Vitamins do not feed the skin in any way from the outside in. The amount used is rarely enough to provide much benefit.

Vitamin A, Retinyl Palmitate, and Retinol: These ingredients are frequently found in cosmetics nowadays. Retinol and retinyl palmitate are derivatives of vitamin A. Vitamin A is also the source for the prescription drug Retin-A. This association with Retin-A misleads many consumers into believing that products containing these ingredients can provide the same or similar benefits to the skin as Retin-A can. None of those claims are true. For the most part, vitamin A, retinyl palmitate, and retinol are simple antioxidants and help prevent possible free-radical damage. They may also have some benefits in terms of allowing moisture to penetrate the skin, but that's about it. The amount used is rarely enough to provide much benefit.

Water: Dry skin or mature skin contains an increased number of dried-out skin cells. Water rehydrates these cells. Whether it is fancy water from the Swiss Alps or natural spring water, demineralized water or water extracted from plants or flowers, water is water, and it is what you need to have on your face, or in your skin care product, if a moisturizer is going to have any effect on your face.

Witch Hazel: This compound is about 15 to 20 percent alcohol. It is considered to be a mild skin irritant. Many products that claim to be alcohol-free contain witch hazel.

WHAT I WAS LOOKING FOR

Facial cleansers: When it came to facial cleansers, I was interested primarily in how genuinely water-soluble they were. I expected facial cleansers to rinse off easily without the aid of a washcloth and be able to remove all traces of makeup, including eye makeup. Once a water-soluble cleanser is rinsed off, it should not leave skin feeling either dry or greasy and filmy feeling. And it should never burn the eyes or irritate the skin.

Toners: The main consideration when it came to toners, astringents, fresheners, tonics, or any other liquid meant to refresh the skin after the cleanser is rinsed off, was that they contain no irritants whatsoever. These products were evaluated on that basis alone. Claims of closing pores or refining the skin are not realistic, so I was looking primarily for toners that left a smooth, soft feeling on the face without irritation.

Exfoliators: When it came to scrubs I looked for products with the least amount of irritants (you can only exfoliate so much skin before you start ripping it off and causing irritation). If you want to use an alpha hydroxy acid product for exfoliation, which I consider to be an excellent idea, I indicated which ones had a high enough percentage of AHA to make a difference on the skin.

Moisturizers: In spite of all the complications surrounding wrinkle creams and moisturizers, this category was actually quite easy to review. Wrinkle creams and moisturizers all do the same thing, so I expected the same thing from all of them: they had to contain ingredients that can smooth and soothe dry skin. All the other claims are exaggerated and misleading. I indicated which products contained the best or latest water binding moisturizing ingredients. I also listed the ingredients that I thought were more hype than proven, such as brewer's yeast, bee pollen, vitamin B, Nyad, and plant extracts. I was also interested in what order the "good" ingredients were listed on the container. Often the percentage of the best ingredients in a product is so negligible that it is practically nonexistent. Just because an ingredient is in there doesn't mean there's enough to make a difference.

Important: When you check the ingredient list of a product, you should realize that the first five to ten ingredients-the ones most abundant in the formulas-are those that affect your skin the most. Ingredient labels are organized in descending order. The most significant ingredient is listed first, the next most used is listed second, and so on. For the most part, the ingredients I listed for each product follow the sequential order in which they appear on the product's ingredient label. (For further information regarding ingredient descriptions, please refer to Ruth Winter's A Consumer's Dictionary of Cosmetic Ingredients, third edition, and Rodale's Illustrated Encyclopedia of Herbs.)

Facial masks: Most facial masks contain clay-like ingredients. They absorb oil and, to some degree, help exfoliate the skin. The problem with many of these products is that they contain additional irritating ingredients. Although your face may initially feel smooth when the mask is first rinsed off, after a short period of time the drying effect it has on the skin creates problems. As a rule I don't recommend either clay facial masks or masks that peel off the skin, which in essence do the same thing in terms of exfoliation. The few clay masks on the market that contain emollients and moisturizing ingredients can still be too drying for dry skin and can cause oily skin to break out. Although I feel that facial masks are in the unnecessary group of products, for those who are interested I've pointed out the ones that do not contain any additional irritating ingredients except for the clay.

Specialty products: Because I didn't want to waste your time or mine, I did not review any cellulite products, neck or throat firming creams, or body firming lotions, because they don't come close to living up to their claims. They are always standard moisturizers with great advertising copy. If you want to waste your money on these products, anything I tell you about them won't change your mind.

> *Remember that on ingredient lists, the closer a specific ingredient is to a preservative (such as methylparaben, propylparaben, ethylparaben, disodium EDTA, urea, and imidazolidinyl urea) or fragrance, the less likely there is any significant amount of it present in the product.*

Caution: Although the cost of cosmetics often fluctuates from store to store and because cosmetics companies often change prices every six months, the prices listed below may not be accurate. Use the prices as a basis for comparison, but realize that they might not accurately reflect what you find at the store. Cosmetics companies also change or reformulate their product lines, sometimes in a minor way and sometimes extensively. Three cases in point: Origins was introducing an entire new line of foundations just as this book was going to press; Visage Beaute had just been bought by Revlon and was undergoing major changes; and Artistry by Amway was changing almost 50 percent of their skin care and makeup products. Any time there are changes of this nature, I will report on them in my newsletter.

For the most part only the English names of foreign-produced products are used. The French and Italian names are pretty, but they don't tell you anything about the product if you don't speak the language.

Acne-Statin

I am extremely skeptical about cosmetics products that claim to get rid of acne, eliminate blackheads, or dry up oil. What I know from personal experience and from the thousands of letters I receive each year from women the world over (not to mention interviews with cosmetic chemists and dermatologists) is that these over-the-counter products don't work, particularly not as well as they would lead you to believe. The truth is, you can't cure acne or dry up oil with over-the-counter, nonprescription medications. Over-the-counter products work for only about 40 percent of a given population (some suggest it is even less than that), and by "work" I mean reduce flare-ups, not cure. What about the 60 percent who don't benefit? Well, they jump from one product to the next, hoping to find something that works.

Most over-the-counter products contain ingredients that help peel the skin (exfoliate dead skin cells), such as salicylic acid; other cosmetic scrub agents to unclog pores; benzol peroxide to kill the bacteria that can be causing blemishes to erupt; and/or drying agents such as alcohol to eliminate the oil. Well, drying ingredients definitely don't work (if anything they tend to encourage more oil), benzol peroxide and salicylic acid can cause extreme irritation, and so can some scrubs.

Where does Acne-Statin *($34.90 for 4 ounces)*, a face wash and moisturizer all-in-one product, fit in with all of this? Well, to be perfectly honest, I'm not sure. Because Acne-Statin doesn't list ingredients on their label, much of what is inside is a mystery and hard to evaluate. Due to a grandfather clause in the FDA's mandatory ingredient listing rules, Acne-Statin doesn't have to list any of their nonactive ingredients. However, what they do have to list are the active ingredients. What isn't a mystery then, is that Acne-Statin contains 0.5 percent triclosan, 0.15 percent methylparaben, and 0.1 percent propylparaben. These active ingredients (which make up a mere 0.75 percent of the product) are a rather expensive joke, because they aren't in the least bit unique or special and they can't really do anything for acne, particularly in these teensy amounts. Triclosan, methylparaben, and propylparaben are standard cosmetic preservatives found in lots of cosmetics. The other 99.25 percent of the product, the inactive ingredients, is covered by the FDA's grandfather clause.

All of Acne-Statin's claims, like those of other cosmetic products, sound sweeping and astoundingly impressive. But as consumers, we are given only advertising and hype to base our decision on. The ingredient list, the only verifiable truth on any cosmetic product, is kept a secret. What they are really telling us is that a product that is 0.75 percent normal cosmetic preservatives and 99.25 percent inactive, standard cosmetic ingredients (what else can they be if they are not listed and this is not a drug but a cosmetic?) is supposed to take care of acne. Simply not possible. Also, if this product has been so astoundingly successful for so many years (long enough to be covered by the grandfather clause), why did no one hear about it before these television ads? If acne was being cleared up with such success over the years, surely this company would be famous.

One more point. In the course of several phone calls to Acne-Statin to find out more about the ingredient list, I got some pretty strange reactions. Most of the people who answered the phone were shocked that the active ingredients listed totaled only 0.75 percent of the product, and they didn't know what the ingredients were or what they did on the skin. No one knew why the other 99.25 percent of the ingredients weren't listed or what they did for the skin either. What everyone repeatedly assured me about was how wonderful this product is and the credibility of the physician who formulated it. Meanwhile, I kept saying, "Then why not list the ingredients like thousands of other products do?" Finally some executive assistant called me back and explained the grandfather clause to me. He also tried to explain the exclusivity of the formula, but I simply reiterated my position: "There are a lot of exclusive formulas out there, but they all list their ingredients, even those that have been around longer than you and can get away with the grandfather clause as well." The conversation ended there.

Adrien Arpel

Foam Cleanser *($19 for 8 ounces)* doesn't quite take off all the makeup and leaves a film behind on the face.

Freeze-Dried Embryonic Collagen Protein Cleanser *($20 for 4 ounces)* contains mostly water, a long list of thickeners, animal protein, detergent cleanser, standard water binding agent, more thickener, and preservatives. This is only an OK cleanser, although a bit on the greasy side. I'm of the opinion that collagen, which in this case is tissue from an animal fetus, is useless, particularly in a cleanser, because it is washed off and can't do anything for the skin. There isn't much in this product anyway.

Sea Kelp Cleanser *($19.50 for 4 ounces)* contains mostly water, mineral oil, thickeners, petrolatum, thickeners, kelp, pumice (scrub agent), more thickeners, algae, and preservatives. This cleanser is really a fairly greasy scrub. For the little amount of sea kelp you're getting, it isn't much of a sea kelp cleanser.

Coconut Cleanser *($19.50 for 4 ounces)* contains mostly water, safflower oil, and propylene glycol, and very little coconut. It will not rinse off without the aid of a washcloth.

Honey Almond Scrub *($18.50 for 8 ounces)* contains mostly glycerin, almonds, thickeners, lemon oil (which can irritate the skin), more thickeners, collagen, animal protein, oils, and preservatives. It will help slough skin, although baking soda mixed with a little water will do the same thing for a lot less. Protein and collagen serve little purpose in a cleanser.

Lemon & Lime Freshener *($17.50 for 8 ounces)* is an alcohol-free freshener containing mostly water, standard water binding agent, aloe, vitamin C, emulsifier, fragrance, balm mint oil, herbal and fruit extracts, and preservatives. It can be soothing to the skin, however, the balm mint oil can be irritating to some skin types.

Herbal Astringent *($17.50 for 8 ounces)* contains no alcohol. It is mostly standard water binding agent, emulsifiers, and preservatives. Very ordinary, although it can be soothing to the skin.

Bio Cellular Night Cream *($37 for 1.25 ounces; $52 for 2.75 ounces)* contains mostly water, synthetic oil, honey, thickeners, standard water binding agents, more thickeners, linseed extract (can be an irritant), emulsifier, RNA, DNA, and preservative. This is a an OK moisturizer, but there is only a tiny amount of RNA and DNA. RNA and DNA can't affect skin cells in any significant way, but they sound very impressive.

Swiss Formula Day Cream #12 with Collagen *($30 for 1 ounce; $48.50 for 2 ounces)* is a very emollient, rich moisturizer. It contains water, standard water binding agent, mineral oil, collagen, lanolin, thickeners, oils, placenta (doesn't say whose), brewer's yeast (source of vitamin B), and preservatives. It claims to be nongreasy, but that doesn't jive with the inclusion of mineral oil and lanolin, both fairly greasy ingredients. Placenta and brewer's yeast won't affect wrinkles in any way, shape, or form.

Vital Velvet Moisturizer *($22.50 for 2 ounces)* contains mostly water, standard water binding agent, lanolin, thickeners, mineral oil, more thickeners, oils, collagen, and preservatives. This is a fairly emollient moisturizer and works well for extremely dry skin only.

Moisturizing Blotting Lotion *($22 for 2 ounces)* contains water, mineral oil, standard water binding agent, thickeners, lanolin, water binding agent, lard, thickeners, egg oil, and preservatives. This is a very rich moisturizer, best for someone with extremely dry skin.

Morning After Moisturizer, SPF 20 *($30 for 1 ounce)*. I wouldn't put this on in the morning after, I would put this on *before* going out in the morning. This is a good, basic, lightweight sunscreen/moisturizer. The collagen, elastin, and the good water binding ingredients are far down on the ingredient list.

Eyelastic Lift *($40)* is a two-part product. You're supposed to mix the **Puff Deflator Capsules** *(0.5 ounce—45 capsules)* with the Eyelastic **Lift and Firm Creme** *(0.5 ounce)*. It won't lift the eye anywhere. The Puff Deflator (do you believe that name?) contains mostly synthetic oil, standard water binding agents, synthetic oil, placenta extract, and preservatives. This ordinary list of ingredients makes for an OK moisturizer, but that's about it. Placenta extract can't make your skin one hour younger. The Lift and Firm Creme contains mostly water, standard water binding agent, synthetic oils, oat flour, thickeners, algae, thickener, honey, elastin, more thickeners, and preservatives. The ingredients work as a paste on the skin (basically flour and honey) with some moisturizing ingredients. It also contains a preservative that is considered a potential carcinogen.

Skinlastic Lift *($40 for 1.7 ounces—18 vials)* contains mostly water, protein, glycerin, plant extract, standard water binding agent, thickener, protein, thickener, preservative (possible skin irritant), plant extracts, and preservatives. Protein in a moisturizer won't lift the skin, but this is a good, although absurdly expensive, moisturizer.

Flower Petal and Botanical Extract Masque *($22.50 for 4 ounces)* contains water, standard water binding agent, emulsifier, plant extracts, thickeners, fragrance, and preservatives. Well, there are definitely some plants in here, but not much. It won't hurt, but it also won't do much.

Flower Petal Mini-Facial in a Jar *($29.50 for 4.5 ounces)* contains mostly water, synthetic oil, a long list of thickeners, flower petals, standard water binding agent, plant extracts, more thickeners, and preservatives. There are definitely some plants in here, but not much. It won't hurt, but it also won't do much.

Sea Mud Mask *($24 for 4 ounces)* contains water, clay, alcohol, thickeners, standard water binding agent, talc, more thickeners, oat flour, and preservatives. There's no sea mud in here. Bentonite is clay from the southwestern United States. This is just an ordinary clay mask, and the alcohol can be an irritant.

Freeze-Dried Collagen Protein Moisture Lock Masque *($25 for 4 ounces)* contains mostly water, a long list of thickeners, protein (calf skin), standard water binding agent, and preservatives. Calf skin? Give me a break.

Freeze-Dried Protein Lip and Laughline Peel and Salve *($38.50 for 1 ounce peel and 0.25 ounce salve)* is a two-part system. The peel contains mostly water, wax, thickeners, allantoin, collagen, and preservatives. The salve ingredient list reads much like one for an emollient lipstick, with castor oil, petrolatum, and lanolin. This won't get rid of laugh lines and it isn't vaguely worth this steep price tag, but it can feel good over the lips.

Lipline Cream *($22 for 0.5 ounce)* contains mostly water, mineral oil, thickener, almond oil, protein, thickener, petrolatum, glycerin, thickeners, protein, more thickeners, oils, thickeners, and preservatives. This is a good moisturizer, but it won't do anything special for the lips. Protein in a moisturizer won't build the skin from the outside in.

Underglow Line Minimizing Moisturizer *($35 for 1.25 ounces)* contains mostly water; thickener; glycerin; standard water binding agents; aloe; thickeners; vitamins E, A, and D; vegetable oil; and preservatives. This is an overpriced but good lightweight moisturizer. It won't change the wrinkles on your face.

Almay

Moisture Balance Cleansing Lotion for Normal Skin *($5.25 for 7.25 ounces)* is a somewhat greasy cleanser that does not rinse well without the aid of a washcloth and leaves some makeup behind. If you have normal skin you will find this cleanser somewhat greasy, but if you have extremely dry skin and use a washcloth (which I don't recommend because of irritation) it is passable.

Deep Cleansing Cold Cream *($3.50 for 4 ounces)* is a traditional cold cream that needs to be wiped off and will leave the skin feeling greasy. I don't recommend wipe-off cleansers.

Cold Cream Cleansing Bar *($2.25 for two 4-ounce bars)* is standard soap that contains mineral oil to help cut the irritation from the soap. However, the soap is still irritating.

Sensitive Skin Foaming Cleanser *($3.50 for 7.75 ounces)*. Like many cleansers, this one contains a gentle detergent usually found in shampoos. I found it to be too drying on the skin, although it did rinse off easily and may be good for someone with extremely oily skin.

Anti-Bacterial Foaming Cleanser *($3.50 for 7.75 ounces)* is a standard detergent cleanser that contains menthol and sodium chloride, which can burn the eyes and irritate the skin.

Oil-Control Complexion Scrub *($6.50 for 4 ounces)* is basically a detergent cleanser with abrasive scrub particles. It can be irritating to some skin types and it won't stop or control oil.

Non-Oily Eye Makeup Remover Lotion *($3.75 for 2 ounces)* is OK, but the preservative is rather high up in the ingredient list and can irritate the eyes.

Moisture Renew Cleansing Cream for Dry Skin *($4.50 for 4.75 ounces)* does not wash off easily and can leave a film behind on the face.

Moisture Renew Balance Toner for Dry Skin *($5.25 for 7.25 ounces)* contains mostly water and alcohol, and can irritate the skin.

Moisture Balance Toner for Normal Skin *($5.25 for 7.25 ounces)* contains ingredients almost identical to those in the toner above, and it too can irritate the skin.

Stress Cream *($10 for 1.9 ounces)* contains good moisturizing ingredients and many of the latest components designed to keep water in the skin. It is a fine moisturizer that contains mostly water, propylene glycol, mineral oil, butylene glycol, a glycerin-like ingredient, and petrolatum. The product can't counteract stress as the name implies, but it will improve dry skin.

Stress Eye Gel *($7.50 for 0.5 ounce)*. This lightweight gel contains an interesting assortment of ingredients that include water, a gel-like ingredient, butylene glycol, an amino acid, allantoin, aloe vera gel, hyaluronic acid, and sodium PCA. All these should feel soothing around the eye and keep moisture in the skin without leaving it feeling greasy. Unfortunately, this product also contains witch hazel, which can be too irritating for the delicate skin around the eye.

Anti-Irritant *($1.25 for 0.3 ounce)* contains mostly water; petrolatum; thickeners; aloe vera; healing agent; vitamins A, C, and E; and preservatives. This is a good moisturizer for dry skin. I wouldn't call it an anti-irritant, but it is soothing.

Replenishing Lotion *($6 for 1.8 ounces)* is a lightweight moisturizer for normal to slightly dry skin. It contains mostly water; standard water binding agents; thickeners; water binding agent; vitamins A, C, and E; soothing agent; thickeners; and preservatives.

Moisture Renew Cream for Dry Skin *($6.50 for 2 ounces)* is a lightweight moisturizer that contains water, mineral oil, propylene glycol, thickeners, and sodium PCA. It is a good moisturizer, although it would be better for normal to dry skin. It doesn't contain enough emollients to really soothe extremely dry skin.

Moisture Renew Lotion for Dry Skin *($6.50 for 3.35 ounces)*. This lightweight moisturizer is similar to the cream above, but in lotion form.

Moisture Balance Eye Cream for Normal Skin *($5 for 0.5 ounce)*. This very rich cream works better for extremely dry skin than it would for normal skin. It contains petrolatum, lanolin oil, mineral oil, propylene glycol, water, and paraffin.

Moisture Balance Night Cream for Normal Skin *($5.50 for 2 ounces)* contains mostly water, mineral oil, standard water binding agent, thickeners, and preservatives. A below-average moisturizer with uninteresting ingredients.

Moisture Balance Cleansing Mask for Normal Skin *($4.50 for 2.5* *ounces)* is a standard clay mask that contains mostly water, clay, alcohol, more clay, thickeners, and preservatives. This won't balance the skin and it can be quite drying for most skin types.

Oil-Control Clay Mask for Oily Skin *($4.50 for 2.5 ounces)* contains water, clay, preservative, detergent cleanser, slip agents, more clay, and preservatives. This won't control oil and it is potentially irritating.

Alpha Hydrox by Neoteric

Alpha Hydrox Lotion and Alpha Hydrox Face Creme are two of the more reasonably priced as well as effective alpha hydroxy acid products on the market. While other companies often hedge on telling you how much AHA their product contains, Alpha Hydrox is more than forthcoming. The AHA ingredient they use is glycolic acid, considered one of the best. If you are interested in trying an AHA moisturizer, I encourage you to start here. The prices and product quality are excellent and the AHA percentage is 8%. One word of caution: To capitalize on the attraction of their excellent AHA moisturizers, they also retail several other products, calling the line a Skin Treatment System. The other products are not anywhere near as impressive as the moisturizers, and too many AHA products on the face can be overkill, producing irritation.

Alpha Hydrox Lotion *($8 for 6 ounces)* contains mostly water, glycolic acid, pH balancer (can be an irritant), water binding agent, thickeners, petrolatum, more thickeners, and preservatives. This is a very good AHA moisturizer for all skin types.

All Body Lotion *($8 for 6 ounces)* contains mostly water, glycolic acid, water binding agent, pH balancer (can be an irritant), thickener, petrolatum, more thickeners, and preservatives. This is a very good AHA product for the face and the body.

Face Creme *($8 for 2 ounces)* contains mostly water, glycolic acid, water binding agent, thickeners, pH balancer (can be an irritant), more thickeners, and preservatives. This is a very good AHA moisturizer for normal to dry skin types.

Oil-Free Facial Formula *($8 for 4 ounces)* contains water, alcohol, glycolic acid, pH balancer (can be an irritant), and preservative. I never recommend alcohol on the skin because it can be too drying and irritating. The benefits of the AHA can be lost to the irritation.

Oil-Free Facial Gel *($8 for 4 ounces)* contains water, alcohol, water binding agent, glycolic acid, pH balancer (can be an irritant), thickener, and preservative. Almost identical to the Oil-Free Facial Formula, it is also too drying and irritating for almost all skin types..

Foaming Face Wash *($5.50 for 6 ounces)* is a standard detergent face cleanser that does not contain AHA. It can be a good cleanser for someone with normal to oily skin, but may be too drying for other skin types.

Hydrating Eye Gel *($9.50 for 0.5 ounce)* is an overpriced gel that contains mostly water, water binding agents, aloe vera, thickeners, and preservatives. It's OK but not worth the price tag.

Toner-Astringent *($5.50 for 8 ounces)* contains mostly water, alcohol, witch hazel, water binding agent, glycolic acid, chamomile extract, soothing agent, menthol (a skin irritant), and preservatives. The chamomile and soothing agent can't counterbalance the irritation caused by the alcohol and menthol.

Aveda

When it comes to "natural" skin care and makeup products, the Aveda line has enough herbs, vegetables, fruits, and flowers to satisfy any botany lover's dreams. On the other hand, regular consumers, distracted by the aura surrounding botanicals, are intrigued but left out in the cold by "infusions" of horsetail, ginseng, comfrey, and juniper, not knowing why they are putting any of that stuff on their face. The products sound good and the ecology-oriented marketing is quite imposing. Taking care of the environment and using "natural and pure" ingredients, even if we don't know what they do for the skin, seem like the right things to do and use. Of course, when they are charging $18 for 4 ounces of skin lotion, companies forget to mention the standard cosmetic ingredients that are really the substance of the product. Furthermore, plants are just plants when mixed into cosmetics and retain little if any of their original form.

More often than not, when you see a long list of herbs and plants, what you are really purchasing is a rather expensive tea. Helpful for the skin? After these herbs have been cooked and preserved in a cosmetic, they don't even contain much of whatever constituted their original promised benefit. Plus there is absolutely no independent evidence that proves any of the exaggerated claims you'll read on product labels. But "natural" products are very seductive, and it is hard not to conclude that you will have naturally perfect skin if you use them. To make it all even more seductive, Aveda publishes an impressive little booklet (on recycled paper) that describes at length some of the benefits bestowed by the plants used in their products. The descriptions are exquisite, bordering on hypnotic. After reading it you will want to cover yourself in these historic potions and elixirs. It takes a lot of willpower to remember that plants mixed into a cosmetic are not in a pure form, and even if they were, there is no research that indicates that the herbs can do what the descriptions claim. Their boast is "2500 years of research," but there are no Romans or ancient Egyptians around to show us their test results.

Aveda is a high-priced fancy cosmetics line with all the natural botanical trappings plus the magnetism of select, boutique distribution. Mostly found in upper-end department stores, hair salons, and the main Aveda store in New York City, this is a cosmetics line with a great deal of marketing chic. The products state that "Only distributors, salons, and licensed professionals who or which have received essential education may sell Aveda products." Very impressive. But exactly what is "essential education"? I have received letters from several salon owners who sell Aveda who wanted me to explain what these products can and can't do. The marketing is designed to appear exclusive, but the reality is just the opposite.

Some of these products are definitely worth your attention. And if you are interested in plants, this line is the king of the hill. By the way, "infusion" and "aqueous extract" are fancy terms for plant water (tea).

Purifying Cream Cleanser *($18 for 5.5 ounces)* is supposed to be a water-soluble cleanser, but after rinsing it leaves a film on the face, requiring a washcloth to get it all off. This product is best for someone with very dry skin. It primarily contains a tea of white oak bark and witch hazel (which can be irritating), thickeners, glycerin, oils, detergent cleansers, oil, fragrance, more oils, vitamin E, and preservatives.

Purifying Gel Cleanser *($16.50 for 5.5 ounces)* is a fairly typical sudsing facial cleanser that contains a tea of chamomile, lavender, and rosemary. The next ingredients are typical foaming detergent cleansers (some of which can be irritating). It may be good for some oily skin types.

Cleansing Scrub *($16.50 for 5.5 ounces)* primarily contains white oak bark and witch hazel as the tea water, thickeners, jojoba meal as the scrub agent, more thickeners, detergent, jojoba oil, detergent cleansers, oils, and more thickeners. It's an OK scrub that can prove irritating for most skin types. (This product is presently being discontinued.)

Exfoliant *($14 for 5.5 ounces)* is a liquid toner that contains lavender water (can be an antiseptic on the skin), chamomile (which can be antiseptic, but can cause allergic reactions in sensitive people), lemon balm (antiseptic properties), witch hazel and alcohol (both can be quite irritating on the skin), and salicylic acid (which peels the skin and can be an irritant). For most skin types this product can prove to be quite irritating.

Deep Cleansing Herbal Clay Masque *($18 for 4.5 ounces)* is for the most part just a standard clay mask that contains kaolin as its primary ingredient. White oak bark, witch hazel, and aloe comprise the tea water, and there are some oils, standard thickeners, and a detergent cleanser. As a clay mask it may be more gentle than most, but it can still prove irritating for sensitive skin and too greasy for oily skin.

Toning Mist *($13.50 for 5.5 ounces)* is a fairly irritating product that contains primarily a tea of white oak bark, witch hazel, and aloe, and peppermint, rosewater, alcohol, grapefruit extract, and glycerin. The glycerin won't soothe the irritation caused by the witch hazel, white oak bark, peppermint, alcohol, and grapefruit extract.

Skin Firming/Toning Agent *($16.50 for 5.5 ounces)* contains rosewater, an herb called Echinacea (which can soothe the skin, but how much of its original properties are still present in a cosmetic is highly questionable), soothing agent, a slip agent, and preservative. This is a good irritant-free toner, but it won't firm anything.

Miraculous Beauty Replenisher *($17.50 for 1 ounce)* is basically a blend of several oils, including jojoba, rose (which contains vitamin C), sour orange, lavender, fennel, geranium, chamomile, borage, and vitamin E. All of these ingredients can be soothing to the skin, but it is a relatively overpriced blend of oils, when any one of these alone, in its pure form, can be applied to the skin for the same effect and much more cheaply. For normal to dry skin only.

Hydrating Lotion *($24 for 5.5 ounces)* contains a tea of chamomile, lavender, rosemary, and comfrey; glycerin; thickeners; and rice and jojoba oil. Several of the thickeners in this product are possible irritants. It can be good for normal to slightly dry skin that isn't sensitive.

Beautifying Formula *($17 for 2 ounces)* contains jojoba, rosemary, lavender, and bergamot oils. Bergamot and lavender oil are possible skin irritants when exposed to sunlight. The oils are soothing on the skin if you stay out of the sun.

Calming Nutrients *($17 for 2 ounces)* contains jojoba, rose, borage, and vitamin E oils. A lot of money for oils that can't feed the skin. These are just oils with fancy names and a high price tag.

Energizing Nutrients *($17 for 2 ounces)* contains jojoba oil, herb oils, borage oil, vitamin E, and vitamin A. You can't feed the skin from the outside in. These are just oils that can feel good on dry skin, nothing more.

Deep Cleansing Herbal Clay Masque *($20 for 4.5 ounces)* contains mostly Echinacea and hyssop water (tea with soothing properties), clay, thickeners, more clay, fragrance, vitamin E, rice oil, thickeners, and preservatives. This is a standard clay mask with some herb water thrown in, but because of the rice oil it may not be as drying as some clay masks.

Intensive Hydrating Masque *($29 for 5.5 ounces)* contains mostly a tea of aloe, kelp, lavender, and rosewater; glycerin; thickener; water binding agent; soothing agent; protein; and preservatives. There is also a "tissue respiratory factor." Skin breathes without the help of any topical ingredient, but doesn't it sound very healthy for skin suffocated by pollutants? Great gimmick.

Avon

Avon's list of skin care products reads like an epic novel; the list goes on forever. There are some good products in here but not many. Unfortunately, this isn't a very sophisticated group of moisturizers. Of course, that observation doesn't include the now-famous Anew moisturizer (Nova in Canada), Avon's own alpha hydroxy acid product, one of the first on the market. This little AHA moisturizer (which has now become three different products, each with a different concentration of AHA) grossed over $30 million for Avon in its first year. Is it worth the fuss? And what about Avon Skin So Soft—is it the bug repellent skin wonder of the decade?

Avon's consumer information from their ordering number—(800) 233-2866—and consumer information center number—(800) 445-2866—was actually quite helpful. No matter how many products I requested ingredient lists for, they provided them without hesitation or question. Thank you, Avon, for great customer service. I still wish Avon's products were better. This is as true for this group of products as for the ones I reviewed in the March issue of *Cosmetics Counter Update*. I didn't like many of them. How disappointing. Many were done in by poor ingredient combinations and lists (preservatives often came before the really worthwhile ingredients, which means you don't get much of the good stuff, and irritating and drying ingredients are included in moisturizers). The final decision is up to you, but Avon just isn't the bargain I was hoping for.

Anew Perfecting Complex for Chest and Neck *($15.50 for 3.4 ounces)* is an AHA moisturizer that contains about 2 percent glycolic acid. It contains water; slip agent; glycerin; glycolic acid (AHA); ammonium glycolate; vitamins A, B, and C (all antioxidants); herb extracts; oils; thickener; and preservatives. This is an excellent emollient moisturizer. The claim that it can slough skin is misleading: there isn't enough AHA. But it is still a good product for a nighttime moisturizer and can be used on the face as well as the body.

Anew Perfecting Complex for the Face *($15.50 for 3.4 ounces)* is an AHA moisturizer that contains about 4 percent glycolic acid. The ingredients are water, thickeners, slip agent, emollient, AHA, thickener, AHA, thickeners, vitamins A and E (antioxidants), standard water binding agent, herb extracts, oils, and preservatives. It will indeed slough skin, and works well as a mild AHA product. It is somewhat thicker than the cream for chest and neck, but it is still emollient and lightweight.

Anew Perfecting Complex for the Hands and Body *($15.50 for 3.4 ounces)* is an AHA moisturizer that contains about 10 percent glycolic acid. It is very similar to the other two Anew products and is the one I prefer for the face as well as the rest of the body because of its higher AHA content. It may be too strong for some skin types, but it is worth a try.

Daily Revival Gentle Cream Cleanser for Dry Skin *($6 for 6 ounces)* contains mostly water, mineral oil, petrolatum, thickeners, preservative, more thickeners, preservative, another thickener, preser-vative, and fragrance. The remaining ingredients are herb extracts and aloe vera gel, which are inconsequential considering their placement after the preservatives. This is really a wipe-off cleanser that is too greasy to rinse off. It would be appropriate for someone with extremely dry skin, but it doesn't really clean that well.

Daily Revival Oil-Clearing Wash for Oily Skin *($6 for 6 ounces)* contains water, slip agent, glycerin, detergent cleanser, herb extracts, thickener, detergent cleanser, preservatives, fragrance, and coloring agents. An OK cleanser for someone with normal skin, but it doesn't rinse well enough for someone with oily skin.

Daily Revival Foaming Facial Wash for Normal to Combination Skin *($6 for 6 ounces)* contains water, detergent cleansers, thickeners, vitamin B (antioxidant), herb extracts, fragrance, preservatives, and coloring agents. This cleanser leaves a slight film on the skin and doesn't foam all that well. A good possibility for someone with dry skin.

Daily Revival Mild Cleansing Bar for Normal/Combination Skin *($2.75 for 3 ounces)* contains sodium tallowate (can irritate the skin and cause blackheads), detergent cleanser, water, more detergent cleansers, glycerin, fragrance, thickeners, lanolin (can cause an allergic reaction), sesame oil, salt (skin irritant), preservative, and a long list of herb extracts and oils that are too insignificant to matter. This bar soap is hardly mild, and someone with combination skin would not be pleased with the inclusion of lanolin and so many oils.

Daily Revival Softening Toner for Normal/Combination Skin *($6 for 6 ounces)* contains water, slip agent, coloring agent, preservatives, citric acid (for pH balance), fragrance, herb extracts, and coloring agents. The herb extracts are too far down in the ingredient list to be significant. This product is mostly water, preservatives, and little else. It won't soften the skin, but it may irritate with that much preservative.

Daily Revival Active Moisture Lotion for Normal/Combination Skin—SPF 6 *($7 for 3 ounces)* is mostly water, glycerin, thickeners, mineral oil, thickener, petrolatum, preservatives, more thickeners, and then a long list of additional ingredients such as herb extracts and water binding ingredients that are really inconsequential, since they come after the preservatives.

Daily Revival Oil-Free Moisture Lotion—SPF 6 *($7.50 for 3 ounces)* is indeed oil-free, but it contains a lot of alcohol (the second ingredient), which is very drying and irritating. Calling this product a moisturizer is a joke.

Daily Revival Fragrance-Free Moisture Lotion—SPF 6 *($7 for 3 ounces)* contains water, glycerin, thickeners, mineral oil, stabilizer, more thickeners, petrolatum, preservatives, more thickeners, and more preservatives. After the preservatives is a long list of herb extracts and water binding ingredients in amounts too minute to be significant. This is not a great moisturizer; it would work for people with normal skin, but why would they need it, particularly given the small amount of sunscreen?

Daily Revival Super Moisture Creme for Dry Skin—SPF 6 *($7.50 for 2.5 ounces)* contains water, thickener, grape oil, sunflower oil, glycerin, thickeners, stabilizer, preservative, skin soother, more thickeners, and a long list of herb extracts, liposomes, water binding agent, and vitamins A, B, and E (antioxidants) at the end of the ingredient list and almost too insignificant to make a difference. This is a very emollient and rich moisturizer for dry skin. It could be excellent as a nighttime moisturizer, but may be too emollient under makeup.

Daily Revival Eye Care Creme *($6.50 for 0.5 ounce)* contains water; slip agents; thickeners; mineral oil; more thickeners; grape oil; more thickeners; squalane (shark oil); thickener; herb extracts; liposomes; vitamins A, B, and C (antioxidants); water binding agent; vitamin E (antioxidant); and preservatives. An excellent moisturizer for normal to dry skin, for the entire face and not just the eyes. What a shame there is only 0.5 ounce. Ignore the name, which incorrectly discourages use all over the face.

Maximum Moisture Super Hydrating Complex *($9.50 for 2 ounces)* is not a great moisturizer. Calling it super hydrating is misleading. It contains a strange list of ingredients, including a tiny amount of sunscreen; cornstarch, which can be drying; lots of thickeners; preservatives listed toward the top of a long list of ingredients; and quaternium-15, a particularly irritating preservative that comes before some of the more important ingredients that would be more helpful to the skin. A few herb oils are nice, but not enough to make up for the rest.

Cellulite Contour Beauty Treatment *($8.50 for 6 ounces)* doesn't really deserve an evaluation, right? It won't do a thing to affect cellulite, right? It isn't worth the money at any price. This mediocre moisturizer contains mostly glycerin and mineral oil, with lots of thickeners and fragrance and preservatives too high up in the ingredient list, but that's about it.

Banishing Cream Skin Lightener with Sunscreen *($6 for 3 ounces)* is a mediocre moisturizer composed mostly of petrolatum. PABA, the sunscreen, is rarely used anymore because of the high risk of skin irritation. It also contains hydroquinone, a very caustic ingredient that supposedly can lighten skin. I am skeptical about this, as I have yet to find any conclusive evidence that indicates it works. They also make a **Banishing Stick** that is slightly more emollient than the cream; it lacks the PABA sunscreen, but the same problems exist with the hydroquinone.

Shine Solution 8-hour Oil Controlling Liquid *($8 for 3 ounces)* contains mostly water, alcohol, talc, more alcohol, zinc oxide, calcium carbonate (better known as chalk), a very irritating preservative, and salicylic acid (peels the skin and is a strong irritant). This won't control oil, but it will severely irritate the skin, causing it to potentially be more oily and dried out at the same time.

Blemish Solver Medicated Touch Stick *($5.50 for 0.3 ounce)* is similar to the Shine Solution Liquid above, with all the same problems and warnings.

Eye Perfector with Liposomes *($6 for 0.6 ounce)*. Typically I like moisturizers that contain liposomes, but this rather pricey little product contains fairly irritating ingredients to place around the eye, including witch hazel (the second ingredient) and quaternium-15 (an irritating preservative). The rest of it is OK and would be a good lightweight moisturizer for the eyes if the other two ingredients weren't present.

Visible Advantage *($10 for 1 ounce)* is supposed to enliven tired, dull-looking skin. It contains mostly water, alcohol, oil-like ingredients, fragrance, some herb extracts (tea water), salicylic acid (peels the skin and is a known skin irritant), and witch hazel. There is no advantage to using this product unless dry irritated skin is an advantage.

Vertical Lip Line Smoothing Cream *($7.50 for 0.5 ounce)* contains mostly water, thickeners, petrolatum, glycolic acid, thickener, a form of vitamin A, more thickeners, a form of vitamin E, some herb extracts, and oils. This is a mini-version of Avon's Anew for the Face. You don't need this extra product; simply use Avon's Anew around your lips. It won't erase the lines, but it can feel smoother.

Pore Reducer Beauty Treatment Mask *($6.95 for 3 ounces)* is basically a clay mask (bentonite) that contains alcohol and rice starch with some glycerin. It won't reduce pores—nothing can do that—but it can dry out and irritate the skin.

Skin Refiner and Gentle Action Scrub *($7 for 2 ounces)* contains mostly water, vegetable oil, mineral oil, thickener, alcohol, beeswax, glycerin, more thickeners, and aluminum silicate as the scrub particles. This product would be fairly greasy and the alcohol could irritate the skin.

Dramatic Firming Cream for Face and Throat *($10 for 1.5 ounces)* is an OK moisturizer for dry skin. It won't firm anything, the ingredients are mediocre, and the price is fairly high for the amount you get. It contains mostly water, thickeners, apricot oil, arnica oil, wax, more thickeners, and preservatives.

BioAdvance Skin Lotion and Fortifier *($17 for 0.85 ounce of the skin lotion and 0.12 ounce of the fortifier)* are two separate components of one product you mix together. Why it doesn't come premixed is strange: there is nothing about the ingredients that can't work together, although the instructions suggest you should purchase a new supply every month. Obviously you're supposed to believe the miraculous properties of this line minimizer are destroyed over time. The ingredients don't bear this out—there's enough preservative in here to make it last for quite a while. The fortifier contains a form of coconut oil, alcohol, thickener, several forms of vitamin A, vegetable oil, and preservatives. The lotion contains water, a form of acrylate (a strong thickening agent), petrolatum, preservative, more thickeners, and preservatives. It seems the only thing unique about this is the vitamin A, but that can't change a wrinkle, and the alcohol can irritate the skin.

BioAdvance 2000 Skin Lotion and Fortifier *($20 for 0.85 ounce of the skin lotion and 0.12 ounce of the fortifier).* For all intents and purposes this product is identical to the BioAdvance product above. The 2000 version is supposed to be for older skin. They should have at least changed the ingredient list to be more convincing about this really being a different product.

Moisture Shield SPF 15 *($9.50 for 1.5 ounces)* is a very expensive (given the amount you get) but standard chemical sunscreen with a good SPF rating. Petrolatum and alcohol are high up in the ingredient list, a confusing combination for most skin types.

Collagen Booster *($10 for 0.85 ounce)* is a very misleading name. First, you can't boost collagen from the outside in with any cosmetic; second, the main ingredient is alcohol, which makes this product quite irritating and drying; and third, the last ingredient is collagen, which means there isn't much in here. This product is a waste of money.

Advanced Night Support *($10 for 0.85 ounce)* contains water; a form of acrylate; thickener; standard water binding ingredients; vitamins A, B, C, and E; and vegetable oil. It also contains quaternium-15, an irritating preservative. If you believe these vitamins will do something for your face, go ahead, but a lot of other products contain them for a lot less and they're based in a nice emollient. This one isn't.

Nurtura Replenishing Cream *($7 for 2 ounces)* is actually a good moisturizer for dry skin! Basically it contains water, vegetable oils, glycerin, several thickeners, a small amount of sunscreen, and preservatives. It isn't great, but it's one of the better moisturizers in Avon's product line.

Avon Moisture Therapy Body Lotion *($4.49 for 7 ounces)* is a very good moisturizer for dry skin that could easily be used on the face. It contains mostly water, mineral oil, thickeners, rice oil, lanolin oil, more thickeners, and preservatives.

Skin So Soft Hand and Body Lotion *($3.45 for 8 ounces)* is a mediocre moisturizer that contains mostly water and thickeners and absolutely no oils or emollients. It is reputed to keep mosquitoes off the skin (although Avon does not endorse this use). It didn't work for me up in Alaska (where it is sold on the roadside as an insect repellent). It also didn't do anything for my dry skin.

Skin So Soft Bath Oil *($9.99 for 16 ounces)* is just mineral oil with some standard cosmetic slip agents, fragrance, and preservatives. You could buy mineral oil for less and use your favorite cologne instead.

Avon Essentials Skin Balancing Lotion *($4.99 for 3 ounces)* contains mostly water, thickeners, sunflower oil, more thickeners, vitamin E, more thickeners, and preservatives. It won't balance anything, but it would be a mediocre to OK moisturizer.

Avon Essentials Hand and Body Lotion *($4.99 for 8 ounces)* is actually a decent moisturizer and can be used on the face for dry skin. It contains water, thickeners, petrolatum, apricot oil, more thickeners, vitamin E, more thickeners, castor oil, more thickeners, and preservatives.

Vita Moist Face Cream *($2.99 for 3.5 ounces)* is an OK moisturizer for dry skin. It contains mostly water, mineral oil, thickeners, petrolatum, more thickeners, and preservatives.

Rich Moisture Face Cream *($4.79 for 7 ounces)* has alcohol listed as the third ingredient. No one could confuse alcohol as being anything but drying, right? How could Avon have missed the obvious.

Avon Clearskin Antibacterial Scrub *($2.99 for 2.5 ounces)* contains mostly water, slip agent, vegetable oil, mineral oil, thickener, glycerin, more thickener, alcohol, detergent cleanser, menthol, and a blue salt coloring agent. As a scrub it is OK, but the oils are not great for anyone with oily skin, and the menthol and alcohol are irritating.

Avon Clearskin Maximum Strength Cleansing Pads *($3.49 for 42 pads)* contains salicylic acid (skin irritant and peeling agent), water, alcohol, witch hazel (skin irritant), an antiseptic, preservative, fragrance, menthol (skin irritant), aloe, and vitamin E. Too strong and drying for most skin types, particularly in association with any of the other Clearskin products.

Avon Clearskin Astringent Cleansing Lotion *($3.49 for 8 ounces)* contains alcohol, antiseptic (can be irritating), water, slip agents, antiseptic (can be irritating), isopropyl myristate (can cause breakouts), and coloring agent. This is too drying and irritating for most skin types; the inclusion of isopropyl myristate is a mystery.

Avon Clearskin Foaming Facial Cleanser *($3.29 for 4 ounces)* contains water, detergent cleansers, coloring agent, preservatives, salt (skin irritant), and menthol (skin irritant). Can be irritating for most skin types, but may be OK for younger skin.

Avon Clearskin Clarifying Mask *($3.49 for 3 ounces)* contains water, a cosmetic plastic, alcohol, an ingredient that turns the mask hard, preservative, and coloring agent. Just a drying mask that can cause more problems for skin.

Avon Clearskin Vanishing Cream *($3.39 for 0.75 ounce)* contains water, slip agent, thickener, preservative, sodium hydroxide (caustic detergent), and benzoyl peroxide (suspected carcinogen). Too strong for most skin types, and I do not recommend using benzoyl peroxide.

Avon Clearskin Overnight Acne Treatment *($3.49 for 2 ounces)* contains salicylic acid (skin irritant and peeling agent), water, alcohol, and thickeners. It will peel the skin and dry it out terribly. Not a great thing to wake up to in the morning.

Basis

Basis Facial Cleanser *($5.50 for 8 ounces)* is a standard detergent cleanser that contains sodium hydroxide. This would be drying and possibly irritating for most skin types.

Basis Intensive Hydrating Oil *($5.50 for 8 ounces)* contains mostly mineral oil, avocado oil, and preservative. This would be a good oil for extremely dry skin, but it is not hydrating.

Basis Overnight Recovery Creme *($7 for 1.6 ounces)* contains mostly water, mineral oil, petrolatum, glycerin, thickeners, AHA, and more thickeners. This is an OK moisturizer for dry skin, but it is not a good AHA product because of the low percentage of AHA.

Basis Soap for Combination Skin *($2 for 3 ounces)* is a standard bar soap with the addition of clay and petrolatum. The petrolatum cannot overcome the irritation caused by the soap, and the clay would be even more drying for already dry areas of the face.

Basis Soap for Normal to Dry Skin *($2 for 3 ounces)* is almost identical to the Combination Skin soap but minus the clay. This standard bar soap is too drying and irritating for most skin types, in particular dry skin.

Basis Soap for Sensitive Skin *($2 for 3 ounces)* is almost identical to the previous two soaps. Like most soaps it is irritating for most skin types and it is one of the last things I would recommend for sensitive skin.

Beauty Without Cruelty

Many companies proudly boast that they do not test their products on animals. However, it isn't often clear whether or not the products contain animal ingredients or whether the ingredients individually were ever tested on animals. Some companies, including The Body Shop, have a self-imposed five-year "grandfather clause," which means that they will use ingredients previously tested on animals as long as the testing took place five years prior to the date the raw ingredient was purchased. Beauty Without Cruelty is one of the few companies with a strict, rigorously defined position concerning animal testing. None of their products are tested on animals, they contain no animal by-products, and none of the ingredients they use has been tested on animals since 1965. The ethics of this company in this regard are admirable. Their moisturizers (and prices) are quite good, and they are now being carried in drugstores such as PayLess and Drug Emporium. You can also order direct by calling (707) 769-5120. Beauty Without Cruelty may be something to take a look at for those particularly interested in truly cruelty-free cosmetics.

Aloe and Olive Cleansing Cream *($5.83 for 8 ounces)* is a fairly standard wipe-off cleanser that can leave the face feeling fairly greasy. It contains mostly water; thickeners; coconut oil; a humectant (propylene glycol, which can be irritating); olive oil; aloe vera (listed as a moisturizing ingredient; it is no more moisturizing than water, but it can soothe skin); thickeners; vitamins A, E, and D; some herbs; and preservatives.

Foaming Herbal Face Wash *($4.49 for 8 ounces)* is OK but it can be quite drying. It contains a small amount of balm mint and peppermint oil, which can burn the eyes and irritate sensitive skin types.

Lemon and Sage Cleansing Emulsion *($5.83 for 8 ounces)* is an OK water-soluble cleanser. However, it does leave a slight film on the skin and the lemon oil can irritate the eyes.

Gentle Herbal Face Wash *($4.49 for 8 ounces)* is a good face wash. It can be drying for some skin types, but overall would be a consideration for someone with oily skin.

Gentle Loofah Face Scrub *($4.50 for 5 ounces)* isn't what I would call gentle. It contains mostly water, walnut shells, detergent cleanser, thickeners, loofah powder (which is more scrubbing material), thickeners, herbs, and preservatives. It would work as a scrub, but it would also be quite drying and irritating for many skin types.

Camomile Freshener (Alcohol-free) *($4.49 for 8 ounces)* contains water, witch hazel (which can be an irritant and does contain some alcohol), aloe vera, a humectant (propylene glycol, which can be irritating), a cleansing agent, menthol and camphor (both can irritate the skin), herbs, and preservative. The name makes it sound gentle, but there is actually very little chamomile in this product and many of the ingredients can be irritating.

Cool Peppermint Freshener (Alcohol-free) *($4.50 for 8 ounces)* is almost identical to the Camomile Freshener above except for the addition of peppermint, which can be a skin irritant.

Oil-Free Hand and Body Lotion *($4.50 for 16 ounces)* contains mostly water, aloe vera, glycerin, thickeners, vitamin E, a soothing agent, herbs, and preservatives. This wouldn't be great for dry skin, but it would be soothing and lightweight.

Oil-Free Hydrator with NaPCA *($4.99 for 4 ounces)* is a lightweight moisturizer that contains water, NaPCA (a water binding ingredient), humectant (glycerin), thickener, cocoa butter, and preservatives. This would be good for dry skin, but the cocoa butter can cause breakouts in certain skin types.

Aloe and E Moisture Cream *($6.25 for 2 ounces)* is a good emollient moisturizer, best for someone with dry skin. It contains mostly water, glycerin, safflower oil, thickeners, vitamin E, a water binding agent, almond oil, more vitamin E, herbs, vitamins A and D, a small amount of sunscreen (but not enough to protect the skin adequately), and preservatives.

Oil-Free Moisturizer *($6.32 for 2 ounces)* is mostly water, humectant (propylene glycol, which can be irritating), thickener, a water binding agent, vitamin B$_6$, thickener, vitamin E, thickener, a soothing agent, liquified protein (a water binding agent), vitamins A and D, herbs, a small amount of sunscreen, and preservatives. This would be a good lightweight moisturizer, but there isn't enough sunscreen to protect the skin adequately.

Oil-Regulating Lotion—Natural Oil Control *($4.99 for 4 ounces)* contains water; aloe vera; a humectant (propylene glycol, which can be an irritant); thickeners; vitamin E; a soothing agent; liquified protein; water binding agent; vitamins E, A, and D; and preservatives. It can't decrease oil production, and the thickeners can cause breakouts. However, it could be considered a lightweight moisturizer for someone with normal to combination skin.

Preventative Age Cream *($7.29 for 2.2 ounces)* contains almost all the same ingredients as many of the above moisturizers. Why aren't any of those advertised as preventing aging? And the other ones are cheaper, too. If you claim a product prevents aging, I guess there are those who are willing to pay more for it.

Purifying Clay and Rye Flour Mask *($4.99 for 2.5 ounces)* contains water, glycerin, zinc oxide, clay, rye flour, more clay (from Jordan—Jordanian clay is not better than clay from anywhere else), thickener, herbs, vitamin E, live yeast, and preservatives. This heavy, thick mask won't purify anything, and there isn't enough yeast in it to raise a doughnut.

The Body Shop

Pineapple Facial Wash *($9.70 for 3.5 ounces)* is an OK water-soluble cleanser that can take off all the makeup but leaves a slightly greasy film on the face.

Viennese Chalk Facial Wash *($5.75 for 2.5 ounces)* contains calcium carbonate (chalk), thickener, water, lanolin, and fragrance. The chalk is supposed to exfoliate, but it doesn't rinse off very well, nor does the lanolin. This could really clog pores in many skin types, and it doesn't remove makeup very well at all.

Milk Protein Cleansing Bar *($5.95 for 3.5 ounces)* is actually a fairly gentle cleanser for a bar, but the coloring agents listed are not for use around the eyes, so I would not recommend this product to be used on the face at all.

Aloe Face Soap *($3.70 for 3.5 ounces)* is a standard soap that also contains aloe vera. It can still be drying and irritating for most skin types.

Cucumber Cleansing Milk *($4.90 for 4.2 ounces)* contains mostly water, glycerin, mineral oil, thickeners, cucumber extract, and lanolin. It must be wiped off with either a washcloth or tissue. It definitely leaves a greasy residue on the skin. This product also contains 2-bromo-2-nitropane-1, 3 diol and triethanolamine, which is believed to be a carcinogenic combination.

Passion Fruit Cleansing Gel *($4.90 for 4.2 ounces)* is an OK water-soluble cleanser that can be slightly irritating to sensitive or dry skin types.

Orchid Oil Cleansing Milk *($4.90 for 4.2 ounces)* contains mostly water, rosewater, sweet almond oil, and oil of orchid. This cleanser must be wiped off with a washcloth or tissue and leaves a greasy residue on the skin.

Glycerin & Oatmeal Facial Lather *($7.75 for 1.7 ounces)* is an OK water-soluble cleanser, however, it does contain sodium hydroxide, which can be very drying and irritating to the skin.

Blue Corn Cleansing Cream *($9.95 for 3.5 ounces)* is an oil-based cleanser that is not water soluble. It leaves a film on the skin and needs a washcloth to remove all traces of makeup. It does contain blue corn tea, but that won't help clean the face. (The blue corn is purchased from Santa Ana, Mexico, in a trade agreement that helped the town buy a new grinding mill. The arrangement is commendable, but there is nothing about blue corn that improves a cosmetic or makes it better for the skin.)

Blue Corn Scrub Mask *($9.95 for 4.3 ounces)* contains mostly water, clay, blue corn powder, thickener, glycerin, alcohol, preservative, alcohol, preservatives, and oils. This is a fairly drying scrub that doesn't rinse off very well.

Blue Corn Water *($5 for 4.2 ounces)* contains mostly water, alcohol, blue corn tea, watermelon juice, slip agent, and preservative. The alcohol makes it too irritating for most skin types.

Blue Corn Lotion *($6.55 for 4.2 ounces)* contains mostly water, oil, blue corn tea, thickeners, glycerin, more thickener, standard water binding agent, and preservatives. This is a good lightweight moisturizer for normal to dry skin.

Orange Flower Water *($5 for 4.2 ounces)* is a toner that contains mostly orange-flower water, but second in the ingredient list is a preservative that is considered to be a problem in cosmetics.

Elderflower Water *($5 for 4.2 ounces)* is a toner containing mostly water, alcohol, castor oil, and elderflower extract. The alcohol makes it too irritating for most skin types.

Honey Water *($5 for 4.2 ounces)* is an irritant-free toner that contains mostly rosewater and preservatives. The amount of preservatives should not be a problem for most skin types.

Aloe Vera Moisture Cream *($8.15 for 1.7 ounces)* is a rich cream containing mostly water, almond oil, glycerin, cocoa butter, thickeners, and aloe vera extract. It should take good care of very dry skin.

Carrot Moisture Cream *($9.40 for 1.8 ounces)* is only for skin types that do not break out. The second ingredient in this cream is isopropyl myristate, which can cause blackheads. Otherwise, this is a lightweight cream that contains water, almond oil, glycerin, thickeners, and carrot oil.

Carrot Facial Oil *($6.90 for 1 ounce)* contains almond oil, hypercium oil (which can cause problems when exposed to the sun), carrot oil, flower oil, wheat germ oil, and olive oil. This would be a great combination of oils if the hypercium oil wasn't so high up on the ingredient list.

Jojoba Moisture Cream *($12.10 for 1.6 ounces)* is only for skin types that do not break out. The second ingredient in this cream is isopropyl myristate, which can cause blackheads. Other than that, this is a rich cream that contains water, jojoba oil, wheat germ oil, thickener, and glycerin, and would be good for dry skin.

Sage Comfrey Open Pore Cream *($7.75 for 1.7 ounces)* contains mostly water, alcohol, witch hazel, and comfrey and sage extract. The alcohol and witch hazel make it too irritating for most skin types.

Glycerin & Rosewater Lotion with Vitamin E *($3.40 for 2 ounces)* is only for skin types that do not break out. The second ingredient in this cream is isopropyl myristate, which can cause blackheads. Other than that, this lightweight, emollient moisturizer contains water, mineral oil, polawax, glycerin, and wheat germ oil. It would be good for someone with very dry skin.

Dewberry 5 Oils Lotion *($6.55 for 4.2 ounces)* contains mostly water, glycerin, thickener, several plant oils, thickener, standard water binding agent, thickeners, and preservative. This is an excellent group of oils and would be great for someone with very dry skin.

White Musk Lotion *($6.55 for 4.2 ounces)* is a lightweight, emollient moisturizer containing mostly water, sweet almond oil, coconut oil, thickener, cocoa butter, and glycerin. It should work well for very dry skin.

Aloe Lotion *($6.55 for 4.2 ounces)* is a rich, extremely emollient moisturizer that contains aloe vera gel, water, wheat germ oil, apricot kernel oil, wax, and water binding agent.

Elderflower Under Eye Gel *($5.95 for 0.4 ounce)* contains elderflower water, witch hazel, glycerin, alcohol, thickener, and preservatives. Witch hazel and alcohol are too irritating to place around the delicate skin of the eye. This ingredient list makes no sense.

Parsley & Mint Face Mask *($9.95 for 3.5 ounces)* contains mostly water, slip agent, alcohol, burdock root (possible irritant), thickeners, chamomile tea, soothing agent, parsley, and preservatives. There's not much parsley in here, but there is alcohol, and that is drying and irritating.

Peanut & Rosehip Face Mask *($9.95 for 3.4 ounces)* contains mostly water, peanut oil, thickeners, glycerin, more thickeners, rose hip pulp, more thickeners, and preservatives. This would be a comfortable facial mask for someone with dry skin.

Under Eye Cream *($6.05 for 0.5 ounce)*. This tiny jar of cream contains mostly water, wax, thickener, rice bran oil, cocoa butter, thickeners, and preservatives. It would be good for someone with dry skin.

Unfragranced Lotion *($6.55 for 4.2 ounces)* is a good lightweight moisturizer for normal to dry skin.It contains water, babassu oil, thickener, glycerin, more thickeners, soothing agent, macadamia nut oil, and preservatives. Babassu oil is similar to palm oil and not anything unique for the skin.

Borghese

Spa Comforting Cleanser *($28.50 for 6.75 ounces)* is an OK water-soluble cleanser that contains mineral oil as one of the first ingredients, so it won't rinse well without a washcloth or tissue. The long ingredient list has all the latest water binding agents, oils, and mineral salts, but they won't help or clean the skin when they're down that far in the list.

Gentle Cleanser Exfoliant *($22 for 2 ounces)* would be a lot more gentle if it didn't contain peppermint oil, which can burn the skin. However, there are plenty of emollients that can soothe the skin and make this cleanser hard to rinse off.

Spa-Soothing Tonic for Sensitive Skin *($25 for 8.4 ounces)* contains mostly water, thickener, slip agent, plant extracts, water binding agents, mineral salts, slip agents, plant oils, and preservatives. This is a soothing irritant-free toner, but because of the oils it is best for normal to dry skin tones.

Gel Delicato *($24 for 7.5 ounces)* contains mostly water, slip agent, several detergent cleansers, and a tiny amount of mineral salts, plant extracts, thickeners, and preservatives. It will definitely take off the makeup, but the detergent cleansers can be harsh on the eyes.

Stimulating Tonic *($25 for 8 ounces)* is a toner that contains mostly water, alcohol, talc, slip agent, and mineral salts. This is a lot of money for alcohol and salt. It would be irritating for most skin types.

Anti-Stress Restorative Creme for Sensitive Skin *($47.50 for 1.3 ounces)* contains mostly water, thickener, standard water binding agents, thickeners, mineral salts, standard water binding agents, more thickeners, plant extracts (tea), good water binding agent, plant oils, more thickeners, and preservatives. It is an OK moisturizer for normal to dry skin, but most of the good ingredients are far down on the list and for this kind of money they should be at the top.

Equalizing Restorative SPF 4 *($37.50 for 1.7 ounces)* contains mostly water, standard water binding agents, a long list of thickeners, mineral salts, plant extacts, more thickeners, vitamin E, plant oils, and preservatives. This is really only a good, but ordinary, moisturizer. The possibly interesting ingredients are down at the end of the ingredient list and don't account for much.

Daily Skin Energy Source *($40 for 1.5 ounces)* contains mostly water, standard water binding agent, thickener, glycerin, more thickeners, petrolatum, more thickeners, amino acids, water binding agents, mineral salts, and vitamins A, C, and E. The rest of the ingredient list goes on for so long that I can't imagine there is even a scant drop of them in here. The first ingredients are just ordinary, and the good stuff is so far down as to be negligible. This is a good moisturizer for normal to dry skin, but there is no energy to be found in here.

Moisture Intensifier *($65 for 1.7 ounces)* contains mostly water, a form of mineral oil, butylene glycol, mineral oil, propylene glycol, mineral salts, and flower oils. This is a lot of money for a very basic lightweight moisturizer. It doesn't even contain any of the latest fad moisturizing ingredients.

Fango Active Mud for Face and Body *($50 for 18 ounces)* is a large jar of mud. The brochure for this jar of clay described it as "Fango Therapy of Montecantini." Montecantini is supposedly some kind of special volcanic clay. The product actually contains water, bentonite (a white clay found in the United States), and a much smaller amount of Montecantini clay. It also contains some mineral salts and some plant oils. It does feel good when you take it off, but that's about it, and dry skin types may find the drying effects of the clay too irritating. As a side note, the special clay from Italy isn't even the main type of mud used, although clay from the good old U.S.A. is the second ingredient. Regardless of whose clay it is, this is a lot of money for mud. There are cheaper clay masks that would do exactly the same thing.

Spa Energizing Moisture Mask for Face and Body *($30 for 8 ounces)* contains mostly water, thickeners, mineral oil, standard water binding agents, more thickeners, eucalyptus oil, menthol, peppermint oil, mineral salts, good water binding agents, thickeners, and preservative. The menthol and eucalyptus and peppermint oils are skin irritants. If your skin isn't sensitive, this could feel quite good on the skin.

Spa Eye Energizing Mask *($22 for 1.7 ounces)* contains mostly water, thickener, standard water binding agents, more thickeners, mineral salts, more thickeners, a nucleic acid, more thickeners, comfrey, standard water binding agent, thickener, vitamins A and E, water binding agents, and preservatives. Once again, most of the good stuff is listed far down in the ingredient list and there is nothing energizing about any of the ingredients.

Spa Lift for Face SPF 8 *($40 for 1.7 ounces)* contains water, slip agent, several thickeners, standard water binding agents, amino acids, vitamins A and E, collagen, thickeners, shark oil, water binding agents, plant oils, and preservatives. This is a good emollient moisturizer with a small amount of sunscreen. It won't lift the face anywhere, but it is a good moisturizer

Spa Lift For Eyes *($40 for 0.9 ounce)* contains mostly water, thickener, standard water binding agents, thickener, mineral salts, soybean oil, collagen, herb extracts (teas), vitamin E, water binding agents, and preservatives. This is nothing more than a good lightweight moisturizer for the eyes, but the price is likely to hurt your vision. Once again, the really interesting ingredients are far down in the ingredient list.

Reenergizing Night Creme *($47.50 for 1.85 ounces)* contains mostly water, several thickeners, standard water binding agents, mineral salts, water binding agents, vitamins A and D, plant oils, soothing agents, water binding agent, more thickeners, and preservatives. This is a good emollient moisturizer for normal to dry skin, but most of the stuff you think you're paying for is at the end of the ingredient list, so it isn't quite as exotic as they want you to believe.

Nighttime Restorative *($55 for 1.8 ounces)* contains mostly water, standard water binding agents, thickeners (including isopropyl myristate, which can cause blackheads), olive oil, sesame oil, apricot seed oil, thickener, water binding agents, vitamin E, mineral salts, more plant oils, thickeners, and preservatives. This is a very good emollient moisturizer for someone with dry skin. The oils and water binding agents are what makes it good; the mineral salts are Borghese's gimmick, nothing more.

"Living Water" Serum *($60 for 1 ounce)* contains mostly water, thickener, mineral oil, standard water binding agents, mineral salts, and water binding agent. This one is beyond me. Mineral oil, standard humectants that you find in a thousand other products, and mineral salts, and it costs $60 for an eyedropper full! What a waste.

Chanel

Cleansing Milk *($30 for 7 ounces)* contains mostly water, mineral oil, water binding agent, thickeners, wheat germ oil, more thickeners, milk protein, fragrance, and preservative (2-bromo-2-nitropane-1, 3 diol, a strong potential skin irritant). It won't rinse off easily without the help of a washcloth, and it also contains isopropyl myristate, which can cause blackheads.

Purifying Clay Cleanser *($23.50 for 8 ounces)* contains water, clay, propylene glycol, mineral oil, and a foaming agent. Clay is not the best ingredient for a cleanser because it is hard to rinse off, and you wouldn't want to use it over the eye area. And why include mineral oil in a product that is meant to absorb excess oil?

Gentle Cleansing Bar *($22.50 for 4 ounces)* is similar to most cleansing bars because it is mostly detergent cleanser and thickener. It can be quite drying to some skin types, but is OK for a bar soap.

Foaming Gel Cleanser *($30 for 7 ounces)* is a good water-soluble foaming cleanser that takes off all the makeup without irritating the skin. There are some oils among the last ingredients, which may not be best for someone with very oily skin.

Gentle Cleansing Cream *($32 for 4 ounces)* is indeed gentle, but it won't rinse off without a washcloth, which isn't very gentle at all. Basically just an expensive wipe-off cleanser.

Gentle Exfoliating Cleanser *($27.50 for 2 ounces)* contains mostly water, mineral oil, detergent cleanser, thickeners, silica (fossil remains), more thickeners, and preservatives (one is 2-bromo-2-nitropane-1, 3 diol, a strong potential skin irritant). It is an OK scrub and somewhat gentle, but the preservative in here is a problem.

Gentle Cleansing Mask *($38.50 for 2.5 ounces)* contains water, clay, witch hazel, clay, water binding agent, thickener, yeast, thickener, more thickeners, and preservatives. Basically just a fairly expensive standard clay mask that can be somewhat drying to some skin types.

Refining Toner *($30 for 7 ounces)* contains mostly water, alcohol, witch hazel, rosewater, plant extracts, slip agents, fragrance, menthol, and preservatives. This is a standard alcohol-based toner that is probably too irritating for most skin types.

Firming Freshener *($30 for 7 ounces)* is an irritant-free toner that contains mostly water, standard water binding agents, lanolin oil, cucumber extract, slip agents, antioxidant, and preservative. This should feel soothing and moist on dry skin if you are not allergic to lanolin.

Total Protection Moisture Cream SPF 15 *($60 for 2.5 ounces)* is an overpriced sunscreen/moisturizer that contains standard cosmetic ingredients of water, thickener, water binding agents, oil, more thickeners, preservatives, and amino acids. It also contains a preservative that is considered a serious problem for skin.

Hydra Systeme Maximum Moisturizing Lotion *($35 for 1 ounce)* has an SPF of 8, which isn't enough to protect you from the sun. It contains water, butylene glycol, and a good soothing agent. There are also two moisturizing ingredients that are supposed to be unique to Chanel. I found no information to suggest these do anything other than retain moisture in the skin, which is good, but not unique.

Firming Eye Cream *($45 for 0.5 ounce)* is an overpriced moisturizer that contains mostly water, rosewater, oil, a long list of thickeners, and preservatives. There is nothing in this cream that can "firm" the skin, but it is a good moisturizer.

Skin Recovery Cream *($90 for 1 ounce)* is an expensive farce. The "recovery" is attributed to the second ingredient in this cream, which is amniotic fluid. I would disagree with any claims about amniotic fluid doing anything special for the skin. The other ingredients are a huge long list of fairly standard cosmetic ingredients, including water, water binding agents, thickeners, protein, amino acids, and oils, just like all the other Chanel products. It is a good moisturizer, but not because of the amniotic fluid and amino acids. The price is what you would really need to recover from at $1,440 a pound.

Day Lift Refining Complex SPF 8 *($45 for 1 ounce)* is Chanel's answer to the alpha hydroxy acid craze, although the company is not forthcoming about the percentage used in their product. When cosmetics companies keep the percentage of AHA a secret, it is always because the amount is usually well under 2 percent (the crucial amount is 8 percent to 15 percent). Nevertheless, this is a very good emollient (although very expensive) AHA product that also contains an SPF of 8, not great, but better than nothing. This product is loaded with a ton of water binding agents. It contains mostly water, thickener, jojoba oil, water binding agents, thickeners, vegetable oil, thickeners, several water binding agents, protein, plant extracts, vitamin E, aloe, several more water binding agents, vitamin A, and preservatives.

Night Lift Cream *($62.50 for 1.7 ounces)* contains mostly water, thickener, water binding agents, macadamia nut oil, protein, thickeners, protein, jojoba oil, more thickeners, herb tea, more thickeners, palm oil, more thickeners, vitamin A, amino acids, fats, and preservatives. This is a good moisturizer, but it won't lift the skin anywhere. Amino acids in a product cannot affect the structure of the skin.

Prevention Serum *($52 for 1.35 ounces)* contains a good sunscreen with an SPF of 15 and mostly water, standard water binding agents, thickeners, protein, more thickeners, collagen, more thickeners, plant extracts, water binding ingredients, and preservatives. This is a lot of money for a fairly basic sunscreen/moisturizer. Its claim to be recommended by the Skin Cancer Foundation is not unique—all sunscreens with a high SPF rating are recommended by most medical associations.

Lift Serum Corrective Complex *($67.50 for 1 ounce)* claims that "independent tests confirm up to 45 percent reduction in the appearance of visible lines and wrinkles after one month's regular use." They follow this with a surprisingly honest assertion: "Each skin is different. You may achieve lesser or even greater results." Greater results can probably happen if your skin is totally parched and you've never used a moisturizer before in your life; but then the results would be the same no matter what moisturizer you used. This product contains some good water binding ingredients, including protein and collagen, but it also has a long list of standard cosmetic thickeners and water binding agents. At more than $1,080 for a pound of this stuff, it should lift your face anyplace you want it to go.

Environmental Purifying Mask *($38.50 for 2 ounces)* contains mostly water, alcohol, thickeners, vitamin E, thickener, herb extracts (tea), vitamin C, and preservative. This won't purify anything, and the alcohol can be irritating to the skin.

Maximum Moisture Mask *($38.50 for 2.5 ounces)* has an SPF of 8 and contains mostly water; mineral oil; a long list of thickeners; water binding agent; fragrance; a group of amino acids; vitamins E, A, and C; and preservatives. A rather unimpressive list of moisturizing ingredients. Amino acids sound good, but can't do much for the skin, and they certainly can't affect the amino acids in the skin cell.

Natural Exfoliating Mask *($38.50 for 2.5 ounces)* contains petrolatum, lanolin, thickener, silica, thickeners, preservative, chalk, and coloring agents. This is a fairly greasy, thick mask. It could possibly be OK for someone with very dry skin who isn't allergic to lanolin.

Charles of the Ritz

Revenescence Liquid *($32 for 4 ounces)* contains mostly water, water binding agent, wax, detergent cleanser, thickener, and preservatives. This is a good water-soluble cleanser for normal to dry skin only, but it can leave a slight film on the face.

Moisture Cream Cleanser *($18.50 for 4 ounces)* is a standard oil-based cleanser that requires a washcloth or tissue to remove all of it.

Revenescence Softening Lotion *($17.50 for 8 ounces)* contains mostly water, alcohol, slip agents, menthol, more slip agents, and preservatives. This is a standard alcohol-based toner that can irritate the skin.

Revenescence 100% Alcohol Free *($17.50 for 8 ounces)* is indeed alcohol-free, but it isn't irritant-free. The third ingredient is potassium chloride, which can be a skin irritant.

Revenescence Moist Environment Night Treatment *($38.50 for 2.2 ounces)* contains mostly water, isopropyl myristate (can cause blackheads), petrolatum, a long list of thickeners, glycerin, water binding agent, and preservatives. This is an OK moisturizer for dry skin.

Special Formula Emollient *($27 for 4 ounces)* isn't anything all that special, but it is a good emollient moisturizer for extremely dry skin. It contains mostly water, lanolin, petrolatum, standard water binding agent, thickeners, and preservatives.

Moisture Intensive Facial .*($20 for 4 ounces)* contains mostly water, thickeners, standard water binding agent, oil, more thickeners, water binding ingredients, menthol, more thickeners, sage, almond oil, and preservatives. I wouldn't call this intense moisture, but it is a good moisturizer.

Revenescence Cream *($30 for 2.2 ounces)* is a very emollient moisturizer for extremely dry skin. It contains mostly water, water binding agent, mineral oil, lanolin, waxes, thickener, fragrance, and preservative.

Age Zone Controller *($30 for 0.8 ounce)* contains mostly water, standard water binding agents, thickeners, collagen, soothing agent, thickeners, and preservatives. This is a lot of money for standard cosmetic ingredients and some collagen. Collagen is only one of many good moisturizing ingredients, and many products contain it. This is too expensive for the amount you get.

Timeless Essence Night Recovery Cream *($35 for 1.7 ounces)* contains mostly water, standard water binding agents, mineral oil, thickeners, oil, more thickeners, vitamin E, almond oil, fragrance, and preservatives. This is a good moisturizer for normal to dry skin, but it isn't timeless and it won't help the skin recover from anything except maybe dryness, which is what most moisturizers do.

Cher's Aquasentials

Now let me get this straight. Cher—one of the few actresses in the world known by only her first name, and famous for her outrageous clothing (or lack thereof)—is now selling cosmetics on television. Cher's new "infomercial" shows her dressed in more clothes than she usually wears, ensconced in a living room set with her family and a skin-care "expert," discussing the creation of her new, simply super skin care products. If you call now, you can join Cher's Skin Care Club for the low price of $95.85 (split into three *easy* payments so you don't know how much you're really spending), which entitles you to receive seven skin care products and the opportunity to spend a lot more on a regular basis. If you don't become a member, these products would cost you $190. Is this for real? Yes, it's for real. So without further ado, let's shut off the television cameras, turn down the special lighting, throw out the natural-sounding script, and look more closely at what you are really buying from Cher's Aquasentials.

Many Aquasentials products supposedly contain a trademarked ingredient called Hydrabond 5000, but it isn't listed as such on any of their ingredient labels. I have struggled to pry loose specific information about this ingredient from the company, but all I got was an incredible runaround and a lot of double-talk instead. No one at the company seems to know where this ingredient is on the label. The supervisor told me that all she knew was what Hydrabond 5000 did: "binds water to the skin, making it look smoother and younger." Advertising rhetoric, and, moreover, nothing crucial, because many ingredients bind water to the skin. What amazes me is the complete lack of reliable information when you call most cosmetics companies. A supposedly major ingredient in these expensive products and the customer-service people don't know what it is? What kind of customer service is that? Without a listing on the ingredient label and without further information from the company, there is no way for me to evaluate it beyond their questionable claim. Now let's get to the real specifics. The first price listed is the so-called retail price, and the second price is the Skin Care Club price.

Eye Makeup Remover *($16 or $8.95 for 1.75 ounces)* is definitely gentle enough for the eye area, but it can dry the skin. It contains a fairly standard coconut oil-based cleansing agent and other water-binding ingredients. For some people, the sixth ingredient, potassium sorbate, may be an irritant.

Facial Cleanser *($15 or $8.95 for 6.7 ounces)* is almost an exact copy of Cetaphil Lotion, only more expensive. You already know how much I like Cetaphil Lotion, so my feelings are the same for this product. Only I prefer the less expensive original version.

Facial Scrub *($20 or $10.95 for 3.5 ounces)* contains mostly water, pumice, thickeners, aloe vera, more thickeners, a form of lanolin, and algae extract. Baking soda mixed with Cetaphil or Cher's Facial Cleanser will do exactly the same thing, and you won't run the risk of reacting to the lanolin. It also contains quaternium-15 fairly high up on the ingredient list, one of the most highly irritating preservatives around.

Facial Toner *($20 or $10.95 for 6.7 ounces)* contains mostly water, water binding agent, slip agent, cucumber extract, castor oil, witch hazel, herb extracts, lactic acid (small amount of AHA), and preservatives. Witch hazel can be irritating but it is far enough down in the ingredient list that it might not be a problem for some skin types. This could be a good irritant-free toner for someone with normal to oily skin.

Continuous Release Moisturizer *($35 or $18.95 for 1.5 ounces)* is a good, lightweight moisturizer for normal to slightly dry skin. It contains mostly water, several thickeners, glycerin, a vegetable oil, more thickeners, preservatives, and more oils. It also contains isopropyl myristate, an ingredient suspected of causing blackheads.

Revitalizing Mask *($35 or $19.95 for 3.5 ounces)* is mostly water, aloe vera, thickeners, clay, chamomile, gelatin, preservatives, more thickeners, slip agents, and a coloring agent. Supposedly this is the product that Cher fell in love with, causing her to purchase the entire line. Well, I guess aloe vera, clay, and chamomile can do wonders for some people, but other than drying the skin and temporarily tightening it, as all other clay masks do, I can't imagine what.

Revitalizing Lift *($29 or $14.95 for 1.5 ounces)* is basically a light gel that dries on the skin and tightens it. If you put on enough it will temporarily tighten the skin for up to an hour or two, but only if you don't move your face very much. It feels somewhat strange, like a layer of plastic on the face, and it can irritate the skin.

Continuous Release Fine Line Serum *($40 or $19.95 for 0.5 ounce)* is basically water, witch hazel, thickener, herb extracts, glycerin, more herbs, preservatives, thickeners, and vegetable oils. The witch hazel can irritate the skin, and the preservatives are unusually high up on the ingredient list, so they might also be irritating to the skin. The product does leave the skin feeling smoother and slightly sticky, but the price is absurdly exorbitant—about $1,280 a pound (full price), to be exact.

Continuous Release Creme Gel *($35 or $18.95 for 1.5 ounces)* is almost identical to the Fine Line Serum. The only difference is its thickness, the result of the addition of standard cosmetic thickeners.

Continuous Release Eye Cream *($40 or $21.95 for 0.5 ounce)* contains mostly water, mineral oils, thickeners, petrolatum, more thickeners, macadamia nut oil, more thickeners, and preservatives. This is a good moisturizer for dry skin, but nothing special enough to warrant the price tag and teeny amount you get.

Christian Dior

Hydra-Dior Cleansing Milk for Dry and Sensitive Skin *($34 for 8.4 ounces)* is a standard mineral oil-based cleanser that is very difficult to rinse off without the use of a washcloth, which is not great for someone with sensitive skin.

Hydra-Dior Cleanser for Oily Skin *($34 for 8.4 ounces)* contains several types of oils—not great for someone with oily skin. This doesn't rinse well, and it leaves a greasy film on the skin.

Equite Gentle Cleansing Bar *($21 for 3.5 ounces)* is a detergent cleansing bar that isn't as drying as most. It can be good for someone with normal to oily skin.

Equite Wash-Off Cleanser *($21 for 6.8 ounces)* is a standard water-soluble detergent cleanser that contains a rather strong detergent. This could be drying for most skin types. It also contains the herb gentian, which contains alcohol and can also be drying to the skin.

Equite Face and Eye Makeup Remover *($21 for 6.8 ounces)* contains mostly water, mineral oil, emulsifier, thickener, plant extract, glycerin, more thickeners, preservatives, and fragrance. It contains the preservative 2-bromo-2-nitropane-1, 3 diol, a strong potential skin irritant, and should not be used near or around the eye.

Eye Makeup Remover Gel *($18 for 2.5 ounces)* This gel contains solvents, which can indeed cut through makeup, but it isn't unique. It contains the same ingredients all eye makeup removers contain: water, polysorbate 80, and peg 20 methyl glucose sesquisterate.

Waterproof Eye Makeup Remover *($18 for 3.4 ounces)* contains mostly water, flower water, and glycerin. It does take off eye makeup, but not easily.

Equite Exfoliating Gel *($25 for 3.6 ounces)* contains mostly water, several standard water binding agents, mineral oil, thickeners, fragrance, preservatives, and, at the very end, silica. This isn't a great exfoliator with the silica so far down at the end, plus the ordinary ingredients don't warrant the steep price tag.

Equite Vitalizing Toner *($21 for 6.8 ounces)* is a standard alcohol-based toner that contains mostly water, alcohol, water binding agents, fragrance, and preservatives. It is too irritating for most skin types.

Hydra-Dior Stimulating Lotion *($34 for 8.4 ounces)* is a standard alcohol-based toner that contains mostly water, witch hazel, alcohol, rosewater, slip agents, fragrance, and preservatives. This isn't stimulating, it is irritating for almost all skin types.

Hydra-Dior Astringent Lotion *($34 for 8.4 ounces)* is a standard alcohol-based astringent that contains mostly water, alcohol, water binding agents, plant extracts, slip agents, fragrance, soothing agents, water binding agents, preservatives, and salicylic acid. The alcohol is too irritating for almost all skin types.

Hydra Dior Skin Freshener for Dry Skin *($34 for 8.4 ounces)* is a good, almost irritant-free toner that contains mostly water, rosewater, witch hazel (can be an irritant), standard water binding agent, more flower-based water, soothing agent, and preservatives. The claim is that the particular "flower waters," which are fairly standard, do special things for the skin. They don't. However, for dry skin types it may be OK, if the witch hazel isn't too irritating.

Equite Alcohol-Free Softening Toner *($21 for 6.8 ounces)* contains mostly water, standard water binding agents, chamomile extract, and preservatives. This is a simple irritant-free toner, nothing special, but good and soothing.

Hydra-Dior Eye Creme *($36 for 0.5 ounce)* claims that it can "delay the formation of wrinkles." The FDA might take issue with this kind of statement; I know I do. Unless it contains a sunscreen with an SPF of 15 or greater, there is no way this claim can be scientifically substantiated.

Hydra-Dior Extra Rich Night Cream *($50 for 0.9 ounce)* contains mostly water, isopropyl myristate (can cause blackheads), lanolin, wax, oil, glycerin, thickeners, fragrance, preservatives, soothing agents, and more preservatives. The vitamins A, C, and E are at the very end of the ingredient list and are negligible. This is a good emollient moisturizer, but the standard ingredients are shockingly overpriced at about $1,600 a pound.

Resultante Revitalizing Wrinkle Cream *($78 for 1 ounce)* contains mostly water, oil, thickeners, mineral oil, and some of the latest moisturizing ingredients farther down in the ingredient list. This is a good moisturizer, but the $78 price tag and misleading name are hard to swallow.

Capture Complex Liposome for the Eyes *($34 for 0.5 ounce)* contains mostly water, glycerin, and thickeners, plus a little animal thymus extract. I like liposomes as a skin care ingredient, although there are much less expensive moisturizers on the market that contain the same thing. Animal thymus extract has no proven abilities to do anything special for the skin, but it may simply sound good on the label.

Capture Complexe Liposomes for the Face *($70 for 1.7 ounces)* contains mostly water, glycerin, thickeners, slip agents, preservatives, and fragrance. This is a good moisturizer, and liposomes are a great way to keep moisturizer in the skin, but there are less expensive versions of this at both the drugstore and at other cosmetics counters.

Capture Lift Complexe Liposomes Night Treatment for the Face *($55 for 1 ounce)* contains mostly water, standard water binding agents, thickeners, preservatives, thickener, fragrance, and more preservatives. The preservatives are just too high up in this ingredient list, and could cause problems for sensitive skin types. All of the good stuff is too far down in the ingredient list.

Resultante Eye Care Cream *($68 for 0.5 ounce)*. For a whopping $3,264 a pound you get mostly water, isopropyl myristate (can cause blackheads), thickeners, glycerin, more thickeners, a small amount of sunscreen, wheat germ oil, elastin, collagen, fragrance, and preservatives. It contains quaternium-15, considered to be one of the most irritating preservatives. This isn't even a very good moisturizer! I'm speechless.

Resultante Throat Cream *($76 for 1 ounce)* contains mostly water, oil, thickener, mineral oil, thickeners, animal thymus extract, lanolin, more thickeners, fragrance, and preservatives. There isn't anything in here that is better for the neck than it would be for your face or elbows, and you can ignore the animal thymus—it can't do anything special for the skin.

Icone for All Types of Dryness *($44 for 1 ounce)* contains mostly water, oil, thickener, glycerin, more thickeners, sunscreen, standard water binding agents, more thickeners, water binding agent, preservative, and fragrance.

There are more ingredients after the fragrance, some of them good, but not in large enough amounts to count. This is a good but not great moisturizer, and not worth the absurd price tag.

Equite Instant Radiance Purifying Mask *($28.50 for 2.5 ounces)* contains mostly water, standard water binding agents, thickeners, preservative, fragrance, water binding agent, and more preservatives. This would be an OK mask but it contains 2-bromo-2-nitropane-1, 3 diol, a very irritating preservative.

Hydra-Dior Cleansing Masque for Oily Skin *($34 for 1.9 ounces)* contains mostly water, magnesium, clay, glycerin, thickeners, plant extracts, protein, and preservatives. A fairly standard clay mask, but less irritating than most. The herbs are thrown in to make it look like you're getting something more than clay.

Clarins

Clarins, a high-end department store cosmetics line from France, has been around for some time, but of late has gained rapid recognition. There are a couple of reasons for this increased attention, the major one being Clarins' prominent advertising campaign in fashion magazines over the past year. Clarins' packaging and merchandising also play a large role. Other department store cosmetics lines are dramatically encased in dark, slick packages or in more subtle, muted shades of gray and peach; Clarins' bright red-and-white packaging with gold trim and occasional splashes of yellow and green is a refreshing change.

Besides Clarins' stand-out packaging and French breeding (as far as Americans are concerned, Europeans always know more about skin care; in Europe, the sales pitch is how much the Americans know—it just depends which line you're selling and where), this company is also capitalizing heavily on the "botanical" craze of the '90s just like everyone else. Their ingredient lists of usual and unusual herbs, flowers, and vegetables are a veritable jungle, with the typical far-out promises that accompany these ingredients. Like Aveda, Origins, The Body Shop, Nu Skin, Saturnia, and dozens of other cosmetics lines, Clarins wants you to believe that a little herb concentrate can do wonders for your skin. According to *Rodale's Illustrated Encyclopedia of Herbs*, many of the extracts used in Clarins products (as well as other botanical-type lines) are potentially irritating. For example, according to *Rodale*, coltsfoot is potentially carcinogenic, and sage and chamomile extracts can cause skin irritation. Always keep in mind that "natural" and "good" are not the same thing; many natural things in the environment are bad for the skin. Do not be misled by the catch-all phrases "natural and pure" or "botanicals": they tell you nothing of value about the product.

The quote in one of the Clarins brochures says: "Clarins promises no miracles, only effective results [from] time-proven natural extracts." Yet claim after claim sounds like miracles. This line even has "bust firming" products. Other quotes that sound fairly miraculous to me are: "maintains firm facial features, takes advantage of the beneficial toning action of facial expressions while helping to reduce apparent slackening," and "refines skin texture, firms skin tone."

Let me make several points perfectly clear: There are no cosmetic ingredients that can do any of those things. Corn poppy, horsetail, carrot, and coltsfoot extracts are not going to do anything extraordinary to the skin when it comes to wrinkles or skin tone. (Just for your information, there is no beneficial anti-wrinkling effect from facial expressions either. Just the opposite is true; facial expressions sag the skin.) As is always true with cosmetics, the so-called *"effective"* or *"natural"* ingredients are combined with a much longer list of standard cosmetic ingredients. By the way, when I called Clarins to see if I could review any of the *"efficiency tests"* they claim prove their products' reliability, I was put on hold forever and then turned down. So much for reliability.

Despite what you may be thinking, I do like some of Clarins' products. What I am disturbed by are the exaggerated, complicated claims used to sell absurdly expensive products. They also sell more types of product than any woman should ever have to smear over her face and body. Below is a breakdown of almost all of Clarins' lengthy and rather expensive product inventory.

Gentle Facial Peeling *($24 for 1.4 ounces)* has a clay base, wax and thickeners, and a list of several herbal extracts. For the most part this is a relatively nonirritating peel, but the clay and wax ingredients can clog pores and can be quite drying.

Face Treatment Cream for Dry or Reddened Skin *($23.50 for 1.7 ounces)* is a good, although extremely expensive, emollient moisturizer that contains mostly water, mineral oil, vegetable oils, thickeners, rice bran oil, a small amount of sunscreen (not enough to protect the skin), lanolin oil, water binding agents, preservatives, and herb extracts. The least they could do is put the herb extracts before the preservatives; there are almost no herbs in this product to speak of.

Face Treatment Cream for Combination Skin Prone to Oiliness *($23.50 for 1.7 ounces)* is somewhat similar to the Face Treatment Cream for dry skin. The first and major ingredients are water, mineral oil, vegetable oils, thickeners, and a small amount of sunscreen (too small to provide adequate protection). The difference between this cream and the one for dry skin is the inclusion of witch hazel, sage, lemon, and grapefruit extracts, which can all be quite irritating to the skin. Also, someone with oily skin would not be thrilled with the amount of oil in this product, which is considerable.

Face Treatment Cream for Dehydrated Skin *($23.50 for 1.7 ounces)* is a good moisturizer for dry skin and very similar to the other two Face Treatment Creams. The first ingredients are similar except for the addition of shea butter, which is extremely emollient. The herb and vegetable extracts, which are farther down in the list, include cucumber (cools the skin) and horsetail, which has some healing properties but not in this small quantity.

Face Treatment Oil for Dry or Reddened Skin *($29 for 1.4 ounces)* contains hazelnut, sandalwood, cardamom, parsley seed, hayflower, and lavender oils. Sandalwood, parsley, and lavender oils can all cause skin irritation, which isn't great for someone with reddened skin.

Face Treatment Oil for Combination Skin Prone to Oiliness *($29 for 1.4 ounces)* contains hazelnut oil, geranium oil, fragrance, rosemary oil, lotus extract, chamomile oil, and sage oil. The claim here is that it helps balance surface oils. I got several different answers about what is meant by "balance." What the ingredients can do is add oils to the skin, and the chamomile, rosemary, and sage oil can irritate the skin. There is a high risk that someone with oily skin could end up with oilier, more irritated skin.

Face Treatment Oil for Dehydrated Skin *($29 for 1.4 ounces)* contains hazelnut oil, patchouli oil (mint), rosewood oil, fragrance, and orchid extract. The patchouli oil and fragrance can be irritating to the skin.

Eye Makeup Remover Lotion *($14.50 for 3.4 ounces)* contains water and flower waters, an oil-type cleansing agent, table salt, and preservatives. One of the preservatives—benzalkonium chloride—is an ammonium-based detergent that is very irritating and, according to several sources, can cause conjunctivitis when used in eye lotions. Table salt is also extremely irritating. Don't ask me why they put it in an eye makeup remover, but they did.

Eye Contour Balm *($25 for 1.7 ounces)* contains water, humectant, wax-like thickeners, flower extracts, serum protein (animal blood), and more thickeners. Not a bad product, but not great, and amazingly overpriced.

Eye Contour Gel *($25 for 0.7 ounce)* is mostly water, flower extracts, witch hazel, thickeners, and preservatives. Because of the witch hazel, this product can irritate the skin around the eyes. They claim it is soothing to the skin, but I doubt it.

Skin Beauty Repair *($35 for 0.5 ounce)*. At these prices—$1,120 a pound—you would think you were buying gold. You're not. What you are buying is shark oil; thickeners; avocado, soybean, lavender, marjoram, and peppermint oils; and preservatives. Marjoram, peppermint, and lavender oils can cause skin irritation. One of the claims is that this product will help restore a natural glow, but that's true only if you consider artificially reddened skin natural.

Gentle Night Cream for Sensitive Skin *($42 for 1.7 ounces)* contains mostly water, mineral oil, lots of thickeners, hazelnut oil, preservatives, soothing agents, vitamins A and E, and more preservatives. This is a good moisturizer, but remarkably expensive for fairly ordinary ingredients.

Gentle Day Cream for Sensitive Skin *($32 for 1.7 ounces)* is almost identical to the night cream, minus a few thickeners. Why it is $10 less is anyone's guess.

Multi-Active Day Cream *($24 for 1.05 ounces)* is a good moisturizer that contains mostly water, thickeners, aloe vera gel (which is mostly water), more thickeners, safflower and borage oils, and preservatives. Borage is a plant that contains tannin (like tea) and can be irritating to the skin.

Revitalizing Moisture Cream with "Cell Extract" *($40 for 1.7 ounces)* contains boring ingredients in contrast to its long, beguiling name. The ingredient list does not include any cell extracts, but cooked and preserved dead animal cells can't do anything for the skin, so it is no great loss. Clarins claims this product can promote youthful radiance. It contains mostly water, mineral oil, thickeners, glycerin, petrolatum, more thickeners, a small amount of sunscreen, some herb and flower extracts, more thickeners, and preservatives. As it turns out, this is an OK, but overpriced, moisturizer.

Skin Firming Concentrate *($42 for 1 ounce)* contains mostly water, spleen extract (tissue from the spleen of a dead animal, usually a cow), aloe vera, herb extracts, humectant, more thickeners, serum protein (animal blood), more herb extracts, and preservatives. If you want to believe that spleen, herbs, and blood can firm the skin, nothing I can say will convince you otherwise.

Oil Control Moisture Lotion *($20.50 for 1.06 ounces)* has a somewhat confusing ingredient list that seems to have little ability to do anything for oily skin except maybe make it worse. The main ingredients are water, thickeners, orris root, zinc sulfate, nylon, hawthorn extract, and preservatives. Orris root, zinc sulfate, and nylon can cause skin irritation.

Balancing Night Gel *($20.50 for 1 ounce)* contains water, skin softeners, mimosa bark, orris root, zinc sulfate, thickeners, witch hazel, and preservatives. Mimosa bark, orris root, zinc sulfate, and witch hazel can cause skin irritation and will do nothing to change the oil production of the skin, except maybe make it worse.

Blemish Gel *($12.50 for 0.53 ounce)* contains water, water binding agents, oak root, zinc sulphate (can absorb oil), preservatives, tea tree oil, and witch hazel, in a tiny bottle. Although zinc sulfate and witch hazel can prove irritating to the skin, tea tree oil and oak root can be soothing. Why can't they just leave the ingredients that irritate the skin out of these products altogether?

Absorbant Mask *($16 for 1.7 ounces)* is basically a very expensive clay mask that contains mostly water, clay, thickeners, more clay, more thickeners, some herb extracts, and preservatives. It will absorb oil, but not any better than any other clay mask. Clay is clay, and this clay probably isn't even from France.

Treatment Cream for All Skin Types (*$55 for 1.7 ounces*) contains mostly water, mineral oil, thickeners, plant oils, ginseng extract (soothes skin), protein, and preservatives. This is a good moisturizer, but mostly for normal to dry skin. Proteins in cosmetics work to keep water in the skin, but not as well as mineral oil, which is why mineral oil is usually one of the first ingredients and the other "specialty" ingredients are much farther down the list.

Treatment Cream for Very Dry, Very Devitalized Skin (*$55 for 1.7 ounces*) is a very good emollient moisturizer that contains water, mineral oil, thickener, shark oil, shea butter, thickeners, lanolin oil, proteins, thickeners, and preservatives, but the price tag is very high and very foolish.

Revitalizing Moisture Mask with "Cell Extract" (*$25 for 1.7 ounces*) is mostly water, standard cosmetic-type thickeners, glycerin, and fruit and vegetable extracts (grapefruit and witch hazel extracts can both be irritating to the skin). The all-important *"cell extract"* seems to be cow fetus fat. Of course, they don't call it that, they call it "bovine embryo lipid fraction," but that's what it is. It won't revitalize anyone's skin.

Firming Neck Cream (*$39 for 1.7 ounces*) is a very expensive product that can moisturize your neck but won't firm even one inch of it. The cream contains water, thickener, mineral oil, glycerin, aloe vera (mostly water), detergent, more thickener, safflower oil, spinal protein (protein cells from an animal's spine), and moisture binding ingredients. This is a good moisturizer, but that's about it.

"Cellulite" Control Gel (*$41.50 for 5.3 ounces*), like all "cellulite" control gels, is an absurd waste of money. The quotes around cellulite are Clarins', not mine. These quotes are a way for Clarins to get around the truth-in-advertising laws. Quotes allow any company a great deal of room about how a word is legally defined. In this case what the company legally means by cellulite control is totally different from what they want you to think they mean. You think they are referring to controlling the bumpy fat in your thighs. What they legally mean is only the surface texture of the skin (the appearance of cellulite). But because of the quotes, the interpretation is vague enough that truth-in-advertising laws haven't been breached because the second ingredientin this product is alcohol, which irritates and swells the skin. This irritation may reduce the appearance of the bumps on the surface of the skin for a few minutes. Of course, you could buy a bottle of rubbing alcohol and do the same thing for 89 cents. Aside from all that, you cannot burn or beat up fat from the outside in, so save your money.

Plant Milk for Bust Beauty Tightening and Toning (*$35 for 1.7 ounces*) doesn't even deserve an explanation, but for those of you who are wondering what could possibly be in a product that claims to "tighten" and "tone" your breasts, the ingredients are water; mineral oil; thickeners; fragrance; more thickeners; hop, fennel, and lemon extracts (which can all cause skin sensitivities); and preservatives.

Bust Firming Gel (*$42 for 1.7 ounces*) deserves even less mention than the Plant Milk for Bust Beauty, but here goes anyway. Water, fish protein (skin cells from a dead fish), algae extract (seaweed juice), plant extracts, and thickeners are the miracle ingredients that are supposed to firm your bust. If you believe this product can work, I have a bridge you may be interested in.

Cleansing Milk with Gentian *($22.50 for 8.6 ounces)* is an OK watersoluble cleanser for someone with dry skin, but Clarins recommends it for people with oily or combination skin. After rinsing, a slightly greasy film is left on the skin. This product also contains isopropyl myristate, which is known for causing breakouts, not great for someone with oily or combination skin. Contains strong fragrance.

Cleansing Milk with Alpine Herbs *($22.50 for 8.6 ounces)* is recommended for people with dry to normal skin, but the alpine herbs can all cause skin irritation and drying, which makes it a poor product for this skin type. Contains strong fragrance.

Gentle Foaming Cleanser *($16.50 for 4.4 ounces)* is actually a very good water-soluble cleanser that nicely cleans the face and removes eye makeup without irritating the skin or eyes. What a shame it is so expensive, because it would be a great daily cleanser for someone with normal to oily skin. Contains strong fragrance.

Toning Lotion for Combination or Oily Skin *($19.50 for 8.4 ounces)* is an alcohol-free toner that contains water, aloe, sage and rosemary extracts, slip agents, antiseptic, and more plant extract. The only problem is that two of the plant extracts in this toner (sage and rosemary) can cause skin irritation.

Toning Lotion for Dry to Normal Skin *($19.50 for 8.4 ounces)* is a fairly good irritant-free toner except for the inclusion of phenoxyethanol, one of the last ingredients, which is a derivative of phenol and can be irritating on the skin.

Self Tanning Face Cream SPF 15 *($18.50 for 4 ounces)* and **Self-Tanning Milk SPF 6** *($16.50 for 4 ounces)* are both standard self-tanning lotions, only more expensive. It is good they come with a sunscreen, although SPF 6 isn't enough to protect the body from the sun. The major concern I have is that Clarins' brochures are very confusing about how to handle sun exposure. In essence they give step-by-step information about how to accelerate getting a suntan, not a chemically induced self-tan but one from the sun. They suggest that using their self-tanning creams will avoid sunburn or any photosensitive reaction. First of all, you can't stop a photosensitive reaction with a sunscreen. If you are using something that recommends staying out of the sun, stay out of the sun. You can prevent a sunburn with the SPF 15 product, but the SPF 6 won't work for everyone. They also suggest that once a golden tan is achieved you can move on to a lower SPF number. That is like telling someone that after you've damaged your skin you can damage it even more. Sunburns age the skin and cause skin cancer, and tanning is just as dangerous.

Clarion

Clear Skin Refresher *($6 for 3 ounces)* is very water-soluble and can remove all the makeup without irritating the eyes. This is a good option for someone with normal to oily skin. The skin will feel clean without feeling that dry or taut.

Complexion Bath *($6 for 3.4 ounces)* is a good water-soluble cleanser that can remove all the makeup and doesn't leave a greasy film behind on the skin. Like the Clear Skin Refresher it is good for someone with normal to oily skin.

Moisture Revival *($6 for 3 ounces)* leaves a greasy film on the face and does not reliably remove all the makeup.

Double Defense Moisturizer *($8.50 for 3.3 ounces)* is a good moisturizer that contains water, synthetic oil, slip agent, thickeners, collagen, elastin, vitamin E, water binding agent, and more thickeners. It claims to be many things, such as ultra-pure, noncomedogenic, and nonirritating, and to protect the skin from environmental damage. "Pure" is a relative term (pure by whose standards?); "noncomedogenic" and "nonirritating" depend totally on your skin and how you react. What is true is that it has an SPF of 15, which will definitely protect your face from the sun.

Restorative Smoothing Creme *($6.79 for 2 ounces)* contains mostly water, glycerin, thickener, petrolatum, synthetic oil, several more thickeners, elastin, more thickeners, fragrance, collagen, and preservatives. The claim is that the elastin and collagen will restore the skin, but both these ingredients are far down on the list. It also contains sodium hydroxide (before the collagen), which can be very irritating to the skin.

Clear Moisture (Oil-Free) *($6.38 for 3.3 ounces)* is another of those oil-free products that isn't really oil-free. The third ingredient is dimethicone, which is a synthetic oil much like petrolatum. Other than that this is indeed a very lightweight moisturizer, and it feels quite soft on the skin. It should be great for someone with normal to combination skin.

Skin Harmonizer (Oil-Free) *($8.50 for 3.3 ounces)* is an OK moisturizer that is made up mostly of standard water binding agents, thickeners, slip agents, and preservatives.

Pure Moisture *($8.50 for 3.3 ounces)* is a very emollient moisturizer that contains water, thickener, glycerin, mineral oil, petrolatum, more thickeners, synthetic oil, more thickeners, and preservatives. One of the preservatives is potassium hydroxide, which can be particularly irritating to the skin.

Moisture Revival *($6 for 3.4 ounces)* contains mostly water, a long list of thickeners, and several preservatives. This is a mediocre moisturizer without much moisture or water binding ingredients.

Infinite Moisture *($7.13 for 2 ounces)* contains mostly water, mineral oil, thickener, glycerin, petrolatum, more thickeners, collagen, elastin, and preservatives. This is a good emollient moisturizer.

After Sun Revitalizing Creme *($4.50 for 3.1 ounces)* can't revitalize sun-damaged skin, but it is a good moisturizer whether or not you sit in the sun. It does contain sodium hydroxide, which can be irritating to some skin types.

Clean and Clear by Johnson & Johnson

Facial Cleansing Bar *($2.69 for $3.75 ounces)* is a standard bar soap that can be drying for most skin types.

Foaming Facial Cleanser *($3.13 for 8 ounces)* is a typical water-soluble detergent cleanser. However, it contains sodium chloride, which can be an irritant, and quaternium-15, considered to be one of the most irritating preservatives. This would irritate the eye area.

Foaming Facial Cleanser for Sensitive Skin *($3.13 for 8 ounces)* is more gentle than the cleanser above, but it still contains quaternium-15, which I would never recommend to someone with sensitive skin.

Blemish Fighting Pads *($3.99 for 50 pads)* contains camphor, clove oil, eucalyptus oil, peppermint oil, alcohol, and salicylic acid. This contains almost every irritating ingredient I can think of. It won't fight blemishes, but it will make the skin red and irritated.

Blemish Fighting Stick *($4.99 for 1 ounce)* is almost identical to the pads above, and the same warnings apply.

Oil-Control Astringent *($3.13 for 8 ounces)* is almost identical to the two products above, and the same warnings apply. This product can't control oil; in fact, it can make the skin worse.

Sensitive Skin Astringent *($3.13 for 8 ounces)* contains mostly water, water binding agents, eucalyptus oil, and clove oil. This would cause havoc on someone with sensitive skin.

Skin Balancing Moisturizer *($3.13 for 4 ounces)* contains mostly water, a long list of thickeners, coloring, fragrance, more preservatives, and a small amount of salicylic acid. A mediocre moisturizer that won't balance anything.

Skin Balancing Moisturizer for Sensitive Skin *($3.13 for 4 ounces)* is the same as the moisturizer above but without coloring or fragrance. The salicylic acid should have been eliminated too, as it can irritate sensitive skin.

Clinique

Wash-Away Gel Cleanser *($14.50 for 5 ounces)* is an interesting water-soluble cleanser that cleans the face and all the makeup off without irritation or any sensation of dryness. This one is worth checking out if you have normal to oily skin.

Water-Dissolve Cream Cleanser *($14.50 for 5 ounces)* leaves a greasy film behind on the skin and doesn't take off all the makeup without the help of a washcloth.

Rinse-off Foaming Cleanser *($14.50 for 5 ounces)* is a very strong detergent-based cleanser that can irritate and dry the skin, plus it definitely can burn the eyes. This is too strong for most skin types.

Crystal Clear Cleansing Oil *($11 for 6 ounces)* is a wipe-off cleanser that contains mostly mineral oil and a small amount of vitamins E and A. The salesperson said it wouldn't leave an oily residue on my face, but it did.

Extremely Gentle Cleansing Cream *($9.50 for 3.5 ounces; $17.50 for 10 ounces)* is a traditional cold cream product (requires wiping off) that contains mostly mineral oil, water, beeswax, petrolatum, thickeners, and preservatives. Wiping off makeup is bad for the skin.

Quick Dissolve Makeup Solvent *($14.50 for 8 ounces)* contains mostly water, mineral oil, slip agents, thickener, plant and nut oils, more thickeners, and preservatives. You are supposed to use this water-soluble cleanser to take off your makeup before you use soap. Two products to clean the face always seems like one too many to me. If soap cleans your face this is an unnecessary step, and if the Makeup Solvent cleans your face you shouldn't need the soap. If you can't use the soap over your eyes, then a water-soluble cleanser that works over the entire face would be the fastest and easiest way to clean your face.

Rinse-Off Eye Makeup Solvent *($10 for 4 ounces)* contains mostly water, detergent cleanser, and slip agents. It will take off eye makeup and leaves no greasy residue.

Clean-Up Stick *($9.50 for 0.06 ounce)* is an interesting way to clean up leftover makeup or makeup mistakes, but a cotton swab and moisturizer or cleanser will do the same thing—for a lot less money.

7 Day Scrub Cream *($9.50 for 2 ounces; $14.50 for 3.5 ounces)* contains mostly mineral oil, water, beeswax, sodium borate (antiseptic), and ozokerite (a wax-like thickener). This is a very thick, heavy product that can cause the same problems it's trying to eliminate, because beeswax and ozokerite can cause skin to break out.

Gentle Exfoliator Rinse-Off Formula *($12.50 for 3 ounces)* contains mostly water, mineral oil, a long list of thickeners, a long list of plant extracts, soothing agent, vitamin E, more thickeners, and preservatives. This is a gentle exfoliator with very little abrasive in it, but I wouldn't call this rinsable. The mineral oil leaves a residue on the skin.

Clarifying Lotion 1, 2, 3, and 4 *($14.50 for 12 ounces)* all contain varying degrees of alcohol, acetone (nail polish remover), benzalkonium chloride, and menthol, which are all extremely irritating to the skin. Clarifying Lotion 4 is even stronger than the first three. All of these are beyond irritating (even the one for sensitive skin contains alcohol and witch hazel). It is amazing to me that Clinique still sells four toners with alcohol and none that are irritant-free.

Dramatically Different Moisturizing Lotion *($18.50 for 4 ounces)* contains mostly water, mineral oil, sesame oil, standard water binding agent, thickeners, petrolatum, and preservatives. This is a good, basic lightweight moisturizer for normal to dry skin, although it isn't "dramatically different" from other emollient moisturizers on the market.

Advanced Care Moisturizer *($32.50 for 1 ounce)* contains mostly water, standard water binding agents, thickeners, mineral oil, plant oils, more thickeners, algae extract, vitamins A and E, more thickeners, and preservatives. The literature calls it a "youth-keeper." It won't keep youth in the skin, but it is a good, reliable moisturizer for dry skin.

Sub-Skin Cream *($38.50 for 2.6 ounces)* contains mostly water; collagen; thickeners; oil; standard water binding agents; more thickeners; soothing agents; vitamins A, C, and E; more thickeners; and preservatives. This is a very good moisturizer, but it won't tighten or firm the skin; it will just keep dry skin at bay.

Daily Eye Benefits *($25 for 0.5 ounce)* contains mostly water, cucumber extract, ivy extract, glycerin, thickeners, aloe vera, petrolatum, standard water binding agents, amino acids, and preservatives. The cucumber and ivy extracts are supposed to reduce puffiness around the eye; maybe they could in a pure form, but not mixed in a cosmetic. This is a good lightweight moisturizer with an incredibly high price tag. Slice up a cucumber and see if that can get rid of puffy eyes before investing in this product at $1,200 a pound.

Moisture Surge Treatment Formula *($18.50 for 2 ounces)* contains mostly water, several good water binding agents, vitamins A and E, water binding agent, plant extracts, thickeners, and preservatives. This is a very good lightweight moisturizer with a nice amount of water binding agents.

Skin Texture Lotion *($18.50 for 1.25 ounces)* contains mostly water, collagen, standard water binding agent, a long list of thickeners, water binding agent, vitamins A and E, soothing agent, more thickeners, and preservatives. This is a good lightweight moisturizer. Collagen is a good water binding ingredient and nothing more.

Turnaround Cream *($27.50 for 2 ounces)* is a great name for a product. It sounds like this cream can turn your skin back to a younger time, but it can't. This average moisturizer contains water, water binding agent, a long list of thickeners, salicylic acid, vitamin E, and preservatives. The major ingredient that supposedly turns the skin around is salicylic acid. It can peel the skin much like Retin-A and alpha hydroxy acids can, and is used in some acne products and foot creams. It is meant to be an alternative to AHA. They must have missed the alpha hydroxy acid bandwagon when they made this one. AHAs are a better skin exfoliant than salicylic acid. Salicylic acid also can't provide the moisturizing benefits that AHAs can.

Very Emollient Cream *($21.50 for 2 ounces)* contains mostly water, oil, water binding agent, thickener, petrolatum, mineral oil, a long list of thickeners, vitamins E and A, more thickeners, and preservatives. This a good emollient moisturizer for dry skin, but it isn't anything unique or special.

Color Me Beautiful

Extra Gentle Cleansing Cream *($12 for 4.2 ounces)* is a standard wipe-off cleanser that leaves a greasy residue on the face.

Very Effective Cleansing Gel *($12 for 4.2 ounces)* is a good cleanser for someone with very oily skin only, but it isn't any more effective than other cleansers of this type.

Skin Conditioning Cleanser *($12 for 4.2 ounces)* doesn't rinse very well (the third ingredient is petrolatum) and requires a washcloth to get it all off.

Gentle Eye Makeup Remover *($12 for 1.6 ounces)* contains mostly water, slip agent, herb extracts, thickener, and preservatives. This is gentle enough and it will take off eye makeup, but the cleansers in this line will do that too.

Instant Eye Makeup Remover Pads *($12.50 for 50 pads)* will take off eye makeup, but so will the face cleansers, so why bother with this step?

Gentle Sloughing Cream *($12 for 1.6 ounces)* contains crushed peanuts, water, honey, clay, thickeners, crushed almonds, plant oil, and preservatives. I wouldn't call this gentle (rub crushed nuts over your face and see how that feels), but it is definitely a scrub.

Exfoliating Scrub *($12 for 1.6 ounces)* isn't much of a scrub, but it is an OK cleanser. It also contains quaternium-15, a very irritating preservative.

Hydrating Mist *($9 for 4 ounces)* contains mostly water, aloe, standard water binding agents, plant extracts, water binding agents, and preservatives (including quaternium-15, which is very irritating). This is a good toner for some skin types.

Hydrating Tonic *($10 for 4.2 ounces)* contains mostly water, aloe, standard water binding agents, and preservatives. This is a very good irritant-free toner.

Purifying Tonic *($10 for 4.2 ounces)* is a standard alcohol-based toner that can irritate the skin, with some fruit oils and chamomile added. It also contains quaternium-15, which is very irritating.

Balancing Tonic *($10 for 4.2 ounces)* contains mostly water, sage extract, plant and fruit oils, witch hazel, water binding agent, slip agent, and preservatives (including quaternium-15, one of the most irritating preservatives). Sage can be an irritant and the oils aren't great for someone with oily or combination skin, but for some skin types this can be OK.

Blemish Zapper *($9 for 0.25 ounce)* contains mostly water, alcohol, talc, zinc, camphor, lavender oil, and preservatives. This won't zap a single blemish, and it can irritate the skin.

Extra Protective Hydrating Complex *($13 for 1.6 ounces)* contains mostly water, standard water binding agents, thickeners, plant oils, protein, a small amount of sunscreen, more thickeners, and preservatives (including quaternium-15, one of the most irritating preservatives). This is a very good moisturizer for dry skin.

Fortifying Eye Cream (*$15 for 1.6 ounces*) contains mostly algae extract, standard water binding agent, a long list of thickeners, soybean oil, marine minerals, plant extracts, elastin, more plant extracts, minerals, water binding agents, animal thymus and tissue extracts, and preservatives. Marine salts and animal parts won't fortify the skin, but still this is a good emollient moisturizer for the entire face, not just the eyes.

Hydrating Mask (*$12 for 1.6 ounces*) contains mostly water, petrolatum, thickeners, shea butter, a long list of water binding agents, cow amniotic fluid, water binding agents, and preservatives (including quaternium-15, which is very irritating). This would feel quite good and emollient to someone with very dry skin.

Intensive Night Care (*$15 for 1.6 ounces*) contains mostly water, algae extract, thickeners, petrolatum, soybean oil, more thickeners, marine salts, plant extracts, more thickeners, animal tissue, more herb extracts, and preservatives. This is a good emollient moisturizer for dry skin, but the marine salts, animal tissue, and herb extracts are there for marketing purposes, not necessarily your skin.

Lightweight Moisture Lotion (*$13 for 1.6 ounces*) contains mostly water; aloe; almond oil; thickeners; sunscreen; more thickeners; plant extracts and oils; vitamins E, D, and A; vegetable oil; more thickeners; and preservatives. This is a good lightweight moisturizer.

Multi-Action Revitalizing Concentrate (*$17 for 1 ounce*) contains mostly water, water binding agent, algae extract, thickener, plant extracts, liposomes, marine salts, thickener, water binding agent, sunscreen, and preservatives (including quaternium-15, which is very irritating). This won't revitalize anything, but it is an OK lightweight moisturizer.

Oil-Free Regulating Fluid (*$13 for 1.6 ounces*) contains mostly water, aloe, thickeners, plant extracts, water binding agent, sunscreen, and preservatives. It won't regulate oil, but it is a good, extremely lightweight moisturizer for someone with minimally dry skin. I wouldn't use it on someone with oily skin.

Regulating Night Therapy (*$12 for 1.6 ounces*) is a good lightweight moisturizer with its share of herb extracts and plant oils. It won't regulate anything, but it will take care of dry skin.

Regulating Mask (*$12 for 1.6 ounces*) is a standard clay mask that also contains alcohol and camphor. This can be very drying and irritating to most skin types.

Cover Girl

Noxzema Original Skin Cream (*$3.33 for 10 ounces*) contains several extremely irritating ingredients, including camphor, phenol, menthol, and eucalyptus. This cleanser would be a problem for most skin types.

Clearly Different Deep Cleansing Face Wash (*$4.50 for 3.5 ounces*) is actually an excellent cleanser for someone with normal to oily skin. It takes off all the makeup and doesn't irritate the eyes or skin. It does contain potassium hydroxide, which can be a problem for some sensitive skin types.

Moisture-Gentle Cleansing Beauty Wash *($4.50 for 3.7 ounces)* doesn't rinse very well or take off all the makeup, and it leaves a slightly greasy residue on the skin, but it could be good for someone with very dry skin.

Noxzema Difrinse Water Soluble Cold Cream *($5.50 for 10 ounces)* is not at all rinsable without the use of a washcloth.

Noxzema Plus Skin Cream *($3.72 for 10.5 ounces)* contains mostly water, glycerin, thickeners, fragrance, more thickeners, castor oil, and preservatives. This is an ordinary moisturizer, not very emollient, but OK for normal skin if you aren't allergic to the fragrance.

Dove

Dove Beauty Bar *($2.17 for 2-4.75 ounce bars)* is a standard soap with some emollients thrown in to cut the irritation and dryness. This is still soap, and quite drying for most skin types.

Dove Beauty Wash *($1.85 for 6 ounces)* is a very drying water-soluble cleanser, and it contains quaternium-15, a very irritating preservative. I would not use this product on the face, and definitely nowhere near the eyes.

EB5

I usually don't like to make fun of people (which is different from critiquing what they make and sell), but does anyone else think that the guy who is supposed to have formulated EB5 Cream and Cleanser, Robert Heldfond, looks like Dr. Zorba on the old *Ben Casey M.D.* television show? Sorry, I just couldn't resist asking. Nevertheless, the claims on the brochure are just as absurd as the ones many other cosmetics companies make. First, you're supposed to believe a pharmacist knows something about formulating cosmetic creams. Pharmacists are trained to deal primarily with prescription drugs; they are not chemists and they are definitely not cosmetic chemists. One of the claims is that EB5 cream is a great daytime cream, yet it doesn't contain a sunscreen. Unless your foundation has a high SPF, this is not a good day cream at all. Another claim is that the 4-ounce jar will last for many months. I guess "many" is relative, but a woman with dry skin who would use this twice a day would be lucky for it to last six weeks. All moisturizers minimize wrinkles, so that's nothing new, but the brochure also states it helps makeup adhere better. Any moisturizer has the exact same ability. There are some good things about this cream, but it isn't as unique as the brochure makes it out to be.

EB5 Facial Cream *($35 for 4 ounces)* contains mostly water, stabilizer, a form of vitamin E, thickener, mineral oil, thickener, vitamin A, vitamin D, and preservatives. This would be a good moisturizer for normal to dry skin, and it contains good antioxidants.

EB5 Facial Cleanser *($18 for 4 ounces)* contains some fairly irritating ingredients high up in the ingredient list and can potentially burn the eyes.

Elizabeth Arden

Visible Difference Deep Cleansing Lotion *($17.50 for 6.7 ounces)* is a good water-soluble cleanser that lathers and rinses well. However, it can be drying to the skin and may burn your eyes. Also, the third ingredient is isopropyl myristate, which can cause blackheads.

Visible Difference Gentle Scrub Creme for the Face *($17.50 for 3.5 ounces)* leaves a somewhat greasy film on the face (the second ingredient is petrolatum), although it might feel good as a scrub for someone with extremely dry, parched skin.

Visible Difference Refining Toner *($15 for 6.7 ounces)* contains mostly water, witch hazel, alcohol, glycerin, and preservative. The alcohol makes it too irritating for most skin types, and one of the preservatives is benzalkonium chloride, which is also a serious skin irritant.

Visible Difference Refining Moisturizer Creme Complex *($47.50 for 2.5 ounces)* contains mostly water, emulsifying wax, glycerin, isopropyl myristate (can cause blackheads), shark oil, beeswax, and preservatives. This is a somewhat heavy moisturizer that might be good for someone with very dry skin.

Visible Difference Refining Moisture Lotion *($28.50 for 1.35 ounces)* would be a good emollient moisturizer/sunscreen except that the sunscreen ingredient is padimate-o, a derivative of PABA, which can be a skin irritant.

Visible Difference Eyecare Concentrate *($30 for 0.5 ounce)* is an ordinary moisturizer that contains mostly water, mineral oil, thickeners, avocado oil, more thickeners, and preservatives.

One Great Soap *($9.50 for 4.5 ounces)* is a surprisingly good soap with good emollients and water binding ingredients. The detergent cleanser used is also milder than most. I would only recommend this for someone with normal to oily skin who likes to use soap.

Extra Control Removing Cleanser *($18.50 for 6.76 ounces)* contains mineral oil and alcohol, a confusing combination for anyone with oily skin. It doesn't clean skin very well, it leaves an oily film on the face, and the alcohol can dry out the skin.

Extra Control Oil Cleansing Astringent *($15 for 6.76 ounces)* contains mostly alcohol, water, slip agent, salicylic acid (peeling agent), menthol, and coloring agents. This is one extremely irritating cleanser that can make skin even more oily than it already is, as well as red.

Extra Control Texturizing Conditioner *($22.50 for 2 ounces)* contains ingredients that I would not ever recommend for someone with oily or combination skin; waxes, mineral oil, and isopropyl myristate (which can cause blackheads) are all at the top of the ingredient list. What could they have been thinking of?

Ceramide Time Complex Capsules *($55 for 0.97 ounce in 60 capsules)* is the most popular product Elizabeth Arden sells, yet these tiny gelatin capsules are more hype than anything else. They contain a standard water binding agent, oil, neural lipid extract (brain fat from an animal), epidermal lipid extract (skin fat from an animal), vitamins A and E, and oil. The ingredients credited with near-wonderous effects are the neural and epidermal lipid extracts. Fat is a good emollient, but there isn't even very much of it in the product. Vitamins A and E are good, but lots of other products include them as well.

Ceramide Time Complex Cream *($45 for 1.7 ounces)* is Elizabeth Arden's attempt at an AHA product. It falls short, with only a small amount of AHA, perhaps less then 2 percent. It is still a good moisturizer that would be very good for the skin, very lightweight and emollient. It's overpriced, but that isn't surprising.

Ceramide Eyes Time Complex Capsules *($37.50 for 0.35 ounce)* contains mostly a standard water binding agent, slip agent, witch hazel (can be a skin irritant, particularly around the eyes), herb extract, apricot oil, fat, vitamin E, water binding agents, and oils. This would be a good lightweight oil to put around the eyes if your skin isn't allergic to the witch hazel—and if you can get over the $1,800 per pound price tag.

Imunage UV Defense Cream SPF 15 *($35 for 1.25 ounces)* contains mostly water, slip agents, a very long list of thickeners, jojoba oil, more thickeners, vitamins E and A, and preservatives. This is an OK lightweight moisturizer/sunscreen that is very overpriced for what you get.

Imunage UV Defense Lotion SPF 15 *($35 for 1.25 ounces)* is almost identical to the cream above, only lighter weight.

Lip Fix Creme *($17.50 for 0.5 ounce)* contains mostly thick waxes, mineral oil, and preservatives. Two of these preservatives, ammonium hydroxide and quaternium-15, can be very irritating. This product won't prevent all lipsticks from bleeding.

Micro 2000 Stressed-Skin Concentrate *($42.50 for 0.85 ounce)* contains mostly standard water binding agents, water, oil, isopropyl myristate (can cause blackheads), jojoba oil, thickeners, minerals, amino acid, more thickeners, and preservatives. This won't help stressed skin any more than any other moisturizer. The ingredient list is just average, nothing special; even the amino acid, which sounds good, is too far down in the list to be significant.

Millenium Hydrating Cleanser *($23.50 for 4.4 ounces)* is an OK water-soluble cleanser that leaves a slightly greasy film on the skin. It also may not remove all traces of makeup.

Millenium Revitalizing Tonic *($22.50 for 5 ounces)* contains mostly water and alcohol. This is too irritating for most skin types.

Millenium Day Renewal Emulsion *($52.50 for 2.6 ounces)* contains mostly water, shark oil, standard water binding agents, thickeners, isopropyl myristate (can cause blackheads), lanolin oil, more thickeners, and preservatives. This is a very rich, emollient moisturizer that should be used only for dry skin. However, if you have a tendency to break out, stay away from this one.

Millenium Night Renewal Creme *($55 for 1 ounce)* contains mostly water, standard water binding agent, shark oil, mineral oil, thickeners, and preservatives. This is a good moisturizer for normal to dry skin, but is absurdly overpriced for very ordinary, boring ingredients.

Millenium Eye Renewal Cream *($35 for 0.5 ounces)* is a very rich, thick moisturizer that contains mostly water, mineral oil, lanolin, thickeners, and preservatives. It will indeed take care of dry skin, but one of the preservatives is benzalkonium chloride, considered to be particularly bad for use around the eyes.

Millenium Hydra-Exfoliating Mask *($27.50 for 2.65 ounces)* is a clay mask that also contains some oil and wax and a silicate. Because of the oil it isn't as drying as most clay masks, but it is still just a rather expensive clay mask.

Skin Basics Skin Deep Milky Cleanser *($18.50 for 6.76 ounces)* is a standard greasy wipe-off cleanser that leaves a film on the skin and doesn't take off makeup very well.

Skin Basics Skin Lotion *($15 for 6.76 ounces)* is a water- and alcohol-based toner that is too drying for almost all skin types.

Skin Basics Beauty Sleep *($32.50 for 2.5 ounces)* is only a basic emollient moisturizer that contains mostly water, mineral oil, thickeners, lanolin oil, thickeners, isopropyl myristate (can cause blackheads), lanolin, more thickeners, and preservatives.

Skin Basics Velva Moisture Film *($35 for 6.76 ounces)* contains mostly water, isopropyl myristate (can cause blackheads), lanolin oil, thickeners, and preservatives (including quaternium-15, which is considered to be a serious skin irritant). This is a very emollient, rich moisturizer for very dry skin, but it can cause blackheads.

Skin Basics Velva Cream Mask *($20 for 3.53 ounces)* is mostly water, thickener, zinc oxide, and preservative. This mostly zinc oxide mask won't do anything for the skin. Phenol is one of the first preser-vatives and it is most definitely a skin irritant.

Soothing Care Gentle Cleansing Emulsion *($23.50 for 7 ounces)* is a mediocre water-soluble cleanser that can't be rinsed off well without a washcloth, which makes this anything but gentle or soothing.

Soothing Care Calming Skin Freshener *($15 for 6.76 ounces)* is a good irritant-free toner that contains mostly water, glycerin, slip agents, soothing agent, and preservatives.

Soothing Care All Day Shielding Moisturizer *($21 for 3.3 ounces)* is a basic, ordinary lightweight moisturizer that contains mostly water, mineral oil, thickeners, avocado oil, a long list of thickeners, and preservatives. One of the preservatives is quaternium-15, a possible skin irritant.

Soothing Care Overnight Soothing Cream *($32.50 for 2.5 ounces)* is a basic moisturizer for normal to dry skin that contains mostly water, mineral oil, thickeners, isopropyl myristate (can cause blackheads), shark oil, thickeners, petrolatum, soothing agent, and preservatives (including quaternium-15).

Soothing Care Comforting Cream Pack *($20 for 3.53 ounces)* contains mostly water, cornstarch, wax, zinc oxide, mineral oil, thickeners, and preservatives. These ingredients aren't what I would call comforting or necessarily beneficial for the skin in any way.

Spa For The Face SPF 15 *($18.50 for 1 ounce)* is one of the many "spa" products on the market that are overhyped past the point of absurdity. This standard moisturizer/sunscreen contains mostly water, a long list of thickeners, standard water binding agents, aloe vera, more thickeners, and preservatives. There are some herbs too far down on the ingredient list to even mention.

Special Benefit Cleansing Cream *($25 for 8 ounces)* is a rather greasy cold cream-type cleanser that contains mostly mineral oil, wax, petrolatum, lanolin, and preservative.

Special Benefit Orange Skin Cream *($30 for 8 ounces)* is a very heavy, extremely rich moisturizer for parched, dry skin. It contains petrolatum, lanolin, vegetable oil, thickener, and preservatives.

Erno Laszlo

Their brochure states "Erno Laszlo has been the authority in advanced skincare for over 50 years. No one blended the art of cosmetology with the science of dermatology before Dr. Laszlo's time." Great copy, except that Erno Laszlo was never licensed to practice medicine in this country and there were those who said he was never really a medical doctor in Eastern Europe, where he was from, although the brochure makes it sound like he was a dermatologist. In his time, Erno Laszlo's claim to fame was prescribing skin care regimes for wealthy women who could afford to visit his clinic and spa. What he was truly best known for was his belief in using old-fashioned bar soap (dry-skin types would first cover their face in oil before using soap), then splashing the face 30 times with a basin full of the soapy rinse water, followed by splashing the face 30 times with scalding hot water. When that was done you would finish by soaking the skin with apple cider vinegar. Laszlo claimed that nothing cleaned better than hot water and soap, but because soap's alkaline content destroyed the skin's pH level, apple cider vinegar was needed to restore it.

(I should mention that I never agreed with this skin care regime, although I have to admit I always admired its originality and concept. My feeling is that hot water is too damaging to the skin, irritating it and causing capillaries to surface as small spider veins on the face. I also feel bar soap is too drying and irritating for the skin. We just aren't that dirty to require such an intense twice-a-day cleansing. I think it causes more problems than it helps. The notion of restoring the skin's pH level is a good idea after soap has stripped it off, but I would suggest that if you cleaned the face gently, without destroying the pH balance, you wouldn't need to use anything to restore it.)

After Erno Laszlo's death in the late '70s, Colgate-Palmolive bought the rights to use the doctor's name and develop the line any way they wanted. Are the current products in alignment with Laszlo's original skin care theories? For the most part the skin care routines still include the bar soap and splashing with soapy hot water and then clean hot water. The rest of the routine is loosely based on the good doctor's concepts. The toners are all alcohol-based, just like other toners on the market. Although I find this skin care routine less complex than most, I am amazed at how much money a cosmetics line can charge for bar soap, alcohol-based toners, and fairly standard moisturizers.

pHelitone Gentle Eye Makeup Remover *($17 for 3 ounces)* does remove eye makeup, but because of the salt and preservatives it contains it can burn the eyes.

Sea Mud Soap *($22 for 6 ounces)* contains standard soap ingredients of tallow and sodium cocoate, with a little sea mud thrown in. It's still just soap, and the mud only makes it more drying and leaves a slight film on the skin once it's rinsed.

Special Skin Soap *($22 for 6 ounces)* contains standard soap ingredients of tallow and sodium cocoate, with an additional detergent cleanser and a small amount of oil. This is still a fairly drying, average bar soap.

Active pHelityl Soap *($22 for 6 ounces)* is just standard soap ingredients that you find in all soaps, with some oil and glycerin added. This is a lot of money for a very ordinary bar of soap.

Hydraphel Cleansing Bar *($14 for 3 ounces)* is a standard bar soap with some good emollients, but it is still just a very expensive standard bar soap.

pHelityl Lotion *($42 for 3 ounces)* contains mostly water, thickeners, mineral oil, vegetable oil, more thickeners, and preservatives. It's good, light-weight, and emollient, but overpriced for a mineral oil-based moisturizer.

Conditioning Preparation *($29 for 8 ounces)* contains alcohol, water, fragrance, and preservative. This is almost pure alcohol, and very irritating to the skin.

Light Controlling Lotion *($27 for 8 ounces)* contains mostly water, alcohol, slip agents, and fragrance. The alcohol is too irritating for most skin types.

Regular Controlling Lotion *($27 for 8 ounces)* contains mostly water, alcohol, talc, glycerin, fragrance, and coloring agents. The alcohol makes this product too irritating for most skin types.

Heavy Controlling Lotion *($27 for 8 ounces)* contains mostly alcohol, water, talc, glycerin, thickener, and coloring agents. The alcohol is too irritating for most skin types.

Heavy Normalizer Shake It *($29 for 8 ounces)* contains mostly water, alcohol, talc, more alcohol, glycerin, and coloring agents. The alcohol makes this product too irritating for most skin types.

Total Skin Revitalizer *($50 for 1 ounce)* is a lightweight emollient moisturizer that contains water, several standard water binding ingredients, soothing agents, slip agents, thickeners, fragrance, and preservatives. This won't revitalize the skin, but it will keep it moist, just like any other moisturizer.

Total Skin Revitalizer for Eyes *($42 for 0.5 ounce)* contains mostly water; a long list of thickeners; grape oil; herb extracts; witch hazel (can be a skin irritant); glycerin; vitamins A, E, and C; more thickeners; and preservatives. This is a good emollient moisturizer, but the witch hazel can be a problem for sensitive skin types.

Total Skin Revitalizer for Night *($60 for 1 ounce)* contains water, water binding agents, vitamins A and E, herb extracts, thickener, protein, oil, a long list of thickeners, and preservatives. This is a good lightweight emollient moisturizer for the face, but the price tag can make it painful.

Active pHelityl Cream *($45 for 4 ounces)* contains mostly petrolatum, safflower oil, thickeners, fragrance, thickeners, and preservatives. This is a standard, emollient petrolatum-based moisturizer. You're paying a lot of money for Vaseline.

pHelityl Cream *($52 for 2 ounces)* contains mostly water, thickeners, mineral oil, more thickeners, petrolatum, and preservatives. This is a fairly standard emollient moisturizer for normal to dry skin. Can you believe they're charging that much for mineral oil and petrolatum?

pHelitone Replenishing Eye Cream *($41 for 0.5 ounce)* contains mostly water, thickener, petrolatum, herb oil, slip agent, thickeners, soothing agent, vitamin E, thickener, mineral oil, more thickeners, and preservatives. Pricey for a jar of petrolatum, don't you think?

pHelitone Firming Eye Gel *($30 for 0.5 ounce)* contains mostly water, castor oil, soothing agent, a long list of herb extracts (tea), thickeners, and preservatives. This won't firm anything, but it will feel light and emollient around the eyes if you aren't allergic to the herbs.

Hyrdraphel Complex *($52 for 2 ounces)* contains mostly water; mineral oil; waxes; mink oil; slip agents; sesame oil; thickener; herb oil; thickeners; vitamins A, C, and E; and preservatives. This is a good standard emollient moisturizer, but mink oil is only an oil, nothing special, and doesn't warrant the steep price tag.

Hydraphel Emulsion *($44 for 2 ounces)* contains mostly water, mink oil, a small amount of sunscreen (not enough to protect adequately from the sun), thickener, shark oil, thickeners, herb oil, more thickener, mineral oil, more thickeners, fragrance, and preservatives. There are antioxidant vitamins in here, but too far down in the ingredient list to be significant. Other than that, this is a good emollient moisturizer with a small amount of sunscreen. Mink oil is not a skin wonder, but it is a good oil, like a dozen other good oils.

Hydraphel Skin Supplement *($29 for 8 ounces)* contains mostly water, standard water binding agents, soothing agent, preservative, water binding agent, and preservatives. This is a good lightweight irritant-free toner.

Daily Moisture Protection Lotion SPF 15 *($45 for 2.5 ounces)* is a good emollient moisturizer/sunscreen that contains mostly water; standard water binding agents; thickeners; mineral oil; more thickeners; water binding agent; borage oil; herb extracts; vitamins A, E, and C; more thickeners; and preservatives. The herbs are a popular addition but won't do much for the skin. Is it worth the price tag? Hardly.

Hydra-Therapy Skin Vitality Treatment *($64 for 6 applications)* is a two-part system that is almost embarrasing, it is so amazingly overpriced. You mix an ordinary liquid with a simple powder that is mostly salt and apply it to the face, let it set, and then rinse. The liquid contains water, slip agent, soothing agent, slip agent, and preservatives, very typical cosmetic ingredients. The powder is made out of magnesium carbonate (powder), sea salt, silica (sand), mineral salt, and calcium (powder). See: ordinary, but absurdly expensive.

Sea Mud Mask *($30 for 4 ounces)* is basically a standard clay mask (kaolin is the second ingredient) with a smaller amount of some clay from the sea as well as other standard thickeners and slip agents. Is sea mud good for the skin? Not any better than any other mud, and even that's highly questionable.

Estee Lauder

Fruition, Triple Reactivating Complex *($42.50 for 1 ounce)* is at the top of Estee Lauder's skin care list because of its outstanding popularity. This is Estee Lauder's alpha hydroxy acid product, but it contains less than 2 percent AHA. It's an OK lightweight moisturizer but not a great AHA product. They recommend wearing it under a regular moisturizer, which is fine, but there are better AHA products on the market that don't require an extra moisturizer.

Instant Action Rinse-Off Cleanser *($16.50 for 6 ounces)* does not rinse off easily without the use of a washcloth. The cleansing agent is mild, so this product can be good for dry skin.

Facewash Self-Foaming System *($16.50 for 6 ounces)* is a fairly drying water-soluble cleanser that may also irritate the eyes.

Rich Results Hydrating Cleanser *($18.50 for 4 ounces)* contains a gentle cleansing agent, but it also contains mineral oil, wax, and other oils that make it hard to rinse off without the aid of a washcloth.

Re-Nutriv Extremely Delicate Cleanser *($32.50 for 7 ounces)* is more like a traditional cold cream than anything else. The very greasy formula contains mostly mineral oil, water, beeswax, petrolatum, shark oil, thickeners, lanolin, and preservatives.

Tender Creme Cleanser *($25 for 8 ounces)* is a cleanser that needs to be wiped off with tissue or a washcloth. It tends to leave a slightly greasy film on the skin and does not take off makeup all that well.

Micro-Moisture Cleansing Bar *($17.50 for 5 ounces)* is a standard bar soap made of tallow and sodium cocoate. It also contains alcohol, which adds to the drying effect of the soap. However, it also contains some oils, which help counteract some of the dryness. This could be OK for some normal skin types who prefer using bar soap.

Micro-Refining Bar Cleanser *($17.50 for 5 ounces)* is practically identical to the soap listed above except for a different coloring agent (this one is blue) and a few different oils. The evaluation is the same.

Solid Milk Cleansing Grains *($18.50 for 3.5 ounces)* contains mostly corn flour, thickeners (one is PVP, a possible irritant), chalk, nonfat dry milk, fragrance, detergent cleanser, soothing agent, and preservatives. This is OK as a scrub but not worth the money for some flour, chalk, and dry milk.

Gentle Eye Makeup Remover *($12 for 3.3 ounces)* is indeed a gentle eye makeup remover, although a gentle water-soluble cleanser should be able to do the same thing without having to wipe and pull at the eye with an extra product.

Gentle Action Skin Polisher *($18.50 for 4 ounces)* is supposed to be a water-soluble scrub, but it doesn't rinse well. The scrub action is mild and the other ingredients are standard thickeners, mineral oil, mild detergent cleanser, and preservatives. This could be good for someone with dry skin, but it isn't any more effective than baking soda mixed with a water-soluble cleanser.

Gentle Protection Tonic *($13 for 6.75 ounces)* is a mild skin toner with very soothing ingredients, including allantoin and ammonium glycyrrhizinate (which doesn't sound soothing, but is). It does contain horse chestnut extract and menthol, which is a mild antiseptic that can be irritating to some skin types.

Mild Action Protection Tonic *($22 for 13.5 ounces)* is a toner containing mostly alcohol. I would not call it mild, I would call it irritating.

Re-Nutriv Gentle Skin Toner *($27.50 for 6.5 ounces)* is an alcohol-free toner that contains mostly gentle ingredients except for arnica extract. It can be irritating, but it can also have mild antiseptic benefit on the skin.

Skin Defender Sensitive Skin Protector *($45 for 0.9 ounce)* contains a small amount of sunscreen plus water, protein, slip agents, water binding agents, vitamin A, more protein, shark oil, thickeners, and preservatives. Protein won't change the skin; it is just a good water binding ingredient. This is a good moisturizer with some interesting ingredients, nothing more or less, and the price tag is staggering for what you get.

Advanced Night Repair *($70 for 1.75 ounces)* is a good moisturizer that contains mostly water, thickeners, shark oil, water binding agents, soothing agent, vitamin A, preservative, thickeners, more preservatives, and coloring agents. It also contains a small amount of sunscreen, which doesn't make sense for use at night, and there isn't enough for daytime protection either. This won't repair anything, but it is a good lightweight moisturizer for dry skin.

Advanced Suncare SPF 15 No Chemical Sunscreen *($18.50 for 4 ounces)* is one of the better nonchemical sunscreens on the market, although, like all titanium dioxide-based sunscreens, it can feel thick and slightly sticky on the skin.

Eyzone Repair Gel *($35 for 0.5 ounce)* contains mostly water, standard water binding agents, thickeners, more water binding ingredients, and preservatives. I was told it would last six months because you use so little, but you would have to use none for this amount of product to last that long. This is good for dry skin, but it won't change wrinkles or do anything unique for the skin.

Time Zone Moisture Recharging Complex *($50 for 1.75 ounces)* contains mostly water, algae extract, standard water binding agents, collagen, thickeners, water binding agent, vitamins A and E, proteins, more thickeners, and preservatives. This is a good moisturizer but it can't reprogram the skin. Collagen and proteins cannot affect the structure of the skin; they are simply good water binding ingredients.

Future Perfect Micro-Targeted Skin Gel *($30 for 1 ounce)* has a great name. Sounds like you can place it over a wrinkle, zero in, and, *poof*, get rid of it. Not possible. However, this is a very good lightweight emollient moisturizer that contains mostly water, thickeners, standard water binding agents, vitamins A and E, water binding agent, more thickeners, herb oils, and preservatives.

In-Control T-Zone Solution *($16.50 for 1.75)*. The ingredients in this product won't change your oily skin. If anything, the salicylic acid can irritate and may cause the skin to produce even more oil.

Equalizer Oil-Free Gel *($27.50 for 1.75 ounces)* is supposed to "monitor" and "disperse" excess oil concentration, but it simply can't do that. The ingredients are water, alcohol, slip agents and thickeners, clay, talc, more slip agents, more thickeners, and preservatives. None of those ingredients can disperse or monitor oil, although the clay and talc can absorb some of it. The alcohol can irritate the skin, making it oilier.

Skin Perfecting Lotion *($27.50 for 6 ounces)* is an ordinary lightweight moisturizer with none of the interesting ingredients in the creme counterpart listed below. It contains a small amount of sunscreen that isn't enough to protect adequately from the sun, plus lots of thickeners and some standard water binding ingredients, and far down in the ingredient list a negligible amount of collagen and aloe.

Skin Perfecting Creme *($35 for 1.75 ounces)* is a lightweight moisturizer with one of the longest ingredient lists I've ever seen. If you are looking for every state-of-the-art moisturizing ingredient, look here: collagen, vitamins, herb extracts, plant oils, proteins, and amino acids, all fairly high up in the ingredient list. This would take care of dry skin and your worry that you might be missing out on the latest skin care ingredients (except for AHA).

Re-Nutriv Creme *($45 for 1 ounce; $235 for 16.75 ounces)* contains mostly water, standard water binding agents, mineral oil, more thickeners, water binding agents, and preservatives. This is a very emollient moisturizer for extremely dry skin.

Re-Nutriv Creme Lightweight *($45 for 1 ounce; $235 for 16.75 ounces)* is almost identical to the creme above, but indeed lighterweight. The suggestion is to use this for normal to oily skin, but I think it is too emollient for the latter skin type.

Re-Nutriv Firming Eye Creme *($42.50 for 1 ounce)* contains mostly water, amino acid, water binding agents (including collagen), several thickeners, lanolin oil, algae, thickener, collagen, elastin, water binding agent, vitamins A and E, mineral oil, more thickeners, and preservatives. This won't firm the eye area, and amino acids and collagen cannot change your skin, but it is a very good emollient moisturizer.

Non-Oily Skin Supplement *($37.50 for 3.25 ounces)* isn't exactly oil-free because the fifth ingredient is squalane, or shark oil. Still, this is a good lightweight moisturizer that contains mostly water, water binding agents, aloe, herb extracts, a long list of thickeners, and preservatives. In spite of not being oil-free it is still a good lightweight moisturizer and could be good for someone with normal to slightly dry skin. I would not recommend it for someone with oily skin unless they also had problems with dry skin.

Counter-Blemish Lotion *($12 for 0.45 ounce)* contains alcohol, thickener, and salicylic acid. This won't stop a blemish or cure one, but it can be irritating to most skin types.

Almond Clay Mask *($18.50 for 4 ounces)* contains mostly water, thickeners, clay, more thickeners, almond meal, more clay, salicylic acid (possible skin irritant), more thickeners, and preservatives. This is a fairly standard clay mask with the addition of a gritty substance (almonds) and a peeling agent (salicylic acid) that can be quite irritating to most skin types.

Rose Refining Mask *($18.50 for 1.75 ounces)* contains mostly water, slip agent, mineral oil, thickeners, petrolatum, shark oil, more thickeners, salicylic acid, soothing agent, more thickeners, a long list of herbs (tea), menthol, more thickeners, and preservatives. This is an interesting mask that contains a strong peeling agent (salicylic acid), but also mineral oil and petrolatum meant to keep skin from peeling. Rather confusing, but it could possibly work as an exfoliator for someone with dry skin, although not as well as an alpha hydroxy acid product.

Triple Creme Hydrating Mask *($27.50 for 2.5 ounces)* contains mostly water, slip agent, almond oil, standard water binding agent, thickener, shark oil, more thickeners, rice oil, more thickeners, water binding agents, more thickeners, and preservatives. These are good moisturizing ingredients, so they would feel good if left on the face for a while.

Eucerin

Eucerin Cleansing Bar *($4 for 3 ounces)* is a somewhat gentle bar soap with a standard soap base but more gentle detergent cleansers. It would be good for someone with normal to oily skin.

Eucerin Cleansing Lotion *($6.60 for 8 ounces)* is a very drying water-soluble cleanser that can irritate the skin and eyes.

Eucerin Creme *($7.39 for 4 ounces)* is an extremely rich, almost heavy moisturizer that contains mostly water, petrolatum, mineral oil, thickeners, and preservatives. This would be best for someone with extremely dry skin.

Eucerin Daily Facial Lotion SPF 20 *($7.45 for 4 ounces)* is an OK light-weight daytime moisturizer/sunscreen (good sunscreen) that contains water, slip agent, mineral oil, thickeners, slip agents, thickeners, and preservatives. One of the preservatives is sodium hydroxide, which can be a skin irritant.

Eucerin Moisturizing Lotion *($7.99 for 16 ounces)* contains mostly water, mineral oil, isopropyl myristate (can cause blackheads), several thickeners, and preservatives. This is just thickeners and mineral oil, which makes it a mediocre moisturizer.

Eucerin Plus Alpha Hydroxy Moisturizing Lotion *($5.47 for 6 ounces)* is a mineral oil-based moisturizer with several thickeners, some standard water binding agents, and about 5 percent AHA. This is an OK AHA moisturizer, but just OK.

Fashion Fair

Deep Cleansing Lotion *($14.25 for 8 ounces)* is a fairly greasy cleanser that would need to be wiped off. It is mineral oil-based and contains lanolin, which is suited better to a moisturizer for very dry skin than to a cleanser.

Skin Freshener I *($11.50 for 6 ounces)* contains mostly alcohol and is very drying, not to mention irritating, to the skin.

Skin Freshener II *($11.50 for 6 ounces)* has basically the same ingredients as Skin Freshener I and can be just as drying to the skin.

Deep Pore Astringent *($13.25 for 8 ounces)* is similar to the Skin Fresheners; the alcohol is just too irritating for most skin types.

Oil Free Moisturizer *($19.50 for 4 ounces)* is indeed an oil-free moisturizer that contains mostly propylene glycol (water binding agent) and thickeners. It also contains isopropyl myristate (fourth ingredient), which can cause blackheads.

Eye Cream *($18.50 for 0.5 ounce)* is a somewhat thick moisturizer that contains very emollient ingredients of water, slip agent, mineral oil, thickeners, plant oils, and preservatives. It also contains some collagen, elastin, vitamins, and amino acids, but they come after the preservative so the amount is negligible. Nevertheless, this is a good moisturizer for dry skin but might be too heavy for around the eye.

Moisturizing Lotion *($18.50 for 4 ounces)* is a basic moisturizer containing mostly water, standard water binding agent, petrolatum, several thickeners and preservatives. This is just an OK, average moisturizer, nothing special.

Moisturizing Creme *($18.50 for 4 ounces)* is an emollient moisturizer that would work well on dry skin. It contains mostly water, thickeners, mineral oil, sesame oil, aloe vera, standard water binding agents, more thickeners, and preservatives.

Flori Roberts

Melanin Cleanser *($13 for 8 ounces)* is a fairly greasy wipe-off cleanser that contains mostly water, thickener, mineral oil, lanolin, and preservatives.

Oil Free Astringent "40" *($12 for 8 ounces)* is an alcohol-based toner that also contains camphor and menthol, making it too irritating for most skin types.

Oil Free Skin Freshener *($12 for 8 ounces)* is almost identical to the astringent above, minus the camphor and menthol. It is still too irritating for most skin types.

Optima Refining Lotion Oil Free *($14 for 8 ounces)* contains mostly water, standard water binding agent, witch hazel, slip agent, protein, and preservatives. The witch hazel can be a skin irritant and one of the preservatives is quaternium-15, which can also be a serious skin irritant.

T-Zone Oil Block *($12.50 for 2.3 ounces)* is mostly alcohol; alcohol won't change the oil on your face but it can irritate your skin and make blemishes look redder.

Melanin Moisturizer *($13 for 4 ounces)* contains mostly water, thickener, glycerin, petrolatum, more thickeners, and preservatives. This fairly standard petrolatum moisturizer would be good for someone with dry skin, but nothing special for women of color.

My Everything Creme *($25 for 3.25 ounces)* contains mostly water, standard water binding agents, isopropyl myristate (can cause blackheads), shark oil, beeswax, nut oils, vitamin A, soothing agents, and preservatives. This would be a good emollient moisturizer for someone with dry skin who isn't prone to breakouts.

Blue Indigo Moisturizer *($11 for 2 ounces)* is basically a petrolatum-based moisturizer with only thickeners and preservatives. It's OK, but not great.

Hydrophillic Moisture Complex *($20 for 2 ounces)* contains mostly water, glycerin, mineral oil, thickeners, collagen, preservatives, a tiny amount of AHA, and more preservatives. This is an OK lightweight moisturizer for normal to dry skin.

Optima Gel Cleanser *($15 for 6 ounces)* is actually a fairly good water-soluble cleanser that should work well for someone with oily skin without irritation or dryness.

Double O Soap *($13 for 4 ounces)* is a standard bar soap with many of the same ingredients as the toner below and would be equally as irritating and drying.

Double O Complex for Oily Skin *($15 for 8 ounces)* contains mostly alcohol, water, peppermint oil, clove, eucalyptus, camphor, and benzoic acid. This toner is an extremely drying product with more irritants in one bottle than most.

Forever Spring

Connie Stevens the actress promotes this line as the reason she looks so wonderful. Well, Connie, you do look wonderful (at least in the pictures), but it has nothing to do with these products. These are just skin care products with ingredients similar to a hundred others on the market. I also want to state clearly that I find the name of this skin care line, Forever Spring, insulting and childish. Any cosmetics company name that implies you won't get wrinkles if you use their products (like Sudden Youth, Instant Youth, Instant Lift, and so on) is also offensive. Having let off steam about my irritation with the way this line is marketed, I can be more objective now and tell you that some of these products are quite good. (Only the cleanser and exfoliator are a problem.) But the "Time Machine" ($120) they sell is definitely one of the biggest wastes of money presently on the market. This Time Machine is supposed to exercise facial muscles through topical stimulation. Facial muscles, just like body muscles, cannot be artificially exercised to be strengthened or built up. Even if this machine did work, the muscles would simply bulge, not lift skin. Have you ever seen older body builders, with muscles *and* sagging skin? It would be the same thing. In addition, the irritation this machine causes can create damage by breaking delicate surface capillaries. It is also supposed to increase circulation. There are better ways to increase circulation than with electricity. Running up and down your stairs for 20 minutes will not only increase your circulation, it will also help your heart and build energy.

Collagen Facial Cleanser *($14.25 for 4 ounces)* is a fairly standard, greasy wipe-off cleanser, not water-soluble. It contains mineral oil, thickeners, lanolin oil, collagen, and safflower oil. The directions say wipe up, never down. Whether you pull the skin up or down you're sagging it. Never wipe off make-up, and use only water-soluble cleansers.

Honey Almond Apricot Scuffer *($13.25 for 4 ounces)* is an OK exfoliator that uses walnut shells. However, baking soda mixed with a cleanser would do the same thing without clogging ingredients such as lanolin oil and emulsifying waxes. This product also contains the preservative quaternium-15, which can be a skin irritant.

Ambrosia Skin Refresher *($9.25 for 8 ounces)* is a very good irritant-free toner that contains good soothing ingredients: water, standard water binding ingredients, aloe vera, water binding agent, soothing agent, and preservatives.

Skin Quencher *($22.75 for 4 ounces)* is a standard collagen-based moisturizer that is meant to be used with the Time Machine. The moisturizer is emollient and would be good for normal to dry skin. But the Time Machine and this moisturizer won't change your skin; collagen is just a moisturizing ingredient, nothing more, and the Time Machine is just silly.

Ginseng Cream *($21.25 for 4 ounces)* is a very good emollient moisturizer for dry skin, containing mostly water, slip agent, coconut oil, mineral oil, thickeners, ginseng, shark oil, collagen, elastin, vitamin E, slip agent, vitamin A, and preservatives.

Facial Clay *($15 for 4 ounces)* is basically a standard clay mask that contains mostly water, clays, glycerin, protein, thickener, cucumber extract, ginseng (tea), and preservatives. One of the preservatives is quaternium-15, which is considered very irritating. The protein and cucumber sound good, but the amount is negligible in comparison to the clay.

Frances Denney

Basic Line

Creamy Cleansing Lotion *($16.50 for 8 ounces)* is a standard mineral oil-based wipe-off cleanser that leaves the face with a greasy film. The third ingredient is isopropyl myristate, which can cause blackheads.

Quick Foam Cleanser *($16.50 for 8 ounces)* is a water-soluble cleanser that can be quite drying, plus it contains quaternium-15, a preservative that can be a strong skin irritant and should never be used near the eyes

Satin Cleansing Cream *($11 for 4 ounces)* is a standard wipe-off cold cream-type product that is mostly mineral oil and petrolatum. Greasy and messy are the words for how this one works.

Mild Skin Lotion *($15.75 for 8 ounces)* isn't at all mild. Witch hazel and alcohol, which are both quite irritating, are near the top of the ingredient list.

Protective Oil Control *($14.50 for 4 ounces)* is just another alcohol-based product that can't control oil, but it can irritate and redden the face.

Ultimate Protection *($25 for 1.7 ounces)* contains mostly water, slip agents, thickeners, a small amount of sunscreen (not enough to protect the skin adequately from the sun), standard water binding agents, water binding agents, more thickeners, and preservatives. There are some vitamin antioxidants in this product, but they are too far down in the ingredient list to be significant. This is a good lightweight moisturizer, but it does not provide ultimate or even very effective protection from anything but dryness.

Ultimate Repair *($25 for 1 ounce)* contains mostly water, standard water binding agents, castor oil, water binding agents, and preservatives. This is a good lightweight moisturizer, but it won't repair skin, it is just a moisturizer.

Multi-Layer Moisturizer *($17 for 2 ounces)* contains mostly water, vegetable oil, slip agents, mineral oil, lanolin, a small amount of sunscreen (not enough to protect adequately from the sun), thickener, plant oils, and preservatives. This is a very good basic emollient moisturizer for very dry skin.

Multi-Layer Night Cream *($18 for 1.25 ounces)* contains mostly water, thickener, mineral oil, water binding agents, thickeners, slip agent, collagen, soothing agents, elastin, and preservatives. This is a good emollient moisturizer, but not as emollient as the moisturizer above. For very dry skin I would use the Multi-Layer Moisturizer at night and forget the Night Cream.

Neck Cream *($17 for 2 ounces)* contains only cosmetic thickeners and preservatives. This isn't a very good moisturizer and it won't do anything for the neck or any other part of the body.

Eye Cream Concentrate *($18 for 0.5 ounce)* contains mostly water, standard water binding agents, mineral oil, thickeners, avocado oil, collagen, thickener, vitamin E, and preservatives. This is a good emollient cream, but don't expect the collagen to do anything special because it can't.

Fade Away with SPF 15 Skin Lightener *($12 for 1.9 ounces)* is an emollient moisturizer/sunscreen with mineral oil and lanolin. It also contains hydroquinone, which can be quite irritating, as the skin bleach. However, there is evidence that suggests hydroquinone can slightly fade "age" spots.

Sensitive Line

Gentle Cream Wash *($18 for 6 ounces)* contains a lot of herbs, but that doesn't help this cleanser because it doesn't remove makeup very well without a washcloth, which means it isn't very gentle. It can also leave a film on the skin.

Mint Wake-Up Gel Refreshing Cleanser *($14 for 6 ounces)* is an OK water-soluble cleanser that can be drying to most skin types; the spearmint oil can irritate the eyes.

Clean Sweep *($16 for 4 ounces)* contains mostly herbal water, aloe vera, wax, slip agents, detergent cleanser, plant extracts, plant oils, thickeners, slip agents, and preservatives. This is a good water-soluble cleanser for normal to dry skin, but it can leave a slight film on the face. The plants sound good but have nothing to do with cleaning the skin.

Balancing Lotion *($14 for 6 ounces)* contains mostly herbal water, aloe vera, alcohol, glycerin, herb extracts (tea), slip agents, and preservatives. Alcohol is irritating even if you hide it between herbs and aloe vera.

Moisture Infusion *($20 for 4 ounces)* contains mostly herbal water, standard slip agents, canola oil, thickeners, slip agents, sea kelp, more thickeners, more plant extracts, slip agents, plant oils, and preservatives. If you can ignore the plants, what you'll find is actually a very good moisturizer for dry skin.

Nourishing Lotion *($14 for 6 ounces)* contains mostly herbal water, aloe vera, glycerin, more plant extracts, plant oils, vitamin E, slip agent, and preservatives. This won't feed the skin, but it is a very good irritant-free toner if you aren't allergic to any of the plants.

Urgent Nourisher *($24 for 2 ounces)* contains mostly herbal water, thickener, a small amount of sunscreen (not enough to adequately protect the skin from the sun), castor oil, thickeners, standard water binding agents, thickeners, apricot oil, vitamin E, plant oil, plant extracts, vitamin A, thickeners, and preservatives. This can't feed the skin, but it is still a very good lightweight emollient moisturizer.

Oil Balancer *($24 for 2 ounces)* contains mostly herb water, a small amount of sunscreen, standard water binding agents, slip agents, thickener, plant extracts, thickeners, slip agents, and preservatives. This is a good lightweight moisturizer, but it will not control oil in any way, shape, or form.

Oil Terminator *($26 for 2 ounces)* contains mostly herb water, aloe vera, a small amount of sunscreen, castor oil, glycerin, vitamin E, grapefruit and spearmint oil, more herb extracts, and preservatives. This product won't stop oil on your face; if anything, because of the grapefruit and spearmint oil, it will add oil to the skin. Plus, some of the plants in this product, including witch hazel, lemon, and pine, can be skin irritants.

Protecting Lotion *($14 for 6 ounces)* contains mostly herb water, aloe vera, glycerin, plant extracts, soothing agents, vitamin E, slip agents, plant oils, and preservatives. This is a soothing irritant-free toner, but it won't change the skin and the herbs aren't what is soothing the skin.

Tender Eyes *($20 for 0.5 ounce)* is a good lightweight moisturizer that contains mostly herb water, glycerin, standard water binding agent, slip agents, plant extracts, thickeners, and preservatives. The herbs won't nourish or moisturize the skin; the other ingredients, although ordinary, are what counts in here.

Texture Treatment *($18 for 4 ounces)* is a standard clay mask that contains some herb oils, which makes it more soothing than most.

Source of Beauty Line

Cleanser *($17 for 8 ounces)* is a good water-soluble cleanser that can take off all the makeup, but can also be slightly drying for some skin types.

Alcohol Free Freshener *($16 for 8 ounces)* contains mostly water, witch hazel (can be a skin irritant), water binding agents, and preservatives. Although this doesn't contain pure alcohol, witch hazel is still a skin irritant.

Cream *($24.50 for 1.25 ounces)* is a rich, emollient moisturizer for very dry skin; it contains mostly water, mineral oil, thickeners, lanolin oil, petrolatum, more thickeners, vitamins A and E, and preservatives. The vitamins are too far down in the ingredient list to be significant.

Freeman Beautiful Skin

Beautiful Skin Lemon & Yogurt Cleansing Milk *($3.59 for 6 ounces)* is supposed to be water-soluble, but it doesn't rinse very well and leaves a film on the skin.

Beautiful Skin Chamomile & Allantoin Lite Moisturizer *($3.59 for 6 ounces)* contains mostly water, standard water binding ingredient, thickeners, slip agent, chamomile extract, vitamins A and E, and preservatives. This is a good lightweight moisturizer.

Beautiful Skin Apricot & Sea Kelp Facial Scrub *($3.59 for 6 ounces)* is a walnut shell-based scrub that is as good as any on the market; the only problem is it contains the preservative quaternium-15, which can be a skin irritant.

Beautiful Skin Avocado & Oatmeal Facial Masque *($3.59 for 6 ounces)* is a standard clay mask with a small amount of oil, which can prevent it from being too drying. If you want to use a clay mask, this is a good one for an exceptionally reasonable price.

Beautiful Skin Cucumber & Ginseng Peel Off Masque *($3.59 for 6 ounces)* contains mostly water, a plastic-like ingredient, alcohol, clay, plant extracts, and preservatives. The alcohol plus the clay make this too drying for most skin types.

Guerlain

You'd better sit down for this one: Guerlain has one of the most expensive skin care products on the market. Guerlain's **Serennissme Issima** is $170 for 1 ounce. That's about $2,720 a pound. What is in this pricey wonder? Standard cosmetic ingredients and something called *genestum*, which supposedly can tackle all the things that can cause the skin to age. Regardless of what genesium is (and it is a major secret at Guerlain headquarters), Serennissme does not contain a sunscreen. Without a sunscreen it can't handle the number one primary cause of skin aging, and that's sun damage. It does have some good water binding ingredients and some antioxidants, but absolutely nothing you can't find in a hundred other products. What an expensive burn! But expensive is what makes this line so seductive. Not everyone can have it. Will you be $170 more beautiful or younger than someone else? Of course not. Still, for many women the issue isn't effectiveness, rather it is the sense of "being worth it." Perhaps my reviews can refocus that notion. The question isn't whether or not you're worth it, but whether or not it is worth your time and effort to be misled by unreal product claims. Bottom line: Don't worry if you can't afford this line, you're not being left out to wrinkle alone in the cold.

To be fair, I should add that Guerlain is not the most expensive product line at the cosmetics counters. It is definitely up there, but not the worse offender.

Evolution Complete Cleanser *($30 for 8.2 ounces)* is a standard mineral oil-based cleanser that doesn't rinse off well without the help of a washcloth, and it can leave a greasy film on the skin.

Evolution Divinaura Beauty Enhancer *($57 for 1 ounce)* contains standard cosmetic ingredients—water, thickeners, standard water binding agents, thickeners, vitamin E, and water binding agent—and, are you ready for this, gold. How much gold? Six milligrams, which is about 0.000353 ounce. What is this microscopic amount of gold supposed to be for? Stimulating and energizing the skin. The gold can't be absorbed, so I imagine if I rub my gold necklace over my face it should do the same thing.

Evolution Exfoliating Creme for the Face *($34 for 1.6 ounces)* contains mostly water, thickener, mineral oil, more thickeners, oak root (an astringent), more thickeners, and preservatives. This is an OK exfoliator but not great, and it doesn't rinse well.

Evolution Refreshing Tonic Vitale *($30 for 8.5 ounces)* is a standard alcohol-based toner that is too irritating for most skin types. There is nothing refreshing about this toner.

Evolution Specific Eye-Contour Care *($26 for 0.5 ounce)* contains mostly water, thickener, amino acids, lanolin, standard water binding agents, more thickeners, water binding agents, vitamin E, and preservatives. This is a good emollient moisturizer, but the amino acids won't do anything to change a wrinkle.

Evolution Sublicreme No. 1 *($60 for 1 ounce)* contains mostly water, amino acids, slip agents, mineral oil, castor oil, thickeners, vitamin E, DNA, fragrance, vitamin A, and preservatives. This is a good lightweight moisturizer, but don't expect anything unique from the amino acids or the DNA—they can't repair skin.

Evolution Sublicreme No. 2 *($50 for 1.7 ounces)* contains mostly water, thickeners, standard water binding agents, amino acids, more thickeners, a small amount of sunscreen (not enough to protect adequately from the sun), water binding agents, fragrance, and preservatives. There are some more good water binding agents and vitamins in this product, but they are too far down on the ingredient list to be significant. This is a good lightweight moisturizer for normal to dry skin, but nothing very unique or impressive. Just a reminder: amino acids can't rebuild the skin from the outside in.

Issima Creme Cleanser *($42 for 6.8 ounces)* is a standard mineral oil-based cleanser with ordinary thickeners and slip agents. It doesn't rinse well without the aid of a washcloth and can leave a film on the skin.

Issima Anti-Wrinkle Eye Contour Fluid *($50 for 0.5 ounce)* contains water, slip agent, horsetail extract (can be a skin irritant), thickeners, a small amount of sunscreen, vitamin E, elastin, more thickeners, plant extracts, vitamin A, and preservatives. This is a good lightweight emollient, but the price tag is way out of proportion for these average ingredients.

Issima Long-Term Rehydrator *($115 for 1.7 ounces).* should be great for this kind of money. Unfortunately, the ingredients are so ordinary as to almost be funny, but it's too expensive to laugh at. It contains mostly water, mineral oil, thickeners, horsetail extract (can be an irritant), more thickeners, standard water binding agents, vitamin E, elastin (keeps water in the skin), lanolin, a very small amount of sunscreen, thickener, a tiny amount of AHA, and preservatives, the same ingredients you find in a lot of other products for a lot less money.

Issima Midnight Secret *($80 for 1 ounce)* contains mostly water, thickeners, water binding agents, amino acids, mineral oil, vitamin E, lanolin, a long list of thickeners, slip agents, and preservatives. This is a good moisturizer for normal to dry skin, but nothing more. There is no secret inside this bottle.

Issima Moisturizing Lotion *($38 for 6.8 ounces)* contains mostly water, standard water binding agents, fragrance, thickener, and preservatives. It's supposed to be an irritant-free toner, but it contains too much fragrance and sodium phosphate, which can be a skin irritant.

Issima Neck Treatment Creme *($77 for 1.7 ounces)* is an ordinary moisturizer (albeit an expensive one) that contains mostly water, mineral oil, wax, thickeners, wheat germ oil, water binding agents, more thickeners, a tiny amount of AHA, and preservatives.

Serennissme Issima Restructuring Treatment with Active Genesium *($170 for 1 ounce).* See my review in the introductory paragraphs.

Issima Aquamasque *($60 for 2.5 ounces)* contains a long list of thickeners, slip agents, vitamin E, protein, plant extracts, water binding agents, more thickeners, and preservatives. This is a good emollient for the skin but not anything unique or special.

Instant Wrinkle Smooth

Instant Wrinkle Smooth by Glamatone *($7.58 for 0.55 ounce)* is one of the many bogus temporary face-lift products on the market. I'm sure many of you have seen at least one, if not several, of these products. The before and after pictures are nothing less than amazing. If you believed the pictures you could easily assume that no one would ever need a face-lift, the results are so remarkable. One side of the face looks haggard and lined; the nose is prominent. The other side is smooth and lifted, with no jowls or laugh lines, and the nose looks thinner. Imagine, even a nose job. Yet most of these products do the exact same thing: temporarily irritate the skin, causing it to swell, and then a plasticizer dries over it to create the supposedly smooth look. Of course, if you move your face or wait an hour the swelling goes down and you're back where you started. Now here's the rub: I've talked to many dermatologists who suggest that repeatedly irritating the skin around the eyes can make wrinkles worse. My suggestion is don't waste your money on any of these.

Jergens

Advanced Therapy Lotion, Aloe & Lanolin *($3.65 for 20 ounces)* contains mostly water, glycerin, thickener, palm oil, aloe vera, lanolin, standard water binding agents, mineral oil, more thickeners, and preservatives. This is a very emollient moisturizer that would be good for someone with dry to very dry skin. It also contains the preservative quaternium-15 (last ingredient), which can be a skin irritant.

Advanced Therapy Lotion, Daily Care Moisturizer *($3.65 for 20 ounces)* contains mostly water, alcohol, glycerin, thickeners, lanolin oil, avocado oil, and preservatives. Why is alcohol (which is very drying) in the first ingredients of a moisturizer? This product is confused and too irritating for most skin types.

Advanced Therapy Lotion, Extra Dry Skin Treatment *($3.65 for 20 ounces)* contains mostly water, thickener, standard water binding agents, palm oil, thickeners, petrolatum, mineral oil, more thickeners, water binding agents, and preservatives. This is a very emollient moisturizer that would be good for extremely dry skin. It does contain quaternium-15, a preservative that can be a skin irritant.

Advanced Therapy Lotion, Vitamin E & Lanolin *($3.65 for 20 ounces)* contains mostly water, glycerin, thickener, palm oil, thickener, vitamin E, lanolin, water binding agents, mineral oil, more thickeners, and preservatives. This is a very good moisturizer for normal to very dry skin.

Lancaster

Very Mild Cleanser *($25 for 17 ounces)* is a mineral oil-based cleanser with standard thickeners. It is not water-soluble and leaves a slightly greasy film on the skin.

Cleansing Bar *($16 for 3.4 ounces)* is a standard detergent bar soap that can be rather drying on the skin and can irritate the eyes.

Foaming Gel Cleanser *($25 for 17 ounces)* is a water-soluble cleanser that can be drying and irritating to the skin, and also to the eyes.

Very Mild Lotion *($25 for 17 ounces)* contains mostly water, glycerin, witch hazel, slip agents, preservative, plant extracts, and preservatives. The witch hazel can be a skin irritant, so I wouldn't call this very mild, but it can be good for normal to oily skin types who do not have sensitive skin.

Vivifying Lotion *($25 for 17 ounces)* is a standard alcohol-based toner that can irritate the skin. It contains some plant extracts, but that won't counteract the irritation from the alcohol.

Face Exfoliant *($25 for 3.4 ounces)* tends to be greasy and leaves a film on the face, plus it isn't the best exfoliator. It contains petrolatum, lanolin oil, and palm oils, which are not easily rinsed.

Competence Daily Vitalizer Extra Rich SPF 2 *($40 for 1.7 ounces)* isn't all that competent; the sunscreen is only SPF 2, not enough to protect adequately from the sun. Other than that, this is a very good lightweight moisturizer with some good water binding agents, a small amount of elastin, and vitamin E. There is thymus extract in here, but it doesn't provide any benefit for the skin.

Competence Daily Vitalizer Normal SPF 2 *($35 for 1.7 ounces)* is almost identical to the Extra Rich lotion above; the difference is fewer thickeners.

Competence Dynamic Eye Creme SPF 2 *($27.50 for 0.5 ounce)* contains mostly water, thickeners, standard water binding agents, water binding agents, thickeners, vitamin E, and preservative. Plant extracts and thymus extract are also in there, but they come after the preservative, not the best placement, although they don't provide any real benefit for the skin anyway. SPF 2 isn't adequate to protect from the sun.

Competence Eye Science *($40 for 0.5 ounce)* is not even vaguely competent. The third ingredient is alcohol, which is very drying and irritating to the skin, particularly the skin around the eyes.

Competence Fortifying Complex SPF 4 *($45 for 1 ounce)* contains water, glycerin, thickener, jojoba oil, thickeners, yeast extract, thickeners, water binding agents, vitamins C and E, thickener, protein, mineral oil, water binding agents, and preservatives. This is a very good emollient moisturizer for normal to dry skin. Yeast can't provide any special benefit for the skin, but they attribute rejuvenating wonders to it anyway.

Suractif Cleansing Treatment *($35 for 17 ounces)* is supposed to be a water-soluble cleanser, only it doesn't rinse very well. It could be good for someone with very dry skin.

Suractif Preparation Lotion *($30 for 17 ounces)* is an irritant-free toner that is actually quite soothing to the skin.

Suractif Skin Retexturizer *($60 for 1.7 ounces)* contains mostly water, glycerin, palm oil, mineral oil, vitamin E, water binding agents, and preservatives. This is a good emollient moisturizer with a small amount of sunscreen, but it is only a moisturizer, nothing more.

Suractif Facial Treatment *($45 for 1.7 ounces)* contains mostly water, glycerin, thickeners, jojoba oil, standard water binding agents, mineral oil, thickeners, vitamin E, and preservatives. This is a good emollient moisturizer for dry skin, but absolutely nothing special or unique. These are ordinary cosmetic ingredients.

Anti-Stress Eye Mask *($30 for 1.7 ounces)* contains mostly water, glycerin, several thickeners, egg white, elastin, plant extracts, and preservatives.

The egg white tightens the face and the emollients are nice, but this is a lot of money for standard ingredients.

Moisture Mask *($27 for 1.7 ounces)* is a mineral oil-based mask added to thickeners and preservatives. A rather ordinary ingredient list with no special moisturizing properties.

Revealing Mask *($25 for 2.5 ounces)* is a standard clay mask that contains no other moisturizers, water binding agents, or oils, so this would be quite drying on the face.

Lancome

Douceur Demaquillant Nutrix Cleansing Emulsion *($19.50 for 6.6 ounces)* is a fairly greasy cleanser that needs to be wiped off. It contains mostly mineral oil, water, slip agent, egg oil, and vegetable oil. That amount of oil would make any cleanser feel greasy.

Galate Milky Creme Cleanser *($19.50 for 6.8 ounces)* is supposed to be a splash- or tissue-off cleanser for all skin types. It is fairly greasy for oily or combination skin, and it doesn't really rinse off without the use of a washcloth. It also contains isopropyl myristate (third ingredient), which can cause blackheads. However, it may be good for extremely dry skin.

Ablutia Gel Moussante Foaming Gel Cleanser *($19.50 for 6.8 ounces)* is a standard water-soluble cleanser that is fairly gentle and cleans the face well. It can be drying for some skin types and possibly irritate the eyes.

Ablutia Huile Moussante Foaming Oil Cleanser *($19.50 for 6.8 ounces)* is similar to the foaming gel cleanser above, except that the cleansing agents are somewhat more gentle. However, there is only a tiny bit of oil in this cleanser, which won't counteract the dryness of the detergent cleansers.

Clarifiance Oil-Free Gel Cleanser *($15 for 3.6 ounces)* is a very good water-soluble cleanser that takes off all the makeup without irritating the eyes or drying out the skin. Nice going, Lancome.

Exfoliance Delicate Facial Buff *($19.50 for 3.5 ounces)* is an OK exfoliator for the face except that it can be drying for some skin types.

Effacile Gentle Eye Makeup Remover *($15 for 4 ounces)* is an oil-free eye makeup remover that isn't all that gentle. I've had several reports that this is irritating to the eyes.

Clarifiance Alcohol-Free Natural Astringent *($16 for 6.8 ounces)* contains mostly water, alum, preservatives, and slip agent. Basically this is just water and alum (like in styptic pencils). It is alcohol-free, but it doesn't contain anything good or interesting for the skin.

Tonique Douceur Non-Alcoholic Freshener for Dry/Sensitive Skin *($17.50 for 6.8 ounces)* is indeed alcohol-free, but the third ingredient is sodium borate, which is a skin irritant. No alcohol is nice, but irritant-free is what you really want.

Tonique Fraicheur Mild Astringent for Normal/Oily Skin *($17.50 for 6.8 ounces)* is an alcohol-based toner and can be irritating to the skin.

Point Correctif Blemish Stick *($13 for 0.2 ounce)* is mainly water and alcohol. This won't correct blemishes and it is a lot of money for such a tiny amount of alcohol.

Clarifiance Oil-Free Hydrating Fluide *($30 for 2.5 ounces)* is a good lightweight moisturizer that contains mostly water, standard water binding agents, thickeners, preservative, fragrance, and more preservatives. It also contains 2-bromo-2-nitropane 1, 3 diol, a very irritating preservative.

Noctosome Renewal Night Treatment *($42.50 for 1.75 ounces)* is a rich, emollient moisturizer for dry skin. It contains mostly water, nut oil, standard water binding agents, tallow (a thickener that can cause blackheads), vegetable oil, protein, thickener, water binding agents, fragrance, vitamin E, protein, and preservatives.

Niosome Daytime Skin Treatment *($42.50 for 2.5 ounces)* is an OK lightweight moisturizer that contains mostly water, nut oil, protein, thickener, standard water binding agents, a small amount of sunscreen (not enough to adequately protect from the sun), and preservatives.

Renergie Double Performance Treatment *($50 for 1.7 ounces)* contains mostly water, standard water binding agents, petrolatum, thickeners, protein, thickeners, a small amount of sunscreen (not enough to adequately protect from the sun), fragrance, vitamin E, protein, preservatives, egg white, and preservatives. This is a good emollient petrolatum-based moisturizer. It also contains 2-bromo-2-nitropane 1, 3 diol, a very irritating preservative.

Oligo-Major Activating Serum with Trace Elements *($42.50 for 0.84 ounce)* contains mostly water, glycerin, yeast, egg white (serum albumin), standard water binding agents, fragrance, and preservatives. This is an OK lightweight moisturizer, but it doesn't activate cell renewal. The trace elements (zinc, iron, manganese, and copper) are too far down in the ingredient list to matter.

Vivifiance Hydrating Eye Gel *($28 for 0.6 ounce)* contains mostly water, standard water binding agents, soothing agent, and preservatives. All the herb extracts, collagen, and interesting water binding agents are at the end of the ingredient and don't add up to much in this product. It is still a good lightweight moisturizer; the absurd price for the amount you get is the only problem.

Progres Eye Creme *($30 for 0.5 ounce)* is a thick eye cream that contains mostly water, standard water binding agents, petrolatum, thickeners, glycerin, fragrance, and preservatives. It also contains its share of fad ingredients such as amniotic fluid, liver extract, and calfskin extract, but they are at the end of the ingredient list and amount to very little. There is no evidence that these ingredients have any positive or negative effects on the skin. Basically, this cream is a good emollient for dry skin around the eyes or anywhere on the face, but it won't change wrinkles.

Progres Plus Anti-Wrinkle Creme *($42.50 for 1.25 ounces)* is mostly water, shark oil, lanolin oil, thickeners, yeast, more thickeners, fragrance, protein, and preservatives. This is a good emollient moisturizer for very dry skin, but it won't get rid of wrinkles.

Forte-Vital Pour Les Yeux Firming Eye Creme *($36.50 for 0.5 ounce)* contains mostly water, mineral oil, standard water binding agents, thickeners, yeast, protein, fragrance, and preservatives. This won't firm anything, but it is a good mineral oil-based moisturizer with some yeast and protein tossed in for effect.

Forte-Vital Serum Raffermissant Skin Firming Serum *($45 for 0.84 ounce)* contains mostly water, spleen extract, yeast, castor oil, thickeners, fragrance, preservative, more thickeners, and more preser-vatives. This is an OK lightweight moisturizer, but that's about it. Spleen extract won't firm skin, but it is high up in the ingredient list, so if this is what you want, there is plenty of it here.

Nutribel Nourishing Hydrating Emulsion *($46.50 for 4.2 ounces)* is a good, very emollient moisturizer that contains mostly water, jojoba oil, glycerin, mineral oil, grapeseed oil, palm oil, thickeners, water binding agents, fragrance, more thickeners, and preservatives. It also contains 2-bromo-2-nitropane 1, 3 diol, a very irritating preservative.

Nutrix Soothing Treatment Creme *($26.50 for 1.85 ounces)* contains mostly mineral oil, water, petrolatum, lanolin, thickeners, water binding agents, fragrance, protein (way down at the end of the list), and preservatives. This is a lot of money for mineral oil and Vaseline.

Hydrix Hydrating Creme *($32.50 for 1.9 ounces)* is a traditional petrolatum-based moisturizer. It contains mostly water, petrolatum, mineral oil, lanolin, thickeners, shark oil, more lanolin, and preservative. A good moisturizer for very dry skin, but this is a lot of money for Vaseline and lanolin. It also contains 2-bromo-2-nitropane 1, 3 diol, a very irritating preservative.

Trans-Hydrix *($32.50 for 1.9 ounces)* contains mostly water, palm oil, shea butter, mineral oil, thickeners, fragrance, preservative, water binding agents, and more preservatives. This is a good standard emollient moisturizer for dry skin. It also contains 2-bromo-2-nitropane 1, 3 diol, a very irritating preservative.

Hydrative Continuous Hydrating Resource *($22.50 for 1 ounce)* contains mostly water, shea butter, glycerin, standard water binding agents, mineral oil, thickeners, a small amount of sunscreen, more thickeners, fragrance, vitamin E, and preservatives. This is a good emollient moisturizer for very dry skin.

Empreinte de Beaute Deep Cleansing Clay Masque *($21 for 2.5 ounces)* is a basic clay mask that contains mostly water, clay, water binding agents, more clay, thickeners, protein, thickener, and preservatives. For a clay mask this is fine, but it also contains 2-bromo-2-nitropane 1, 3 diol, a very irritating preservative.

Masque No. 10 Hydrating Masque *($21 for 2.2 ounces)* contains mostly water, gum tragacanth (a gel thickener that is a possible skin irritant), a gelatin substance, thickener, and preservatives. There isn't much moisture in here; it is basically just a gel that dries on the face. Not very impressive, but the skin will feel smooth when you take it off, just like it does with most masks.

Durable Minceur Cellulite "Relief" Gel *($42.50 for 6.8 ounces).* The only reason I'm including this is to remind you that there are no creams on the market that can do anything to eliminate cellulite. I imagine that the word *relief* is in quotes on the packaging to obscure the meaning and to help relieve some of the pressure the FDA might put on a claim such as this.

La Prairie

Even if your skin could improve with these products, the prices might kill you. But there are a few women who can afford these prices, so what do they get for their money? The prestige of knowing they can afford the imperial price tag. High-priced skin care lines attract women who think that the dollars they spend give them something special most other women can't afford. To some extent, they're right. Those who can afford it get something other women have to live without: an immense amount of marketing hype and positioning. If you could read the ingredient labels and understand them, you would find their prices as ludicrous as I do. Many of La Prairie's claims are based on the use of ingredients such as placental protein, flower and herb extracts, animal collagen, and amino acids. There is no research that indicates any of these ingredients can alter the skin, but that doesn't stop the claims. To satisfy your own curiosity, I suggest you compare ingredient labels. You will notice that most of the ingredients in the La Prairie products (just like Chanel, Guerlain, Borghese, Yves St. Laurent, and Erno Laszlo products) are fairly standard cosmetic ingredients. The amount of the "specialty" ingredients is almost negligible by comparison.

La Prairie's claim to fame is their Clinic La Prairie in Montreux, Switzerland, where the rich come for injections of sheep placenta extract. Does it make a difference? Of course they say it does, but there are no independent studies that prove their claim. The question I ask myself is why hasn't this supposedly superior skin care wonder come to the United States. If sheep injections work, do it here, there are plenty of people who would love to waste their money, just like in Europe. I suspect the reason they don't is because they would never get away with it under the watchful eye of the FDA.

Essential Purifying Gel Cleanser *($45 for 7.3 ounces)* contains mostly water, detergent cleanser, thickener, slip agent, thickener, detergent cleanser, and preservative. There are some herb extracts, but they are at the end of the ingredient list, too minuscule to matter. This cleanser does rinse off, but leaves a slight film on the skin. It can also irritate the eyes.

Purifying Creme Cleanser *($45 for 6.8 ounces)* is meant to be rinsed off but it requires a washcloth. This cleanser is mineral oil- and petrolatum-based, which means it leaves a film on the skin.

Essential Exfoliator *($45 for 7 ounces)* is a standard facial scrub that contains mostly water, mineral oil, thickener, apricot powder, thickeners, detergent cleanser, and preservative. This is an OK scrub but it doesn't rinse very well and, to say the least, is overpriced for what you get.

Essence of Skin Caviar, Cellular Eye Complex with Caviar Extract *($80 for 0.5 ounce)* contains mostly water, standard water binding agents, protein, glycerin, placental protein, soothing agent, thickener, and preservatives. Well, at least the placental protein is higher up, before the preservatives, but this is still only a lightweight emollient and nothing more. If you want to believe protein can do something for the skin besides work as a water binding agent, that's up to you, but you've been warned.

Skin Caviar *($90 for 2 ounces)* is a lightweight oil contained in small gelatin pellets that break open when you rub them on the skin. Cute idea. These pellets contain mostly standard water binding agents, water, alcohol, vitamins A and E, soothing agents, plant oil, plant extracts, and preservatives. The alcohol is irritating to the skin and negates the possible benefit of the moisturizing ingredients.

Face Complex with Caviar Extract *($80 for 1 ounce)* contains mostly water, standard water binding agents, a small amount of sunscreen, thickener, algae extract, placental protein, water binding agent, vitamins A and E, plant extracts, thickeners, and preservatives. Everything else is typical except for the placental protein, but we've already discussed how inconsequential that is, right?

Age Management Balancer *($65 for 8.4 ounces)* contains mostly water, several standard water binding agents, algae extract, a small amount of AHA (less than 2 percent), water binding agents, plant extracts, and preservatives. This is a good irritant-free toner, but hardly worth the price tag.

Age Management Cream Natural SPF 8 *($125 for 1.7 ounces)* is one of the most expensive sunscreens on the market. It is a nonchemical SPF 8 and it does contain about 2 percent AHA (which isn't much), but other than that it is just an emollient moisturizer with fairly standard cosmetic ingredients. It does contain some good water binding agents and vitamins, but they are too far down in the ingredient list to be significant.

Age Management Serum *($125 for 1 ounce)* contains about 5 percent AHA, which is good but not great; 8 percent would be better. It is a good moisturizer with standard cosmetic ingredients; the interesting ingredients—vitamins, placental protein, extracts, and water binding agents—are far down at the end of list and too minor to matter. What a price tag for a rather ordinary AHA product.

Cellular Refining Lotion *($55 for 8.4 ounces)* is an irritant-free toner that contains mostly water, standard water binding agents, protein, preservative, soothing agent, and more preservatives. There are a few plant extracts, collagen, elastin, and placental extract, but they are at the very end of the ingredient list so the amount is insignificant.

Cellular Purifying Lotion *($55 for 8.4 ounces)* is a standard alcohol-based toner with a small amount of placental protein thrown in, but that can't compensate for the irritation caused by the alcohol.

Cellular Skin Conditioner *($65 for 4.2 ounces)* contains mostly water, mineral oil, glycerin, thickeners, and preservatives. Once again the placental protein is at the very end of the ingredient list, which means there is only a negligible amount of it. This is only a fairly ordinary mineral oil-based moisturizer.

Cellular Balancing Complex *($60 for 1.7 ounces)* contains mostly water, standard water binding agent, a small amount of sunscreen, glycerin, algae extract, standard water binding agents, thickeners, placental protein, several water binding agents, vitamins A and E, and preservatives. This is a good lightweight emollient moisturizer for normal to dry skin. We don't need to talk about the placental protein anymore, do we?

Cellular Night Cream *($95 for 1 ounce)* is a rather rich moisturizer for dry skin; it contains mineral oil, petrolatum, standard water binding agents, thickeners, and preservatives. Again the last ingredient in the listing is placental protein. Other than that, this is a rather boring mineral oil-based moisturizer with no other interesting emollients or water binding agents.

Cellular Eye Contour Creme *($75 for 0.5 ounce)* comes in at almost $2,400 per pound, yet it is nothing more than a petrolatum-based moisturizer. It contains a small amount of collagen, and placental protein is at the very end of the ingredient list.

Cellular Day Creme *($90 for 1 ounce)* is a standard mineral oil-based moisturizer. It contains mostly water, mineral oil, petrolatum, standard water binding agents, thickeners, and preservatives. This is a lot of money for a product that is mostly mineral oil, Vaseline, and nothing else.

Cellular Neck Creme *($105 for 1 ounce)* is practically identical to the Cellular Day Creme except for the addition of collagen and some plant extracts at the end of the ingredient list. It won't do anything special for the neck because the ingredients aren't anything speical.

Cellular Balancing Mask *($55 for six 0.24-ounce treatments)* is a two-part mask that you mix together. The liquid is mostly water, citric acid (an astringent and possible skin irritant), aloe vera, and preservatives. The powder contains mostly sodium bicarbonate (yes, baking soda), clay, thickeners, talc, placental protein, collagen, and fragrance. Minuscule amounts of aloe vera and baking soda are not going to balance anyone's skin.

Cellular Cycle Ampoules for the Face *($240 for seven 0.1-ounce treatments).* This one prices out to about $7,000 a pound! They can't be serious. This is a two-part self-mixed treatment (or joke, depending on your point of view). The liquid contains water, standard water binding agents, polyacrylamide (a thickener that is considered extremely toxic to the skin), and preservatives. The powder contains elastin, placental protein, and salts. A tiny amount of elastin and placental protein mixed with water? Are there really women willing to buy this?

Emergency Tonic *($50 for 1.7 ounces)* is a toner that contains mostly water, mineral oil, alcohol, propylene glycol, placental protein, and herb and flower extracts. It also contains salicylic acid, which along with the alcohol makes this a fairly irritating liquid.

L'Oreal Plenitude

Deep Cleansing Gel *($5 for 5 ounces)*. This foaming cleanser is fairly drying. It contains somewhat strong shampoo-type detergents that can be irritating to the eyes.

Hydrating Cleansing Creme *($6.19 for 6 ounces)* is supposed to be water-soluble but it isn't; it only comes off with the help of a washcloth and leaves a greasy film on the skin.

Foaming Gel Scrub *($5.96 for 4 ounces)* is a fairly drying cleanser that contains alcohol among the first ingredients.

Refreshing Eye Makeup Remover *($6.19 for 4.2 ounces)* does take off the eye makeup, but some of the first ingredients can cause irritation.

Tender Eye Makeup Remover *($6.50 for 4.2 ounces)* is definitely gentler than the Refreshing Eye Makup Remover.

Hydrating Floral Toner *($4.95 for 8.5 ounces)* contains mostly water, standard water binding agent, castor oil, preservative, soothing agent, and preservatives. This is a good irritant-free toner.

Oil-Control Toner *($5.68 for 8.5 ounces)* would be a good alcohol-free toner except that it contains potassium hydroxide, which is a very irritating substance, among the first ingredients.

Oil-Free Protective Daily Moisture Lotion SPF 12 *($5.96 for 1.4 ounces)* contains mostly water, standard water binding agents, thickeners, and preservatives. This is a good lightweight moisturer that is indeed oil-free and contains a decent amount of sunscreen.

Oil-Free Active Daily Moisture *($6 for 1.4 ounces)* is almost identical to the Protective Daily Moisture except it doesn't contain sunscreen. It is an OK lightweight moisturizer.

Protective Daily Moisture Lotion SPF 12 *($6.50 for 1.4 ounces)* contains mostly water, standard slip agent, vegetable oil, standard water binding agents, palm oil, thickeners, and preservatives. This is a good emollient moisturizer for dry skin, with a decent amount of sunscreen.

Hydra Renewal *($8.75 for 1.7 ounces)* is a very good emollient moisturizer for dry skin; it contains mostly water, glycerin, shea butter, standard water binding agents, mineral oil, vegetable oil, a long list of thickeners, preservative, vitamin E, and more preservatives.

Night Replenisher *($8.25 for 1.4 ounces)* is a very emollient moisturizer for dry skin; it contains mostly water, seasame oil, shea butter, vegetable oil, glycerin, lanolin oil, thickeners, elastin, more thickeners, preservative, protein, and more preservatives. Elastin and protein don't do much for the skin, and even if they did, there isn't enough of them to make a difference.

Action Liposomes *($15.75 for 1.7 ounces)* is an emollient moisturizer that contains mostly water, apricot oil, standard water binding agents, thickeners, a small amount of sunscreen, more thickeners, and preservatives. Liposomes are a good way to deliver moisturizer to the skin. It also contains 2-bromo-2-nitropane 1, 3 diol, a very irritating preservative.

Advanced Wrinkle Defense Cream *($8.25 for 1.2 ounces)* contains mostly water, standard water binding agents, thickeners, vegetable oil, a small amount of sunscreen, protein, vitamin A, and preservatives. This is a good lightweight moisturizer that won't protect from the sun or change wrinkles.

Eye Defense *($9.25 for 0.5 ounce)* contains mostly water, jojoba oil, standard water binding agents, protein, thickener, and preservatives. This is a good emollient moisturizer.

Wrinkle Defense Cream *($12 for 1.7 ounces)* contains mostly water, thickeners, castor oil, petrolatum, glycerin, vegetable oil, corn oil, salt, liver extract, protein, and calfskin extract. The liver and calfskin extract provide no special benefits, but the other ingredients will improve dry skin.

Firming Facial Serum *($15.75 for 1 ounce)* contains mostly water, standard water binding agents, thickener, protein, water binding agent, and preservatives. The protein won't do much, but this is a good light-weight moisturizer.

Lubriderm

Body Bar *($1.94 for 4 ounces)* is a standard bar soap with some oils tossed in to reduce the irritation caused by the soap.

Loofah Bar *($1.94 for 4 ounces)* is almost identical to the Body Bar, with a scrub agent thrown in. This can be rough on some skin types.

One Step Facial Cleanser *($3.59 for 4 ounces)* is a good water-soluble cleanser that can be good for someone with oily skin. It does, however, contain the preservative quaternium-15 and the emulsifier sodium hydroxide; both can be quite irritating.

Facial Moisturizer SPF 5 *($6.05 for 4 ounces)* contains mostly water, standard water binding agents, thickeners, and preservatives. This product contains two preservatives (quaternium-15 and dmdm hydantoin) that are considered to be very irritating.

Lotion for Dry Skin Care *($4.70 for 8 ounces)* is a very rich, simple moisturizer for dry skin; it contains mostly water, mineral oil, petrolatum, thickener, lanolin, more thickeners, and preservatives.

M.A.C. (Make-up Art Cosmetics)

M.A.C. claims that these products are "based on dermatologically advanced moisturization concepts [using] noncomedogenic compounds." Although these products don't contain any mineral oil, lanolin, or isopropyl myristate, they have plenty of other ingredients that could make you break out or irritate your skin. There is no such thing as a product that is totally noncomedogenic. Their advanced moisturizing ingredients are not so advanced anymore, and are found in many different products on the market. In fact, lately they've become fairly standard ingredients. Also, all the "latest water binding ingredients" can't do any more for the skin than other moisturizing ingredients can. There are no studies around that can prove they positively affect aging one way or the other. By the way, the lactic acid listed in most of the M.A.C. moisturizers is present only as a moisturizing ingredient or to acid-balance the product, not as an alpha hydroxy acid ingredient.

M.A.C., like many product lines, has taken on the practice of listing each ingredient's source, such as coconut oil, corn, yeast, or vitamin. These identifiers are misleading, because they do not describe the chemical process the coconut or corn went through to become an unnatural-sounding ingredient whose name you don't understand on the label. The preservatives are ignored altogether, with no adequate description of their origins.

I would like to mention that one of the cosmetic chemists at M.A.C. was extremely helpful in my review of these products. Although we disagreed several times (I don't like alcohol in toners, I disagree that a cosmetic can provide oxygen to the skin as a benefit for cell turnover, and I don't accept the use of clay masks as being beneficial for the skin), I was surprised at his willingness to discuss my questions and concerns in a straightforward manner. Of course, he was biased, but with other cosmetics companies I rarely get past public relations departments that can never answer the simplest of my questions, like prices or exact names of products. Thank you, M.A.C, you are a rebel out there in the land of department store cosmetics. Keep up the good work.

Foaming Cleanser *($14 for 4.4 ounces)* is an OK water-soluble cleanser for oily skin, although it may prove to be quite drying. The cleansing agent is potassium hydroxide (caustic potash), which is a strong alkaline detergent. There are several ingredients that are supposed to bind water to the skin, but they won't be all that soothing if your skin is irritated by the potassium hydroxide.

pH Balanced Cleanser *($20 for 8.8 ounces)* is an OK water-soluble cleanser that can clean all the makeup without burning eyes, but it can still be somewhat drying on the skin. There is a long list of water binding ingredients that can help soothe the skin, but most will be washed away before they have a chance.

Exfoliating Cleanser *($16 for 4.4 ounces)* will indeed take off some skin, but the irritation from the potassium hydroxide and the potential for the jojoba wax (the second ingredient listed) to clog pores or cause allergies should be considered.

Eye Makeup Remover *($17.50 for 4.4 ounces)* should be a gentle eye makeup remover, although a detergent cleanser listed among the first ingredients can be too irritating for some skin types.

PA-1 Phyto-Astringent Purifying Toner *($17.50 for 4.4 ounces)* is basically water, alcohol, cucumber extract, and witch hazel (which contains alcohol). The alcohol and witch hazel can be quite irritating to the skin, making oily skin worse. The cucumber extract is supposed to nourish the skin; it can't, but it does produce a nice cooling sensation. The seventh ingredient is whole wheat amino acids, which can help water penetrate the skin but won't prevent the irritation from the other ingredients.

PA-2 Phyto-Astringent Purifying Toner *($17.50 for 4.4 ounces)* is almost identical to PA-1, with some orange and papaya extract added. Both can cause skin irritations, and the alcohol and witch hazel are still a problem for most skin types.

PA-3 Phyto-Astringent Purifying Toner *($17.50 for 4.4 ounces)* is probably a very good irritant-free toner, but witch hazel is still one of the last ingredients. There isn't much of it, but it can be a skin sensitizer. Some of the herb extracts can also produce skin sensitivities, but basically this toner should be fine for most skin types.

PA-S Phyto-Astringent Purifying Toner *($17.50 for 4.4 ounces)* would be a great toner if the second ingredient weren't witch hazel, which can irritate some skin types. The price of all these toners is exorbitant, and they won't purify anything, although there are some good water binding agents in them.

EP-1 Environmental Protective Day Emulsion *($28 for 2.1 ounces)* contains mostly water, thickeners, pollen extract, soybean oil, olive oil, and wheat germ oil, and is a very good, although overly expensive, moisturizer. It has all the trendy moisturizing ingredients, plus SPF 8 sunscreen (not enough protection to keep the sun off the face). The fourth ingredient is pollen extract (a form of oil), which has a slight possibility of causing allergic reactions.

EP-2 Environmental Protective Day Emulsion *($28 for 2.1 ounces)* is a very good moisturizer and almost identical to the EP-1, so the concerns are the same, as is the exorbitant price.

EP-3 Environmental Protective Day Emulsion *($28 for 2.1 ounces)* is a very good moisturizer and almost identical to the EP-1 and EP-2, so the concerns are the same, as is the exorbitant price.

CR-1 Cellular Recovery Night Emulsion *($35 for 2.1 ounces)* is a very good moisturizer and almost identical to the EP-1, EP-2, and EP-3, so the concerns are the same, as is the exorbitant price. The major difference according to M.A.C is the "live yeast extract," which supposedly supplies the skin cells with oxygen, improving cell renewal. It's an unlikely premise that anything in the cream is alive, given the amount of preservatives present and the way cosmetics are formulated. However, like all cosmetics companies, M.A.C. doesn't have to back up their claims with scientific studies, so they can say what they want.

CR-2 Cellular Recovery Night Emulsion *($35 for 2.1 ounces)* is a very good moisturizer, but it can't help your cells to recover. It is almost identical to the CR-1 Cellular Recovery Night Emulsion.

EZR Eye Zone Repair *($35 for 1 ounce)* is a good moisturizer containing a long list of water-binding ingredients and oils. It is very similar to all the other M.A.C. moisturizers. It also has some cucumber, chamomile, and yeast extract. See the CR-1 Night Emulsion for further explanation about the yeast; you already know not to expect much from the plant extracts.

NMF Moisture Regulated Formula *($20 for 4.4 ounces)* contains many of the same ingredients as the other moisturizers, as well as a sunscreen of SPF 8 (not enough to protect the skin from the sun).

VM-1 Vitamin and Mineral Hydrating Mask *($16 for 2.1 ounces)* contains water, clay, glycerin, antiseptic (potential skin irritant), detergent, more clay, alcohol, thickeners, vitamins A and E, and preservatives. This is just a standard clay mask with some extra irritating ingredients that I wouldn't recommend for anyone's skin.

VM-2 Vitamin and Mineral Hydrating Mask *($16 for 2.1 ounces)* contains water, clay, glycerin, sesame oil, standard slip agents, more clay, thickeners, vitamin A, vitamin E, and preservatives. This is a standard clay mask with some oil added to reduce the dryness caused by the clay. For a clay mask this would be OK for some skin types.

$\mathcal{M}$arcelle (Canada Only)

Hydractive Water Rinsable Cleansing Lotion for Normal to Dry Skin *($11.45 for 240 ml)* is an OK cleanser that leaves a film on the face and doesn't take off makeup very well.

Aquarelle Oil-Free Purifying Cleanser for Oily Skin *($8.95 for 240 ml)* doesn't purifying anything, but it does take off makeup nicely without irritating the eyes or overly drying out the skin.

Cleansing Creme *($12.95 for 120 ml)* is supposed to be water-soluble but it leaves a film on the face. It does take off makeup fairly well and could be good for someone with very dry skin

Cleansing Bar *($5.50)* is a standard bar soap with a detergent cleanser that can be drying for most skin types.

Hydrative Hydra-Pure Cleansing Bar *($6.50)* is a standard bar soap with some water binding agent added that won't help counteract the drying effect of the soap.

Scrub Wash *($9.25 for 100 ml)* is a very drying cleanser that contains clay (which isn't very rinsable) and alcohol. It will exfoliate the skin, but there are less harsh ways to do that.

Moisture Lotion *($10.95 for 90 ml)* is an OK but ordinary lightweight moisturizer. The second ingredient is isopropyl myristate, which can cause blackheads, so this product can be a problem for most skin types.

Moisture Cream *($8.50 for 40 ml)* is almost identical to the Moisture Lotion and the same concerns apply.

Eye Contour Gel *($10.95 for 15 ml)* contains mostly water, glycerin, water binding agent, aloe vera, thickener, soothing agent, and preservatives. This would be a soothing lightweight moisturizer for the eye area; it would also be just fine for the whole face, but they don't give you enough to use all over.

Eye Care Cream *($6.50 for 15 ml)* had no ingredient list, so I was not able to evaluate the product.

Clay Mask *($9.25 for 100 ml)* is a standard clay mask that contains mostly water, witch hazel (can be a skin irritant), clays, and glycerin. It would be fairly drying for most skin types.

Moisturizing Peel Off Mask *($9.25 for 100 ml)* had no ingredient list, so I was not able to evaluate the product.

Aquarelle Skin Freshener *($9.95 for 240 ml)* had no ingredient list and the company was not forthcoming with the information, but I suspect from the smell that this is a standard alcohol-based toner.

Anti-Aging Cream *($14.25 for 40 ml)* is a good emollient moisturizer that contains mostly water, several thickeners, elastin, water binding agent, sesame oil, thickener, collagen, water binding agents, vitamin E, and preservatives.

Night Cream *($7.68 for 40 ml)* had no ingredient list, so I was not able to evaluate the product.

Mary Kay

Creamy Cleanser *($9 for 6.5 ounces)* is indeed a creamy cleanser, but it can't be rinsed off without the aid of a washcloth. It also can leave traces of makeup behind.

Deep Cleanser *($9 for 6.5 ounces)* is a water-soluble detergent cleanser that can be too drying for most skin types.

Gentle Cleansing Creme *($9 for 4 ounces)* is a traditional, greasy cold cream product containing mostly mineral oil, water, petrolatum, beeswax, glycerin, and other types of waxes. This might be gentle, but it is also quite heavy, and wiping off makeup is not good for the skin.

Extra Emollient Cleansing Creme *($9 for 4 ounces)* is almost identical to the Gentle Cleansing Creme, only heavier.

Purifying Bar *($11 for 4.2 ounces)* is a standard bar soap that won't purifying anything, but it may dry out the skin.

Gentle Action Freshener *($10 for 6.5 ounces)* is a nonirritating toner that can be somewhat soothing on the skin. It does contain witch hazel, but it is at the very end of the list so it shouldn't pose a problem. Some silk amino acids are also in this product; they may sound good, but even if they could do something for the skin, they come well after the preservatives, so there isn't much in here.

Blemish Control Toner *($10 for 6.5 ounces)* contains mostly water, alcohol, slip agent, more alcohol, menthol, and eucalyptus oil. It also contains salicylic acid. There is no evidence that alcohol or salicylic acid will control blemishes, and both ingredients, as well as the menthol and eucalyptus oil, are extremely irritating.

Refining Freshener *($10 for 6.5 ounces)* contains mostly water and alcohol, which can irritate the skin.

Daily Defense Complex with SPF 4 *($25 for 1.4 ounces)* is an ordinary moisturizer with a minimal amount of sunscreen that can't defend adequately from the sun. There are a few interesting ingredients in here, but they come after the preservatives, so they don't count for much.

Balancing Moisturizer *($16 for 2.4 ounces)* is a good basic moisturizer for normal to dry skin, containing mostly water, mineral oil, standard water binding agents, thickeners, avocado oil, and preservatives.

Enriched Moisturizer *($16 for 1.4 ounces)* isn't all that enriched and isn't all that different from the Balancing Moisturizer. It does contain collagen, but it is far down in the ingredient list and there's not enough to really benefit the skin.

Extra Emollient Moisturizer *($16 for 4 ounces)* is a very rich, somewhat heavy moisturizer for dry skin; it contains mostly water, wax, shark oil, sesame and soybean oil, standard water binding agents, thickeners, collagen, and preservatives.

Extra Emollient Night Cream *($11 for 2.5 ounces)* is a very rich, extremely heavy moisturizer for someone with severely dry skin. It contains mostly petrolatum, mineral oil, several waxes, thickener, more waxes, and preservatives.

Advanced Moisture Renewal Treatment Cream *($19 for 2.5 ounces)* is a good rich moisturizer for dry skin; it contains mostly water, mineral oil, thickener, petrolatum, safflower oil, several thickeners, and preservatives. Some vitamin E, protein, and other lipids are in this product, but they come well after the preservatives so there isn't enough to matter. This is a good moisturizer, but nothing special.

Eye Cream Concentrate *($12 for 0.75 ounce)* is a good emollient that contains mostly water, petrolatum, thickener, safflower oil, mineral oil, more thickeners, and preservatives. Vitamin E, aloe, and collagen are also in here, but they are at the end of the ingredient list, so there isn't enough to matter.

Skin Revival System is a two-part product consisting of **Skin Revival Cream** *($25 for 1.5 ounces)* and **Skin Revival Serum** *($25 for 1.5 ounces)*. This is Mary Kay's answer to the AHA craze. The claims about this product are just short of miraculous, yet as an AHA product it is overpriced and doesn't contain much AHA. One of the salespeople told me it contained about 5 percent AHA, but I couldn't get a firm number from the company. You're supposed to apply the serum, let it dry, and then apply the cream, and then an additional moisturizer if you want. That's more complicated than it needs to be. The cream is mostly a rich moisturizer with less than 1 percent AHA. It also contains Nayad, a yeast that is supposed to soothe the skin. I doubt that, but it's in here if you're interested. The serum contains mostly water, alcohol, AHA, thickener, salicylic acid (a peeling agent), and Nayad. There are plenty of AHA products that contain 8 percent AHA, and don't contain alcohol or salicylic acid, which can both irritate the skin.

Oil-Control Lotion *($16 for 3.4 ounces)* is a lightweight moisturizer that contains mostly standard water binding agents, thickeners, and preservatives. There are no ingredients in this product that can control, change, or affect the amount of oil your skin produces. If anything, it can make the skin feel greasy.

Acne Treatment Gel *($6 for 1.25 ounces)* contains mostly water, slip agent, and benzoyl peroxide (5 percent). The active ingredient is the benzoyl peroxide, a popular ingredient used in dozens of products designed for acne that are a lot cheaper than this product. This product also contains sodium hydroxide, a very irritating form of emulsifier.

Clarifying Mask *($11 for 4 ounces)* is a standard clay mask that can definitely dry the skin.

Moisture Rich Mask *($11 for 1.4 ounces)* is a very emollient cream that contains mostly water, thickeners, safflower oil, more thickeners, standard water binding agent, sesame oil, avocado oil, petrolatum, more thickeners, and preservatives. It also contains an insignificant amount of vitamin A. This should feel very good on dry skin.

Revitalizing Mask *($11 for 2.4 ounces)* is a standard clay mask that also contains a lightweight abrasive. It is thicker than most because it also contains candelilla and carnuba (as in car) wax, so it can also clog pores and be difficult to rinse off.

M. D. Formulations

If you are looking for a serious line of alpha hydroxy acid products, then M.D. Formulations, along with NeoStrata, Murad, Alpha Hyrdrox, and Avon (Avon's Anew), is one of the right companies to look at. Not only is the percentage of AHA over 12 percent for most of the products (8 percent to 15 percent is the optimum percentage for the best and most immediate results), but the line is surprisingly varied and complete. It is also extremely expensive. There is everything from lotions to gels, and creams, cleansers, acne products, shampoos (considered good for dandruff or psoriasis), and even foot and nail treatments in this line, priced from $25 to $60. If you want to exfoliate skin on any part of your body with a concentration of AHA that can really make a difference, you will be impressed by some of these products. Now, before you think I've gotten too carried away and sound like I'm endorsing a product line, M.D. Formulations does contain several products that I think are bad for the skin, and their AHA moisturizers are fairly ordinary except for the AHA content. However, even given those reservations, if you pick and choose right, what you stand to find are some very good AHA products (albeit overpriced, especially when compared to Avon and NeoStrata).

M.D. Formulations is sold directly to physicians for retail sale. For information on the physician nearest you who is selling these products, please call (800) 347-2223. If there isn't a salon or physician near you who sells M.D. Formulations, you can ask them to ship it to you direct by calling that same number. Under the company name Herald Pharmacal, they have created a line of products called **Aqua Glide** and **Aqua Glycolic**, meant to be sold in drugstores, and these are priced from $8.50 to $16. Definitely a price your face can live with. These products were not available before this book went to press, but I will review these in my newsletter as soon as they are available. For more information about these products, you can also call (800) 347-2223.

One word of caution: Any time you use an AHA product that contains over 8 percent AHA, some stinging can occur; also, you should avoid letting it come in contact with the eyes or any mucous membranes. As with any cosmetic ingredient, you may have an allergic reaction to AHA. Slight stinging is expected, but continued stinging is not. Discontinue use if this should happen.

Facial Cleanser with 12% Glycolic Compound *($25 for 8 ounces)* is a problem for most skin types. It is overkill to put AHA in a cleanser that could accidently get too near your eyes or mouth when splashing and cause serious irritation. I would not recommend washing the face or other body parts with this product.

Glycare 5 for Extremely Oily or Acne Prone Skin *($35 for 4 ounces)* is basically an alcohol-based toner that contains 7 percent AHA. I would not recommend using alcohol on anyone's skin, and the alcohol in combination with the AHA can cause extreme irritation. It also contains eucalyptus oil, which is additionally a skin irritant.

Glycare 10 for Extremely Oily or Acne Prone Skin *($35 for 4 ounces)* is almost identical to the Glycare 5, only it contains 12 percent AHA. The same warnings about irritation apply.

Facial Lotion with 12% Glycolic Compound *($45 for 2 ounces)* is basically just AHA with a thickener and preservatives. This is a good basic AHA product for most skin types, however, if you have normal to dry skin you would most likely need to use a moisturizer in addition to the lotion.

Night Cream with 14% Glycolic Compound *($60 for 2 ounces)* is a simple AHA cream of water, thickeners, and preservative. It is an ordinary moisturizing base that probably would not be sufficient for someone with very dry skin.

Smoothing Complex with 10% Glycolic Compound *($35 for 0.5 ounce)* is almost identical to the Night Cream but minus a few thickeners. It is a good overall AHA product.

SPF 20 Sunblock *($25 for 4 ounces)* is a standard SPF lotion that provides good protection. This would be good for someone with normal to dry skin. It does not contain AHA and is very expensive for a standard sunscreen.

Advanced Hydrating Complex-Gel Formula *($40 for 1 ounce)* is a below-average, very expensive moisturizer for the eyes that does not contain AHA. The ingredients are water, alcohol, thickener, water binding agent, thickeners, and preservatives. The alcohol is drying. Although it also contains a good water binding agent and Nayad (yeast), they are at the very end of the ingredient list and the amounts are negligible. If the skin around your eye is dry this won't do much to change it, and it could make it worse.

Advanced Hydrating Complex-Cream Formula *($40 for 1 ounce)* contains mostly water, several thickeners, water binding agent, thickener, and preservative. A good water binding agent and Nayad (yeast) are in this cream but they are at the very end of the ingredient list and the amount is negligible.

Vit-A-Gel with Vitamin A Propionate *($40 for 1 ounce)* contains mostly aloe vera, slip agents, vitamin A, slip agent, thickeners, several water binding agents, and preservatives. If you're looking for a good dose of vitamin A, here it is, but the best part of this product is the lightweight water binding agents. It's pricey for what you get, but it is a good product.

Skin Bleaching Lotion *($30 for 1.5 ounces)* is a standard 2 percent hydroquinone product. Most skin bleaches contain this ingredient. To make it more effective, use it in conjunction with one of the AHA creams or lotions over the discolorations. AHA in combination with 2 percent hydroquinone is reportedly an effective combination.

Benzoyl Peroxide 5% for Extremely Oily and Acne-Prone Skin *($25 for 4 ounces)* is a good benzoyl peroxide toner, but it is rather expensive for a simple 5 percent solution. If you want a benzoyl peroxide product, there are similar solutions for a lot less at the drugstore.

Benzoyl Peroxide 10% for Extremely Oily and Acne-Prone Skin *($25 for 4 ounces)* is identical to the 5 percent solution above except for the proportion of benzoyl peroxide, and the same warnings apply.

Body Scrub *($30 for 8 ounces)* is a mixture of scrub agent, AHA, and detergent cleanser. I'm skeptical that a body scrub containing AHA is worthwhile—after all, the AHA is just washed off. The scrub is effective, but the AHA is probably wasted.

Monteil of Paris

Cleanser Actif *($18.50 for 8 ounces)* cleaned the makeup off well, but unfortunately it also burned the eyes and left the skin feeling slightly dry.

Super Sensitive Cleanser *($18.50 for 8 ounces)* might be good for super-sensitive skin, but it doesn't take off makeup very well and leaves a greasy film on the skin.

Super Sensitive Freshener *($18.50 for 8 ounces)* claims to contain no irritants, however, it contains cetrimonium bromide and sodium phosphate, which can both be irritating to sensitive skin. I wouldn't say this is a bad product, but it isn't quite as super-sensitive as they would lead you to believe.

Super Soft Rinse-Off Cleanser *($18.50 for 8 ounces)* is a good cleanser for normal to dry skin and it is preservative-free, which is a nice touch. It contains detergent cleansers further down in the ingredient list, so it is milder on the skin. It does take off the makeup and rinses nicely.

Freshener Actif *($18.50 for 8 ounces)* contains mostly water, witch hazel, soothing agent, water binding agents, collagen, mineral salts, and preservatives. The witch hazel can be irritating to most skin types.

Decongestant Cleanser Combination *($18.50 for 4 ounces)* is an OK water-soluble cleanser for someone with oily skin. It contains detergent cleanser that can clean off all the makeup, but it also contains a few waxes that can clog pores. It can also be slightly drying. One of the preservatives is dmdm hydantoin, which can be a skin irritant and should not be used around the eyes. ("Decongestant" refers to deep cleaning, but it only cleans skin-deep, which is all you want.)

Decongestant Cleanser Delicat *($18.50 for 4 ounces)* is almost identical to the above cleanser. The difference is minor. This is not a cleanser that would do well on delicate/sensitive skin.

Decongestant Cleanser Fort *($18.50 for 4 ounces)* is similar to the above cleansers and the same warnings apply.

Tonique Combination for Combination Skin *($18.50 for 8.1 ounces)* contains mostly water, witch hazel, standard water binding agents, protein, elastin, salt, water binding agents, plant oils, and preservatives. The witch hazel can be an irritant for most skin types, plus the oils would not make someone with partly oily skin happy.

Tonique Delicat for Dry/Sensitive Skin *($18.50 for 8.1 ounces)* is a very good irritant-free toner that contains mostly water, glycerin, mineral salt, soothing agent, water binding agents, plant oils, and preservatives.

Tonique Fort for Oily Skin *($18.50 for 8.1 ounces)* is a standard alcohol-based toner that contains some collagen, amino acids, and plant oils. The alcohol will irritate the skin and the oils will only make oily skin more oily.

Ice Fundamental Soft Rinse-Off Cleanser *($25 for 3.7 ounces)* is a good water-soluble cleanser for someone with dry skin. It can leave a slight film on the face, but it does take off all the makeup. The algae extract provides no benefits, but it's in here to sound like the sea is cleaning your face.

Ice Fundamental Emulsion *($42.50 for 1.3 ounces)* is an ordinary lightweight moisturizer that contains mostly water, thickeners, and a small amount of algae and grapefruit extract and preservative. This is a good but very ordinary moisturizer. You're paying a lot of money for some algae extract that doesn't provide any benefit for the skin.

Ice Ultimate Cream Concentrate *($47.50 for 1.3 ounces)* contains mostly water, vitamin E, thickener, shark oil, more thickeners, plant extract, petrolatum, more thickeners, fragrance, aloe vera, water binding agents, and preservatives. This is a good emollient moisturizer for dry skin.

Super Moist Beauty Emulsion *($42.50 for 1.3 ounces)* contains mostly water; thickener; lanolin; shark oil; isopropyl myristate (can cause blackheads); thickeners; mineral oil; glycerin; soothing agents; vitamins A, E, and D; protein; collagen; elastin; more thickeners; and preservatives. Everything you can think of is in here, but basically it is just a good emollient moisturizer for dry skin.

Moisture Build Triple Action Emulsion Oil-Free *($32 for 2 ounces)* contains mostly water, standard water binding agent, thickeners, plant extract, several more water binding agents, almond oil, orange oil, and preservatives. Perhaps Monteil should read their ingredient list before they claim their product is oil-free; this one contains oil. Nevertheless, it would be a good moisturizer for someone with normal to dry skin.

Firmant Des Rides *($40 for 8 ounces)* contains mostly water, thickeners, water binding agents, protein, collagen, amino acids, salt, and preservatives. This won't firm the skin or get rid of wrinkles; it's just a good emollient moisturizer for normal to dry skin.

Firming Action Moisture Lotion SPF 2 *($32.50 for 2 ounces)* contains mostly water, mineral oil, standard water binding agents, several thickeners, collagen, elastin, amino acids, vitamin E, safflower oil, soothing agents, thickeners, and preservatives. This is a good light emollient moisturizer for someone with normal to dry skin, but there isn't enough sunscreen to protect the skin from the sun.

Lip Line Defense Dual Phase Treatment Formula *($30 for 0.3 ounce)* is a two-part process. The Gel Phase is applied to the lips and lip area as a mask and then rinsed off with a washcloth. It is supposed to exfoliate the skin, but the washcloth is probably doing most of the work because the ingredients aren't the best for exfoliating the skin. There are definitely better exfoliators on the market than this one. The Cream Phase is an ordinary moisturizer that contains mostly water, mineral oil, and thickeners. Down at the end of the ingredient list is some protein, but that won't help the lines around your lips.

Skin-Stress Relief Dual Phase Balancing System for Oily Skin *($50 for 1.5 ounces of Treatment Gel and Face Creme)* is supposed to coax the skin back to tranquillity. First you apply the gel, and then the cream. The gel contains water, witch hazel, slip agent, thickeners, amino acid, more thickeners, plant extracts, and preservatives. The cream contains water, slip agent, thickeners, mineral salts, more thickeners, vitamin E, more thickeners, and preservatives. If you want to believe plant extracts, mineral salts (table salt), and other standard cosmetic thickeners can calm the face, go for it. Other than that this is a fairly ordinary lightweight moisturizer that comes in two parts. The witch hazel can be a skin irritant.

Skin-Stress Relief Dual Phase Comfort System for Dry Skin *($50 for 1.5 ounces of Treatment Gel and Face Creme)* does not have exactly the same ingredients as the oily skin version, but they are still more alike than different. The basic review remains the same; it is a good two-part moisturizer for dry skin, but it won't calm the skin or fill out wrinkles.

Double-Action Skin Lightening Creme *($25 for 2.1 ounces)* is a standard bleach cream that contains 2 percent hydroquinone, which has some ability to lighten skin discolorations. This also contains a small amount of sunscreen, but other than that it is just a series of thickeners and slip agents.

Moon Drops by Revlon

Like many skin care lines, Moon Drops divides its skin care products into three skin types: Normal/Oily, Normal/Dry, and Sensitive/Delicate. The grouping seems more convenient than it is, but that's true for all skin care lines. Many of the products designed for each skin type don't match or benefit that specific skin type. Pay attention to the product descriptions that follow and ignore their skin care groupings.

Moon Drops Replenishing Cleansing Lotion Normal to Dry *($6.93 for 8 ounces)* is a mineral oil-based cleanser that leaves a greasy residue on the face and requires a washcloth or tissue to remove all the makeup.

Moon Drops Extra Gentle Cleansing Cream Sensitive/Delicate *($6.93 for 4 ounces)* is a wipe-off cleanser that can leave a greasy film on the skin.

Moon Drops Foaming Cleansing Gel—Soap-Free—Normal to Oily *($6.93 for 8 ounces)* is a standard detergent-based cleanser that can take off all the makeup without leaving a greasy film on the skin. It can be drying for some skin types and the menthol can irritate some skin types.

Moon Drops One-Minute Scrub Skin Polishing Normal to Dry *($7.49 for 4 ounces)* is an OK scrub, but it can leave an oily residue on the skin. It could work for someone with very dry skin, but I would not even begin to recommend this for someone with normal skin.

Moon Drops Comforting Toner Sensitive/Delicate *($6.93 for 8 ounces)* is actually a very gentle toner that can be quite soothing and lightly emollient for most skin types. It does contain a small amount of a preservative that can be irritating to the skin, but not enough to be a problem for most skin types.

Moon Drops Softening Toner Normal to Dry *($6.93 for 8 ounces)* is similar to the toner above except it contains some good water binding agents and vitamins A and E. The same critique applies.

Moon Drops Clarifying Astringent Oil Control Normal to Oily *($6.93 for 8 ounces)* is an alcohol-based toner that also contains some chamomile extract and a soothing agent, but that won't compensate for the irritation caused by the alcohol.

Moon Drops Nourishing Moisture Lotion SPF 6 Normal to Dry *($7.93 for 4 ounces)* won't nourish anyone's skin, but it is a good emollient moisturizer for dry skin. It contains mostly water, standard water binding agents, thickeners, petrolatum, vitamins A and E, shark oil, water binding agents, more thickeners, and preservatives. The SPF isn't enough to adequately protect from the sun.

Moon Drops Lightweight Moisturizer SPF 6 Normal to Oily *($7.93 for 4 ounces)* is indeed a lightweight moisturizer that would be quite good if it contained an adequate sunscreen to protect from the sun, but it doesn't. It contains mostly water, standard water binding agents, thickeners, plant extracts, water binding agents, and preservative.

Moon Drops Soothing Moisture Cream SPF 6 Sensitive/ Delicate *($7.93 for 4 ounces)* would be a good emollient moisturizer except that it doesn't contain enough sunscreen to adequately protect from the sun.

Moon Drops Soothing Moisture Lotion SPF 6 Sensitive/ Delicate *($7.93 for 4 ounces)* is an OK lightweight moisturizer, but it isn't all that soothing; the ingredients are similar to many of the moisturizers in this collection. The SPF isn't enough to adequately protect from the sun.

Moon Drops Five Minute Clay Mask Deep-Cleansing Normal to Oily *($7.49 for 4.8 ounces)* is a standard clay mask that can't deep clean but it can help exfoliate the skin.

Moon Drops Three Minute Moisture Pack Skin Calming Sensitive/Delicate *($7.49 for 4.12 ounces)* is similar to many of the other moisturizers in this line. It contains mostly water, thickeners, mineral oil, standard water binding agents, plant extract, soothing agent, more thickeners, and preservatives. This is an unnecessary product if you use any of the other moisturizers in this line.

Murad

Much like M.D. Formulations and NeoStrata, Murad is a line of skin care products that boasts an above-average content of AHA. Most of the products contain 8 percent to 15 percent glycolic acid, which makes these very reliable AHA creams and lotions. Murad also has its share of products that contain alcohol and other irritating ingredients, but for the most part this is an above-average selection of AHA products. I should mention that the price is a bit overstated at around $40 per product, especially when compared to NeoStrata (with a similar AHA content), for around $16 per product.

One word of caution: Any time you use an AHA product that contains over 8 percent AHA, some stinging can occur; also, you should avoid letting it come in contact with the eyes or any mucous membranes. As with any cosmetic ingredient, you may have an allergic reaction to AHA. Slight stinging is expected, but continued stinging is not. Discontinue use if this should happen.

Advanced Combination Skin Formula *($40 for 3.3 ounces)* is a lightweight gel that contains 8 percent to 15 percent AHA and mostly water, alcohol, salicylic acid, water binding agents, aloe vera, vitamins A and E, and preservatives. The alcohol and salicylic acid are both very drying and make this a very irritating gel. The AHA should be enough to exfoliate the skin without the extra irritants.

Advanced Oily Prone Skin Formula *($40 for 3.3 ounces)* is almost identical to the Advanced Combination Skin Formula, but minus some of the good water binding agents. Although I think the alcohol and salicylic acid are too irritating, if you're going to lean in this direction at least go for the one that has some soothing water binding agents.

Advanced Skin Smoothing Lotion *($40 for 5 ounces)* contains about 8 percent to 15 percent AHA and water, standard water binding agents, several thickeners, sodium hydroxide (a strong skin irritant), water binding agent, vitamin E, aloe vera, and preservatives. This is a good AHA product for normal to dry skin, but the sodium hydroxide can be a problem for sensitive skin.

Advanced Skin Smoothing Cream *($40 for 1.7 ounces)* contains about 8 percent to 15 percent AHA and is almost identical to the lotion above. It also has an SPF of 8, which is not enough to protect adequately from the sun. It is still a good emollient AHA product for normal to dry skin.

Murasome Eye Complex 10 *($40 for 0.5 ounce)* contains about 8 percent to 15 percent AHA plus water, several thickeners, standard water binding agent, sodium hydroxide (possible skin irritant), more thickeners, water binding agents, vitamins E and A, water binding agent, soothing agent, and preservatives. It also has an SPF of 8, which is not enough to adequately protect from the sun. This is a good emollient AHA product for the eyes, although the sodium hydroxide can be a problem for those with sensitive skin.

Murasun Spectrum 15 Daily Defense *($18.50 for 3.5 ounces)* is a good emollient sunscreen for the face or body that contains no AHA. It is just a standard SPF 15 product and overpriced when you consider the assortment of other SPF 15 sunscreens on the market for a lot less money.

Advanced Age Spot and Pigment Lightening Gel *($40 for 1.7 ounces)* is a standard 2 percent hydroquinone product that also contains alcohol. Most skin bleaches contain hydroquinone, which can be quite drying, and the alcohol only exacerbates the problem. To overcome the dryness from the alcohol and to make the hydroquinone more effective, use it conjunction with one of the AHA creams or lotions over the discolorations. AHA in combination with 2 percent hydroquinone is reportedly an effective combination.

NeoStrata

It is a strange coincidence that M.D. Formulations, Murad, and NeoStrata, three of the companies that sell a complete line of AHA products, should be lined up alphabetically one right after the other (with only a minor interruption by Monteil and Moon Drops). The question you are probably asking is, What are the differences between these products? Although the people who sell these lines wax poetic about the quality of their AHA complex or compound, the truth is that their AHA content is more alike than different. All of these companies make products with high concentrations of AHA, and their claims are equally impressive. The bottom line is that the results are equal. AHA provides a good consistent exfoliation that reduces the thickness of the skin's outer layer, which can solve many skin problems, including dryness, blemishes, sun damage, and skin discolorations. Which product line should you choose? Good question. NeoStrata is definitely the most reasonably priced of these three, but Avon's Anew and Alpha Hydrox are both very good lines and contenders in this group because they also contain a good percentage of AHA.

As this book went to press, NeoStrata products were not all that easy to obtain. While I am writing these words they are only available through physicians. You can call (800) 628-9904 to find the physician in your area who carries the products. You can also order them via a charge card phone order from Crown Drugs in Philadelphia by calling (800) 852-7696. Starting in 1994, NeoStrata products (the exact same products) will also be in drugstores.

One word of caution: Any time you use an AHA product that contains over 8 percent AHA, some stinging can occur; also, you should avoid letting it come in contact with the eyes or any mucous membranes. As with any cosmetic ingredient, you may have an allergic reaction to AHA. Slight stinging is expected, but continued stinging is not. Discontinue use if this should happen.

Skin Smoothing Cream *($13.50 for 2.5 ounces)* contains 8 percent AHA as well as water, thickeners, standard water binding agents, more thickeners, and preservatives. This is a good AHA product in an OK moisturizing base.

Skin Smoothing Lotion *($13.50 for 6 ounces)* contains 10 percent AHA as well as water, standard water binding agent, thickeners, petrolatum, standard water binding agents, more thickeners, and preservative. This is a good AHA product in a good emollient base.

Solution for Oily and Acne Skin *($10 for 4 ounces)* contains 8 percent AHA as well as alcohol, standard water binding agent, and slip agents. The alcohol is too irritating and drying for most skin types.

Enhanced Gel Formula *($13.50 for 4 ounces)* contains 15 percent AHA as well as water, alcohol, and preservative. The strength of the AHA is good, but the alcohol causes dryness and irritation.

Gel for Age Spots and Skin Lightening *($11 for 1.6 ounces)* is a standard 2 percent hydroquinone skin lightening product, except this one also contains 10 percent AHA. This would be a good product to try over age (sun damage) spots, except the second ingredient is alcohol, which can be drying and irritating to most skin types.

Neutrogena

Neutrogena has been around for a long time, starting back in 1954, when that first clear amber bar of soap was manufactured. How well I remember discovering that bar of soap when I was a teenager. It didn't leave quite the same soap film on the skin as most bar soaps, and the amber color just radiated purity and a deep clean that could get rid of blemishes. I knew that my acne would go away if I diligently washed my face with this little gem. Of course, that wasn't the case. It didn't change my acne one little bit and it dried my skin just like other bar soaps did. Oh well, so much for amber clarity.

In the '90s, Neutrogena has expanded and created a skin care line that has many elements worth considering for all skin types, although their emphasis is still for those women who worry about breakouts. The bar soaps are still here, but so are a couple of OK water-soluble cleansers, a rather good irritant-free toner, and lightweight daytime sunscreens. One point of contention: Several of the products are listed as being noncomedogenic. There is no way a product can know ahead of time what can make someone break out. I have had reactions to many products that claimed they wouldn't cause blackheads or acne. That doesn't make these products bad, it just makes the claim misleading.

Transparent Facial Bar Original Formula *($2.69 for 3.5 ounces)* is a standard bar soap with detergent cleansers that can be drying for most skin types. The first two ingredients are triethanolamine and triethanolamine stearate, which are considered strong skin irritants when present in this amount. This is not a soap I would recommend for any skin type.

Transparent Facial Bar Dry Skin Formula *($2.69 for 3.5 ounces)* is a standard bar soap with detergent cleansers that can be drying for most skin types. The first two ingredients are triethanolamine and triethanolamine stearate, which are considered strong skin irritants when present in this amount. This is not a soap I would recommend for dry skin or any skin type.

Transparent Facial Bar Acne Prone Skin Formula *($2.69 for 3.5 ounces)* is a standard bar soap almost identical to the Dry Skin Formula except for the addition of a few stronger detergent cleansers. This soap would be even more drying and irritating than the one above, and that would be a problem for someone with acne skin.

Transparent Facial Bar Oily Skin Formula *($2.69 for 3.5 ounces)* is a standard bar soap almost identical to the Dry Skin Formula, with the same warnings and problems.

Antiseptic Cleanser *($5 for 4.5 ounces)* contains a large number of ingredients that are too irritating for almost all skin types, including camphor, peppermint oil, eucalyptus oil, and benzethonium chloride. The recommendation on the label is to avoid the eye area as it will burn the skin there, however, it is likely to burn the skin all over the face. I would not recommend this product for any skin type.

Liquid Neutrogena (Fragranced or Fragrance-Free) *($8.69 for 8 ounces)* is a fairly drying water-soluble cleanser that can thoroughly clean the face but would be a problem for anyone with sensitive, dry, or combination skin. Even someone with oily skin may find this irritating.

Oil-Free Acne Wash *($6.49 for 6 ounces)* is a standard detergent cleanser with some herb extracts, except that it also contains salicylic acid. Because this product might get in the eyes I would not recommend using it, because salicylic acid should not get near a mucous membrane.

Facial Cleansing Formula *($8.69 for 8 ounces)* is a water-soluble cleanser that can tend to dry out the skin. It is milder than most, but definitely not for anyone with dry skin.

Non-Drying Cleansing Lotion *($7.77 for 5.5 ounces)* is a good water-soluble cleanser for someone with dry skin; it takes off all the makeup but it does tend to leave a slight film on the skin if not used with a washcloth (which can be quite irritating on the face).

Alcohol-Free Toner *($7.77 for 8 ounces)* is indeed an irritant-free toner that would be quite soothing for most skin types. One of the preservatives is benzalkonium chloride, which can be a skin irritant for those with sensitive skin.

Intensified Day Moisture SPF 15 *($12.69 for 2.25 ounces)* is an OK lightweight moisturizer with a good SPF factor. It contains mostly water, glycerin, thickeners, standard water binding agent, thickeners, and preservatives.

Moisture Non-Comedogenic Facial Moisturizer SPF 15 *($7.80 for 4 ounces)* contains mostly water, water binding agent, petrolatum, thickeners, and preservatives. I find the noncomedogenic claim extremely misleading. Any one of these ingredients (except for water) can potentially cause someone to break out, as I did. This can be a good lightweight moisturizer/sunscreen for normal to dry skin.

Moisture Non-Comedogenic Facial Moisturizer SPF 15 (Sheer Tint and Untinted) *($9.99 for 4 ounces)* is similar to the SPF 15 untinted moisturizer above, and the warning and review are the same.

Night Cream *($13 for 2.25 ounces)* is a rich emollient moisturizer for dry skin that contains mostly water, glycerin, sesame oil, thickener, petrolatum, more thickeners, and preservatives.

Eye Cream *($8 for 0.5 ounce)* contains mostly water, thickeners, mineral oil, petrolatum, water binding agent, and preservatives. This is a good emollient moisturizer for dry skin.

Oil Absorbing Drying Gel for Oily Skin Control *($3.33 for 0.75 ounce)* contains mostly alcohol, slip agents, and preservatives. Alcohol won't control oil; all it can do is dry and irritate the skin.

Neutrogena Chemical-Free Sunblocker SPF 17 *($7.99 for 4 ounces)* isn't really chemical-free, but it is titanium dioxide-based, an excellent way to protect from the sun if you can tolerate the slightly white film it leaves behind on the face.

New Essentials

Please take what I am about to say with a grain of salt. I was really surprised at how much I liked several of the products in this new cosmetics line from Revlon. Although their claims about being hypoallergenic, doctor tested, noncomedogenic, and so on go too far, these products do not contain any fragrance or coloring agents. That is great. In addition, many of the moisturizers contain impressive water binding agents and antioxidants (vitamins A, E, and C), which can be very good for the skin, and the prices won't knock you out.

Extra Gentle Purifying Gel *($15 for 4 ounces)* is a standard detergent cleanser that isn't extra gentle. Besides the possible irritation from the cleansing agents, it also contains menthol, which can cause skin irritation. However, it can be a good water-soluble cleanser for someone with oily skin.

Daily Purifying Lotion *($10 for 6 ounces)* is a standard mineral oil cleanser that can leave a greasy film behind on the skin. It contains mostly water, mineral oil, standard water binding agents, thickeners, water binding agents, thickeners, and preservatives. The ingredients read more like a good moisturizer than anything like a good water soluble cleanser.

Exfoliating Facial Scrub *($15 for 4 ounces)* is a detergent scrub that can be very drying on the skin.

Extra Gentle Moisturizing Eye Makeup Remover *(7.50 for 3.35 ounces)* is only mineral oil, slip agent, and preservatives. You could buy pure mineral oil for a lot less money and it won't contain any preservatives which would make it even more gentle for the eyes.

Extra Gentle Waterproof Eye Makeup Remover *($7.50 for 1.5 ounces)* contains mostly mineral oil, slip agent, thickeners, and a small amount of vitamins A and E, aloe, and preservatives. It is gentle and does remove waterproof eye makeup.

Extra Gentle Oil-Free Eye Makeup Remover *($7.50 for 3.35 ounces)* is indeed oil-free, but the preservatives and one of the cleansing agents make it anything but extra gentle. I would test this one first over the eye and make sure it doesn't cause irritation.

Extra Strength Tonic *($15 for 6 ounces)* contains mostly water, alcohol, slip agents, soothing agents, and preservatives. It also contains salicylic acid, which peels the skin. There are gentler ways to exfoliate the skin than salicylic acid, and the alcohol adds additional unnecessary irritation.

Clarifying Skin Tonic *($10 for 6 ounces)* is a standard alcohol-based toner that contains mostly water, alcohol, slip agents, and preservatives.

Refreshing Eye Gel *($15 for 0.75 ounce)* isn't all that refreshing, but it does contain some good water binding agents and soothing agents, which would feel very good on the skin. It also contains witch hazel, which can be a skin irritant.

Refreshing Skin Tonic *($10 for 6 ounces)* is almost identical to the Refreshing Eye Gel and the same evaluation applies.

Oil Balancing Gel *($18.50 for 3.25 ounces)* can't balance oil, or even change it a little. It contains mostly water, alcohol, slip agents, menthol (a skin irritant), thickeners, and preservatives. This product is dying and can cause skin irritation.

New Essentials Protection SPF 25 *($16 for 2.5 ounces)* is an OK moisturizer with a good strong sunscreen, but it isn't very emollient. It does contain vitamins E, C, and A, which is helpful, but that doesn't help the emollience. However, it is worth a try if you're looking for a good high-rated sunscreen.

Daily Hydrating Cream *($15 for 2 ounces)* contains a small amount of sunscreen that doesn't adequately protect from the sun, plus water, mineral oil, standard water binding agents, petrolatum, thickeners, amino acids, soothing agents, vitamin E, water binding agent, more thickeners, and preservatives. This is a good moisturizer for someone with dry skin.

Hydrating Eye Cream *($15 for 0.75 ounces)* contains mostly water, standard water binding agent, petrolatum, thickeners, soothing agent, vitamins A and E, more thickeners, and preservatives. This is a good emollient moisturizer for normal to dry skin.

Moisture Maximizer *($25 for 1.6 ounces)* contains mostly water, water binding agents, thickeners, and preservatives. This is a good lightweight moisturizer for most skin types.

Moisture Nourishing Night Cream *($20 for 2 ounces)* contains mostly water, several standard water binding agents, safflower oil, mineral oil, petrolatum, thickener, several water binding agents, thickeners, and preservatives. This is a good emollient moisturizer for dry skin.

Vitalizing Night Cream *($27.50 for 1 ounce)* contains mostly water, thickener, petrolatum, standard water binding agents, vitamin E, soothing agent, collagen, and preservatives. This is a good emollient cream, but nothing all that different from any of the moisturizers in this line.

Soothing Lip Treatment *($15 for 0.75 ounce)* contains mostly petrolatum, wax thickeners, several water binding agents, vitamins A and E, and preservatives. It is nothing more than a good emollient lipstick with a small amount of sunscreen, but it should take care of dry lips.

Nivea Visage

Foaming Facial Cleanser *($7.19 for 5 ounces)* is a water-soluble cleanser that can be extremely drying on the skin and may irritate the eyes.

Gentle Facial Cleansing Lotion *($7.19 for 6.8 ounces)* doesn't rinse very well and doesn't take off all the makeup without the aid of a washcloth, which isn't very gentle on the skin.

Hydro-Cleansing Gel *($7.19 for 6.8 ounces)* is a standard detergent cleanser that can be quite drying for most skin types. It does contain a fair amount of glycerin, which can help soothe the skin, but the detergent cleansers can still be a problem.

Alcohol Free Moisturizing Facial Toner *($7.19 for 6.8 ounces)* is a soothing, lightly moisturizing, fairly irritant-free toner. It contains mostly water, standard water binding agents, more water binding agents, perservative, fragrance, amino acids, and more preservatives.

No Oil, All Moisture Hydrogel *($7.19 for 6.8 ounces)* contains mostly water, slip agent, thickeners, water binding agent, and preservatives. This is definitely oil-free and lightweight, which can be good for someone with combination skin.

Daily Facial Moisture Lotion SPF 15 *($9.49 for 4 ounces)* contains mostly water, thickener, mineral oil, more thickeners, glycerin, vitamin E, and preservatives. This is a fairly ordinary moisturizer with a little bit of vitamin E, but the sunscreen is great.

Facial Nourishing Lotion SPF 4 *($6.83 for 4 ounces)* contains mostly water, mineral oil, thickeners, standard water binding agents, more thickeners, vitamin E, and preservatives. This is an OK moisturizer for normal to dry skin, but the sunscreen is not enough to adequately protect from the sun.

Liposome Cream with Vitamin E *($11.99 for 1.7 ounces)* contains mostly water, thickeners, standard water binding agents, vitamin E, alcohol, and preservatives. There is only a tiny bit of alcohol in here, so it shouldn't be a problem for most skin types. This is an OK moisturizer for most skin types. Liposomes are good, but it would be better if this moisturizer and the following ones with liposomes contained more emollients and water binding agents.

Liposome Eye Contour Gel *($9.99 for 0.5 ounce)* contains mostly water, standard water binding agents, thickeners, and preservatives. This won't do anything to reduce puffiness, but it is a good lightweight moisturizer, overpriced for the tiny amount you get.

Liposome Firming Gel Creme *($9.75 for 1 ounce)* is mostly water, thickener, standard water binding agents, more thickeners, and preservatives. This won't firm anything, but it is an OK lightweight moisturizer for normal to dry skin.

Anti-Wrinkle Cream with Vitamin E SPF 4 *($9.49 for 1.7 ounces)* contains mostly water, several thickeners, vitamin E, more thickeners, and preservatives. This is an ordinary moisturizer that can feel fairly thick, it contains only a tiny amount of vitamin E, and the SPF is too small to adequately protect from the sun. This moisturizer can't and won't fight wrinkles or even dry skin very well.

Advanced Vitality Creme *($9.49 for 1.7 ounces)* contains mostly water, thickeners, glycerin, several more thickeners, vitamin E, nut oil, water binding agents, and preservatives. All of the good ingredients are at the end of the ingredient list. This isn't a very advanced moisturizer at all.

Restorative Night Cream *($9.49 for 1.7 ounces)* contains mostly water, thickeners, standard water binding agents, plant oils, vitamin E, fragrance, and preservatives. After the preservative, there are some good water binding agents, but they are too far down in the ingredient list to count. This is a good moisturizer for normal to dry skin.

Nu Skin

Let me start by saying that Nu Skin is not a miracle, a cure, the total answer, or even part of the answer for every woman's skin care needs. Nevertheless, the people who sell this line would lead you to believe it can alter your life as well as your skin. Like all of the other lines I've reviewed, there are some very good products, some that are useless, and some that are simply a waste of money. Plus, as usual, the claims for the products are all highly exaggerated and overstated. What sets Nu Skin apart is its intense direct marketing strategy. As in most multi-level businesses, you meet someone who is selling the line, and if you subsequently buy some of it, you are then asked to sell it. The promise of unlimited financial return sounds like the pot of gold at the end of the rainbow. Because of the multilevel aspect of the sales arrangements, the people who got in at the beginning and can corral more distributors are more likely to make money than those who came in later. Selling isn't as lucrative as getting people to sell for you. The saturation point can come on quick, which is one of the reasons the Federal Trade Commission and the Securities and Exchange Commission have contacted the company (attorney generals in seven states are doing the same). According to the March 1992 issue of *Drug and Cosmetic Industry* magazine, Nu Skin International has responded to complaints and lawsuits in Ohio, Illinois, Michigan, Florida, and Pennsylvania by voluntarily consenting to change some of its marketing and sales policies. One of the problems was that sales reps, in order to keep their commission percentage up, would overbuy cosmetics. After signing agreements with the attorney generals' offices in these states, Nu Skin will refund up to 90 percent of their distributors' unsold products. The company will also monitor their distributors to be sure that 80 percent of their sales are to at least five customers not affiliated with the company. Unfortunately for Nu Skin, in spite of these efforts, Connecticut's attorney general has filed a new lawsuit claiming the company's advertising misleads distributors into believing they will make more than they can. Actual figures indicate that 98 percent of all Nu Skin distributors average about $38 a month in commissions.

(By the way, Nu Skin isn't the only home sales company fighting lawsuits. Herbalife International is having its share of problems. Some of the difficulty is with the FDA, concerning a product that supposedly eliminates cellulite and sundry other false claims. There are also legal questions surrounding one of Herbalife's consultants, who has served a two-year prison term for fraud and conspiracy in a different home sales company.)

Aside from the distribution of Nu Skin, the literature that accompanies the products announces in no uncertain terms that these products are packaged miracles. *"All of the good and none of the bad"* the brochures and accompanying tapes proudly announce. Unfortunately, it depends on how you define "bad." The products do contain preservatives that can be potentially irritating. Some of the products also contain peppermint oil, spearmint oil, witch hazel extract, acetaminde MEA, grapefruit extract, camphor, benzethonium chloride, quaternium-15 (releases formaldehyde), and 2-bromo-2-nitropane-1, 3-diol (a suspected carcinogen), which are all fairly irritating ingredients and known skin sensitizers.

Another difficulty about the phrase *"All of the good . . ."* is that this product line includes almost every gimmick in the book. Some gimmicks are good for the skin, but most are there just for show, covering all the necessary bases of "natural" skin care: royal bee jelly, human placenta extract, aloe vera, vitamins, wheat germ oil, walnut husks, collagen, jojoba oil, and herbal extracts. Rather than arguing the benefits of these ingredients, (although many of you may already know that you cannot feed skin from the outside in and that there is no evidence that any of these function better than other moisturizing ingredients), I want you to understand the placement of these specialty ingredients in these products. Most are located at the bottom of the ingredient list. That means they represent the smallest amount possible. As you may have already guessed and will see as I review each individual item, the first ingredients, the primary components of the product, are fairly standard cosmetics ingredients such as water, thickeners, water binding agents, and plant oils. None of this means there aren't good products in the line, because there are, but they are not the miracles the company would lead you to believe.

I should mention that the one exception is their use of aloe vera. This much-hyped ingredient is often the first or second ingredient listed. Will it do anything special for your skin? I've yet to interview a dermatologist or cosmetic chemist who says it can, and there are absolutely no independent studies or data (from a lab that doesn't sell aloe or aloe-related products) that indicate aloe vera does anything for the skin except provide water and a slight cooling sensation. But a lot of people disagree with me on this one, so it's up to you.

Cleansing Lotion *($10 for 4 ounces)* contains mostly water (part aloe vera and water), thickener, and oils. It leaves the skin feeling clean, although there is a slight oily feeling left after it's rinsed off. It is probably best for someone with dry to normal skin. It also includes human placenta extract, royal bee jelly, and vitamins that get washed off the face, so even if they do something for the skin, they don't stay around very long to do it.

Enhancer *($8 for 2 ounces)* is a lightweight gel that contains mostly water (part aloe vera and water), thickener, glycerin, and hyaluronic acid. These ingredients can nicely retain moisture in the skin, but they won't heal the skin. It also includes peppermint oil, which can cause irritation.

Facial Scrub *($10.50 for 2 ounces)* contains mostly water, aloe vera, glycerin, walnut husks, thickeners, and preservatives. It also contains peppermint oil, which can be irritating to the skin, and there are vitamins at the very end of the ingredient list, which means they are negligible. For the most part this is a good scrub, but it can be irritating for some skin types.

Exfoliant Scrub Extra Gentle *($10.50 for 2 ounces)* contains mostly water (water and aloe vera), glycerin, sea shells (abrasive), thickeners, and peppermint oil. It exfoliates the skin quite nicely, but the peppermint oil does not make this product extra gentle. There are vitamins at the end of the ingredient list, after the preservatives, meaning a minute amount is included.

NaPCA Moisture Mist *($8.50 for 8 ounces)* contains mostly water, aloe vera, NaPCA, and water binding agents. This would feel refreshing on the skin, but the claim that it can control fine lines is not possible.

pH Balance *($8 for 4 ounces)* contains mostly aloe vera, water, witch hazel (can be a skin irritant), water binding agents, human placenta extract, camphor, and preservatives. For some skin types this could be a good toner, but the witch hazel and camphor can cause skin irritation.

Intensive Eye Complex *($40 for 0.78 ounce)* contains mostly aloe vera, thickener, water binding agent, thickeners, shark oil, several water binding agents, soothing agents, collagen, vitamin E, plant oils, and preservatives. This is a good lightweight moisturizer with several good water binding agents high up in the ingredient list, but the only thing intensive about this product is the price.

Rejuvenating Cream *($25 for 2 ounces)* won't rejuvenate the skin, although it can be a good lightweight moisturizer. It contains mostly aloe vera, water, thickeners, standard water binding agent, vitamin E, water binding agents, and preservatives. After the preservatives there is also a list of vitamins, NaPCA, royal bee jelly, and elastin, but there isn't enough of these in here to affect your skin.

NaPCA Moisturizer *($16 for 2 ounces)* is a good lightweight moisturizer that actually contains very little NaPCA. The major ingredients are aloe vera, water, thickeners, vitamin E, water binding agent, preservatives, NaPCA, more preservatives, and vitamins. Remember, ingredients listed after the preservatives don't account for much.

Celltrex *($25 for 0.5 ounce)* is simply a lightweight moisturizer that contains mostly aloe vera, collagen, thickeners, water binding agents, vitamin E, and preservatives. Collagen can't change the skin, it just keeps water in the skin.

Face Lift (with Activator) *($32 for 2 ounces)* is really two separate items you mix together to get the results implied by the name. Basically, the Face Lift powder is egg white, cornstarch (possible irritant), and silica (like sand). The Activator contains water, benzethonium chloride (a skin irritant), aloe vera, soothing agent, and water binding agent. This product swells and irritates the skin and then the egg white and cornstarch temporarily dry it in place, which supposedly makes it look smoother. It doesn't, at least not for long. The irritation around the eyes can be a problem and could possibly cause more wrinkles.

Clay Pack *($11.50 for 2 ounces)* is a standard clay mask that contains mostly water, standard water binding agents, clay, thickeners, and preservatives. Again, like many of the Nu Skin products, the vitamins, royal bee jelly, and human placenta extract are at the end of the ingredient list, meaning you get a tiny amount of them. Besides the clay there are no other irritants or drying agents, so this could be a fairly gentle clay mask.

Glacial Marine Mud *($30 for 12 ounces)* contains only mud from Canada and two preservatives. One of the preservatives listed is 2-bromo-2-nitropane-1, 3 diol, a strong skin irritant. The claim of improved skin tone after rubbing mud over the skin—whether it be from Canada, Italy, or your own backyard—is not possible.

Sunright Accel *($20 for 8 ounces)* claims it can help you get an accelerated tan by enhancing your own melanin production, which is the same as claiming it can help your skin become leathery and get skin cancer faster. There is no such thing as a safe tan from the sun. I do not recommend this product.

Liquid Body Loofah *($10.50 for 8 ounces)* contains mostly water (aloe vera and water), detergent cleansers, and walnut husks. This product is indeed abrasive and can exfoliate the skin. It also contains spearmint oil, which can irritate sensitive skin.

Oil of Olay

Olay is neither plant, nor animal, nor anything else; it is only the name of a product line, but a very convincing name because its popularity remains strong. For the longest time I wondered if people really thought it was some kind of oil derived from an exotic plant. Oil of Olay has quite a product line. It's not very exciting, lacking any state-of-the-art moisturizing ingredients, but there are a few good products to be found.

Facial Cleansing Lotion *($4 for 3 ounces)* is a lightweight cleanser that doesn't quite rinse off without the aid of a washcloth; it can leave an oily residue on the skin.

Foaming Face Wash *($4 for 3 ounces)* does clean the face well, with only a slight drying effect afterward. One of the preservatives is dmdm hydantoin, a strong skin irritant.

Water-Rinsable Cold Cream *($3.99 for 4 ounces)* can't rinse off with water and it leaves an oily film on the face.

Sensitive Skin Foaming Face Wash *($3.37 for 3 ounces)* is an OK water-soluble cleanser that can be drying. It's definitely not the best for sensitive skin: one of the preservatives is dmdm hydantoin, a strong skin irritant.

Refreshing Toner *($4.50 for 7.75 ounces)* contains alcohol, witch hazel, water binding agent, soothing agents, and water binding agents. All the ingredients but the alcohol would have made this a decent toner. Alcohol and witch hazel irritate the skin and negate all the soothing benefits of the other ingredients.

Daily UV Protectant Cream SPF 15 (Fragrance and Fragrance Free) *($6.99 for 1.7 ounces)* is a very lightweight moisturizer with a good sunscreen. It contains mostly water, glycerin, thickeners, and preservatives. Ordinary but adequate to slightly moisturize the skin.

Daily UV Protectant Lotion SPF 15 (Fragrance and Fragrance Free) *($5.99 for 3.5 ounces)* is a very lightweight moisturizer with a good sunscreen that contains mostly water, glycerin, and thickeners. Like the cream above, it isn't anything special, but it is an adequate sunscreen.

Original Beauty Fluid *($5.99 for 4 ounces)* is a very ordinary, rather poor moisturizer that contains only water, mineral oil, and thickeners. There is nothing beautiful about this one.

Sensitive Skin Beauty Fluid *($7.25 for 4 ounces)* is an emollient fragrance-free moisturizer that contains mostly water, thickener, mineral oil, petrolatum, more thickeners, an preservatives. This would be a good emollient moisturizer for dry skin. One of the preservatives is dmdm hydantoin, a strong skin irritant.

Oil-Free Beauty Fluid *($7.69 for 6 ounces)* contains mostly water, glycerin, thickeners, standard water binding agent, more thickeners, and preservatives. This is an ordinary moisturizer that contains more thickeners than anything else, and not worth recommending. One of the preservatives is dmdm hydantoin, a strong skin irritant.

Moisture Replenishing Cream *($7.43 for 2 ounces)* is a fragrance-free cream that contains mostly water, mineral oil, thickeners, standard water binding agents, more thickeners, and preservatives. It is a good lightweight moisturizer.

Intensive Moisture Complex *($7.63 for 1.7 ounces)* contains mostly water, mineral oil, standard water binding agents, a long list of thickeners, and preservatives. This is an OK emollient moisturizer, but it is hardly intensive.

Night of Olay Night Care Cream *($6.91 for 1.7 ounces)* contains mostly water, standard water binding agents, thickeners, and preservatives. This is an OK lightweight moisturizer for normal to dry skin. One of the preservatives is dmdm hydantoin, a strong skin irritant.

Hydro-Night Renewal Gel *($10.99 for 1.7 ounces)* contains mostly water, soothing agent, standard water binding agents, and preservatives. This won't renew anything, but it is an OK extremely lightweight moisturizer for normal skin. One of the preservatives is dmdm hydantoin, a strong skin irritant.

Origins

Origins (like Aveda and The Body Shop) offers skin care systems based on every 1990s fad in the book and then some, including botanicals, essential oils, natural ingredients, recycled packaging (including a recycling service for the empty bottles and compacts at their counters), products that aren't tested on animals, "ancient" skin care treatments, anti-stress formulas, and aroma therapy. The recycling efforts and animal-free testing are both impressive and praiseworthy examples to other cosmetics companies who continue to test their products on animals and don't use recyclable packaging. However, it's the ancient and natural stuff that is the real bait that women get hooked by. The ingredient list is so obscure, it's difficult for even me to see beyond the plants and herbs. Even the salespeople I interviewed didn't know what all those herbs were about. As you might have expected, juxtaposed around the "special" oils and herb extracts are standard skin care ingredients. Plus, many of the "good" ingredients are at the end of list, meaning practically nonexistent.

Origins' basic skin care theory is presented in a very logical manner. Their assertion is that all skin wants to act normal, the way it did when you were young. As we grow up our skin gets confused or behaves badly, not because it wants to, but because it lacks something. If skin is supplied with the correct plants and oils, according to Origins, "nature's memory" can inwardly "retrain" your skin to function like all skin wants to function—normally. What an enticing concept. Of course, the ingredients that supposedly retrain your skin to function normally are derived from the "ancient science of essential oils," which assumes, of course, that people from long ago had great skin because of this special knowledge. It does sound convincing, but, alas, there aren't any ancient people around to prove or disprove those claims. Moreover, you can't retrain the skin; that claim sounds like something the FDA should take a closer look at. But I have to admit this is one of the most original skin care ploys I've ever seen, and that is saying a lot.

In order to review this line without writing an entire book about it, I have summarized most of the plant extracts (which are little more than tea brews) by listing them as just that: plant extracts or plant water. If you want more information about what each of the 30 or so plants listed in these products can supposedly do for the skin (and I feel the claims are not valid when the herbs are cooked and preserved in a cosmetic), contact the company directly (the number is in the appendix) or consult *Rodale's Illustrated Encyclopedia of Herbs*. Having said all that, I still think there are some good products to be found in this line; you just have to read between the lines to find out what they are.

Liquid Crystal *($12 for 5.9 ounces)* leaves a greasy film on the face and takes a lot of cleanser to remove all the makeup without the aid of a washcloth.

Mint Wash *($12.50 for 5.9 ounces)* is a good water-soluble cleanser that doesn't dry out the skin and takes off all the makeup, Unfortunately, it can slightly burn the eyes.

Pure Cream *($12.50 for 6 ounces)* is supposed to be water-soluble but it leaves a greasy film on the face if not used with a washcloth. Plus, the peppermint oil in it can burn the eyes.

Cream Bar *(8.50 for 4 ounces)* is a standard bar soap that also has several oils added. The oils can help reduce the dryness caused by the soap.

Well-Off *($10 for 4 ounces)* is a fairly gentle eye makeup remover.

Swept Away *($15 for 3 ounces)* is a fairly gritty exfoliator that contains jojoba wax and a small amount of peppermint oil; both can be skin irritants. This is supposed to be gentle for sensitive skin, but that doesn't seem to be the case.

Swept Clean *($15 for 3 ounces)* is a very gritty exfoliator that is almost identical to Swept Away except for the addition of menthol (which can be a skin irritant) and charcoal (which can be drying and irritating).

Managing Solution *($15.50 for 5.7 ounces)* is a toner that is supposed to normalize oil production. Plant water, essential oil, aloe vera, vitamin E, slip agents, and preservatives won't change oil production. The oil content of this product won't make someone with oily skin very happy.

Oil Manager *($15.50 for 5.7 ounces)* contains nothing that can stop oil or close pores. It does contain some plant oils, which would be a problem for someone with oily skin. What could Origins have been thinking?

Zero Oil *($10 for 6.4 ounces)* cannot stop oil production; it can absorb some oil, but if you have oily skin it won't even absorb that much. It contains camphor, which can be a skin irritant, and irritations can stimulate oil production. Zero Oil is as misleading a name as they come.

Drenching Solution *($15.50 for 5.7 ounces)* contains mostly plant water, aloe vera, plant oils, vitamin E, thickeners, and preservatives. This is a good soothing toner of sorts, but it won't teach skin to retain water.

Steady Drencher *($20 for 1.85 ounces)* contains mostly plant water, peach kernel oil, aloe vera, olive oil, several thickeners, rice oil, vitamins A and E, plant oils, and preservatives. This is a very emollient moisturizer that will take care of dry skin.

Tuning Solution *($15.50 for 5.7 ounces)* is supposed to rebalance the oily and dry areas of your face. It doesn't contain anything capable of doing that, but it is an OK toner of sorts. It contains mostly plant water, aloe vera, plant oils, vitamin E, thickeners, and preservatives.

Fine Tuner *($20 for 1.9 ounces)* is supposed to even out combination skin. There is nothing in here that can change oily skin, although it does contain some oils that can definitely help dry skin. It also contains shea butter, which can be a problem for someone with oily skin.

Mending Solution *($15.50 for 5.7 ounces)* is almost identical to the Tuning Solution, except this one is supposed to energize look-young systems. The skin doesn't have look-young systems. Amazing that similar products are supposed to do two such disparate things to the skin.

Time Mender *($20 for 1.85 ounces)* contains mostly plant water, standard water binding agents, thickeners, vitamin E, water binding agents, preservatives, and a long list of oils. This is a good moisturizer for dry skin, but the oils don't add up to much coming after the preservatives. The claim is that this product can firm the skin. It can't.

Comforting Solution *($15.50 for 5.7 ounces)* is supposed to help skin defend itself against the environment. It can't do that, however, it is a soothing toner of sorts that contains aloe vera, plant oils, soothing agent, vitamin E, and preservatives.

Constant Comforter *($20 for 1.85 ounces)* contains mostly plant water; standard water binding agents; almond oil; shark oil; several thickeners; vitamins E, A, and B$_6$; water binding agent; and preservatives. There is a long list of oils at the very end of the ingredient list, representing a tiny amount in the cream. This is a good emollient moisturizer for normal to dry skin, but it doesn't calm anything.

Line Chaser *($25 for 0.5 ounce)* can't stop wrinkles in any way, shape, or form, but it is still an OK lightweight moisturizer for normal skin. It contains mostly cucumber water, thickeners, standard water binding agents, and preservatives.

Fringe Benefits *($10 for 1.3 ounces)* contains mostly rosewater, coloring agent, wax (carnuba), thickeners, chamomile extract, more thickeners, water binding agent, yeast, and preservatives. This is a good emollient moisturizer.

Starting Over *($20 for 1 ounce)* is supposed to improve cell renewal; it can't do that, but it is a good moisturizer that contains many of the same ingredients as several other Origins products: plant water, standard water binding agents, thickeners, plant extracts, pine oil (can be a skin irritant), more thickeners, and preservatives.

No Puffery *($20 for 6.4 ounces)* claims it can release trapped fluids and toxins from the skin, but that is not possible. It contains mostly plant water, standard water binding agents, marine plant extract, plant extracts, and preservatives. If you want to believe the plants can suck stuff out of your skin, that's up to you, but you've been warned.

Urgent Moisture *($25 for 2 ounces)* contains mostly plant water, standard water binding agents, thickeners, water binding agents, more thickeners, and preservatives. This is a good lightweight moisturizer for normal to dry skin. It is supposed to perform best in super-dry weather, but it doesn't contain enough antioxidants to protect the skin from serious dehydration.

Clear Improvement *($15 for 2 ounces)* is a standard clay mask that contains mostly plant water, clay, slip agent, thickeners, standard water binding agent, charcoal, more thickeners, and preservatives. The charcoal is supposed to lift impurities out of the pores; it can't do that, but this is an otherwise OK clay mask.

Let The Sunshine SPF 14 No Chemical Sunscreen *($12.50 for 5 ounces)* is one of the better titanium dioxide-based sunscreens on the market. This one is worth a try. There is also Let The Sunshine SPF 7 and SPF 21, both nonchemical sunscreens. The SPF 7 isn't strong enough to protect adequately from the sun, but the SPF 21 is great.

Physicians Formula

This is one of the few cosmetics companies that publishes a list of the irritating ingredients they don't use in their products that often show up in other skin care and makeup products. None of the Physicians Formula products contain lanolin, aluminum sulfate, benzoic acid, bovine extracts, linoleic acid, oil of walnut, salicylic acid, serum proteins, or yeast extract. However, they do use quaternium-15 and phenoxyethanol, two very irritating preservatives. That seems contradictory, but you can't have everything. Even if you don't use the products, you can write to Physicians Formula Cosmetics at 230 South Ninth Avenue, City of Industry, California 91746, to ask for a copy of the information about irritating ingredients, except for the ones they decided to use. When other companies make claims that their products are hypoallergenic, you could easily use this list as a reference guide.

My only other issue with this skin care line is its name. It sounds as if a bunch of physicians got together and designed this line or as if physicians prefer these products to others, but neither is the case. Other than that, some of these products are definitely worth considering. In particular, I liked Physicians Formula's Captyane line of products, which is their version of liposomes, in essence a time-release moisturizer. These are good moisturizers, even though the claims are as exaggerated as it gets.

Deep Cleanser *($4.93 for 4 ounces)* is a standard detergent cleanser that also contains potassium hydroxide, which can be very irritating to the skin. This cleanser can't deep clean, but it can deeply dry out the skin.

Beauty Buffers Exfoliating Scrub *($5.39 for 2 ounces)* is a good exfoliant that isn't as irritating as most.

Captyane Replenishing Eye Complex *($11 for 1.4 ounces)* contains mostly water, mineral oil, thickeners, water binding agents, safflower oil, water binding agent, and preservatives. This is a good emollient moisturizer, but it won't prevent or change wrinkles.

Captyane Replenishing Night Treatment *($11 for 1.4 ounces)* contains mostly water, thickeners, egg yolk, more thickeners, vitamin E, and preservatives. This is a good emollient moisturizer, however, one of the preservatives is quaternium-15, considered a strong skin irritant.

Captyane Replenishing Gel-Cream *($11 for 1 ounce)* contains mostly water, safflower oil, standard water binding agents, shark oil, collagen, thickeners, water binding agents, vitamin E, and preservatives. This is a very emollient moisturizer for dry skin.

Deep Moisture Cream *($7.99 for 4 ounces)* contains mostly water, thickener, mineral oil, glycerin, thickeners, petrolatum, more thickeners, safflower oil, and preservatives. This is an ordinary mineral oil- and petrolatum-based moisturizer, good for dry skin, but boring.

Elastin Collagen Moisture Lotion *($8.49 for 4 ounces)* contains mostly water, thickener, safflower oil, collagen, thickener, mineral oil, water binding agents (elastin), more thickeners, and preservatives. This is a very emollient moisturizer that would be good for dry skin. One of the preservatives is quaternium-15, considered a strong skin irritant.

Extra Rich Rehydrating Moisturizer *($8.49 for 4 ounces)* contains mostly water, thickener, mineral oil, more thickeners, and preservatives. This isn't as rich or as interesting as many of the other moisturizers in this group. It's a poor name considering the mediocre ingredient list.

Gentle Moisture Lotion *($8.49 for 4 ounces)* contains mostly water, mineral oil, thickeners, petrolatum, more thickeners, and preservatives. It is almost identical to the Extra Rich Moisturizer and the same basic evaluation applies.

Enriched Dry Skin Concentrate *($7.99 for 4 ounces)* contains mostly water, thickeners, avocado oil, glycerin, thickeners, vitamins A and E, corn oil, and preservatives. This is a good emollient moisturizer for dry skin.

Oil Control Oil-Free Moisturizer *($8.49 for 4 ounces)* contains mostly water, thickeners, glycerin, soothing agent, more thickeners, and preservatives. This is a good lightweight moisturizer for normal to dry skin. One of the preservatives is quaternium-15, considered a strong skin irritant.

Vital Defense Moisture Lotion SPF 15 *($7.79 for 6 ounces)* is a good moisturizer/sunscreen for dry skin. It contains a long list of thickeners and a small amount of water binding agents. One of the preservatives is quaternium-15, considered a strong skin irritant.

Vital Defense Oil Free Lotion SPF 15 *($7.79 for 6 ounces)* is a good sunscreen for someone with combination skin. It contains some clay, which can absorb a small amount of oil, which is better than nothing. Keep in mind that although this lotion is labeled "oil-free," the wax-like thickeners might make you break out. One of the preservatives is quaternium-15, considered a strong skin irritant.

Emollient Oil *($5.23 for 2 ounces)* contains mostly safflower oil, sesame oil, petrolatum, slip agents, and fragrance. This is a good, very emollient oil, but no more so than using a pure oil from your pantry shelf.

Deep Cleaning Face Mask *($5.39 for 2.75 ounces)* is a standard clay mask that contains mostly water, witch hazel, clay, alcohol, and glycerin. The clay is drying, and the alcohol and witch hazel will only make it worse. This mask won't deep clean, but it can deeply irritate the skin.

Pond's

Cleansing Lotion & Moisturizer In One *($3.40 for 7 ounces)* leaves a greasy film on the skin and doesn't take off makeup very well.

Foaming Cleanser & Toner In One *($3.40 for 7 ounces)* is a good water-soluble cleanser but can be drying for some skin types.

Cold Cream Deep Cleanser *($5.83 for 6 ounces)* is a classic greasy cold cream that needs to be wiped off.

Water Rinsable Cleanser *($4.50 for 5.5 ounces)* is not at all water-soluble. The main ingredients are water, mineral oil, and beeswax. If anything, the cleanser leaves an oily film on the skin.

Water Rinsable Cleanser for Sensitive Skin *($4.50 for 5.5 ounces)* This cleanser is almost identical to the one above, which means it isn't what I would call water-soluble.

Facial Cleansing Foam *($4.50 for 4 ounces)* is a supposedly water-soluble cleanser that contains mineral oil, beeswax, and ceresin, which aren't water-soluble and leave a film on the skin.

Moisturizing Cleansing Bar with Moisture Complex *($1.99 for 3.25 ounces)* is a standard bar soap that has no ingredients that would moisturize the skin. This soap would be quite drying for most skin types.

Oil Controlling Cleansing Bar with Multi-Action Astringent *($1.99 for 3.25 ounces)* is a standard bar soap that also contains alcohol. That won't control oil, and the only action it can provide is dryness and irritation.

Clarifying Astringent *($3.09 for 7 ounces)* is a standard alcohol-based toner that also contains witch hazel, menthol, and eucalyptus, all of which can seriously irritate the skin.

Extra Rich Moisturizer *($4.50 for 3.9 ounces)* is a fairly basic moisturizer that contains water, mineral oil, thickener, petrolatum, glycerin, more thickeners, and preservatives. It can be quite good for dry skin.

Dry Skin Extra Rich Formula *($7.39 for 11 ounces)* is a standard mineral oil- and petrolatum-based moisturizer with thickeners and preservatives. It would be OK for dry skin.

Nourishing Moisturizer Lotion Oil-Free *($7.99 for 3.25 ounces)* can't nourish the skin, but it is a good moisturizer for normal to dry skin. It contains mostly water, glycerin, thickeners, vitamins A and E, water binding agents, and preservatives.

Nourishing Moisturizer Lotion Oil-Free with SPF 15 *($7.99 for 3.25 ounces)* is almost identical to the lotion above except it contains a good sunscreen.

Overnight Nourishing Complex Cream *($5.99 for 2 ounces)* contains mostly water, water binding agents, several thickeners, vitamins A and E, amino acids, and preservatives. This is a good lightweight moisturizer for dry skin, but the vitamins can't feed the skin, they are just good antioxidants.

Dramatic Results Skin Smoothing Capsules with Nutrium *($11.49 for 0.26 ounce)* contains mostly standard water binding agents, shark oil, vitamins A and E, and water binding agents. The results won't be dramatic, but this is certainly good for someone with dry skin.

Revitalizing Eye Gel with Vitamin E *($5.99 for 0.5 ounce)* contains mostly water, witch hazel, slip agent, vitamin E, plant extracts, and preservatives. Witch hazel is a possible skin irritant and a problem in a product meant to be used near the delicate skin around the eye. One of the preservatives is dmdm hydantoin, which can also be a skin irritant.

Prescriptives

Prescriptives is one of the few department store cosmetics lines to be entirely fragrance-free. That is a praiseworthy effort in a sea of competitive products that rely on smell more than quality to sell products. That's not to say I find the rest of Prescriptives' formulations or prices equally exceptional, but the omission of fragrance is a healthy step in the right direction.

Gentle Wash Lotion Cleanser *($16.50 for 7.5 ounces)* is a good water-soluble cleanser for someone with dry skin. It takes off all the makeup, but it can leave a slight film on the skin unless you use a washcloth, which isn't all that gentle.

Soothing Cream Cleanser *($16.50 for 6 ounces)* contains mostly water, mineral oil, glycerin, shark oil, thickeners, vitamins A and E, more thickeners, and preservatives. This cleanser can only be removed by being wiped off. It leaves a greasy film on the face.

Sparkling Clean *($16.50 for 4 ounces)* is an OK water-soluble cleanser that takes off all the makeup and leaves no film on the face. However, it does contain a small amount of lemon and spearmint oils, which can irritate or burn the eye area.

Essential Cleansing Gel *($16.50 for 3.5 ounces)* is a standard detergent-based cleanser that has a few plant extracts. It can be drying for most skin types.

Essential Cleansing Bar *($13.50 for 5.3 ounces)* is a standard bar soap—nothing more, nothing less. It can be drying and irritating to some skin types.

Skin Refining Gel *($17.50 for 3.5 ounces)* contains mostly water, alcohol, slip agents, menthol, soothing agent, and preservatives. This product is supposedly a gentle exfoliant but the alcohol and menthol can cause irritation and dryness.

Skin Refiner *($17.50 for 3.5 ounces)* contains mostly water, mineral oil, slip agents, several thickeners, vitamin E, more thickeners, and preservatives. This is a mild exfoliant that can leave a greasy film on the skin.

Eye Makeup Remover *($15 for 4 ounces)* is a standard eye makeup remover that contains mostly water, slip agents, detergent cleanser, slip agent, and preservatives.

Skin Balancer No Fragrance, Alcohol-Free *($16.50 for 6 ounces)* might not contain alcohol, but it does contain magnesium and zinc sulfate at the beginning of the ingredient list. Both of these can cause allergic reactions and irritate the skin.

Skin Reviver *($16.50 for 6 ounces)* won't revive anyone's skin, but it will cause irritation. It contains mostly alcohol plus some magnesium and zinc sulfate, which can cause allergic reactions and irritate the skin. It also contains salicylic acid, which peels the skin. Basically this is one harsh product for the face.

All You Need Action Moisturizer *($30 for 1.7 ounces)* is hardly all you need, but the name does sound great. It doesn't have an SPF, so it isn't all you need for daytime. It would be fine as a nighttime moisturizer for someone with dry skin, but nothing exceptional. This is Prescriptives' attempt at an alpha hydroxy acid product, but it doesn't contain enough AHA to be considered adequate in that area either. It contains mostly water, standard water binding agents, several thickeners, fruit extracts, water binding agent, vitamin E, plant extracts, and preservatives.

All You Need Action Moisturizer Oil-Free *($30 for 1.7 ounces)* is fairly similar to the moisturizer above, give or take a few plant extracts and thickeners. The same critique applies.

Comfort Cream SPF 6 *($37.50 for 1.7 ounces)* contains mostly water, standard water binding agents, nut oil, thickeners, algae extract, more thickeners, vitamin A, water binding agents, plant extracts, vitamin E, more thickeners, and preservatives. This is a very good moisturizer for someone with normal to dry skin, but I wouldn't call it any more comforting than anyone else's moisturizer.

Flight Cream *($28 for 1.7 ounces)* is supposed to be suitable for skin subjected the rigors of flying conditions. It is only a good standard moisturizer for dry skin, but nothing more, and there is certainly nothing special about it for dry cabin air. It contains mostly water, standard water binding agents, mineral oil, thickeners, algae extract, shark oil, more thickeners, vitamin E, yeast, plant extracts, and preservatives.

Line Preventor *($45 for 1 ounce)* won't prevent lines, although this is a good moisturizer for dry skin. It contains mostly water, standard water binding agents, protein, thickeners, vitamin E, shark oil, plant oil, water binding agents, and preservatives. There is a sunscreen in this product, but it is not strong enough to adequately protect the skin from the sun.

Extra Firm Skin Care Concentrate *($55 for 1.7 ounces)* contains mostly water, standard water binding agents, tissue extract, algae extract, water binding agents, vitamins A and E, plant extracts, and preservatives. Tissue and algae extracts can't firm the skin, but you're supposed to believe they can, which is how they can convince you to spend $55 on this product. Other than that, it is a good moisturizer.

Simply Moisture *($35 for 2 ounces)* contains mostly water, water binding agents, shark oil, several thickeners, vitamins E and A, water binding agents, grape oil, aloe vera, lots of thickeners, mineral oil, and preservatives. This is a good lightweight moisturizer for normal to dry skin. It also contains a sunscreen, but not enough to adequately protect from the sun.

Multi-Moisture Pure Hydrating Cream *($37.50 for 1.9 ounces)* contains mostly water, standard water binding agents, water binding agents, thickeners, vitamin E, and preservatives. This is a good lightweight moisturizer for normal to dry skin. It also contains a small amount of sunscreen, but not enough to adequately protect from the sun.

Eyewear *($35 for 0.5 ounce)* consists of mostly water, water binding agent, thickener, mineral oil, shark oil, thickeners, algae extract, standard water binding agents, several water binding agents, vitamins A and E, thickeners, plant extracts, and preservatives. It is a good moisturizer for normal to dry skin. Don't expect much from the algae extract; it can't do much for the skin.

Anti-Blemish *($12.50 for 1 ounce)* is just another alcohol-based blemish product with a little salicylic acid thrown in to help peel the skin. It does contain some glycerin and a soothing agent, but that won't counteract the irritation from the other ingredients, and alchohol or salicylic acid won't change a blemish on your face.

Principal Secret

Yes, Victoria, there is still money to be made from being beautiful. When your television series ended and other jobs weren't pending, convincing women that they can look like you, or that what you know about being an American beauty will help them (for three easy payments), turned out to be quite lucrative.

Everyone wants to know about Victoria Principal's products—you should see the letters I get. (We all need to stop watching late-night cable TV.) More accurately, they're Madame Aida Thibant's products, but no one has heard of her, so who would buy them? Actually, I shouldn't say no one has heard of her, because according to the pamphlet she is world-renowned and often quoted, although no quotes or credits are provided, nor even the address of her Beverly Hills salon.

Why are we so interested in a product line named after Victoria Principal? Maybe it's because she was Bobby's wife and she put up with all those Ewings year after year. What else could qualify her to let us in on her skin care secrets? All this celebrity secrecy (do Cher or Connie Stevens know about this?) is only $89.95 (for six overpriced products that you definitely don't need) or $59.85 (for three very overpriced products you don't really need either). But wait! There is a bargain in all of this. If you join The Principal Secret Skin Care Club, you can save money: $10 off the total purchase.

If you think I sound cynical it's because I am. I've said it before, but it needs repeating: *Celebrities are not skin care or makeup experts, they are actresses who have signed a good contract to represent a product line.* Believing that they have discovered the perfect products and are sharing them with you is just not living in the real world. The name is what you are being lured by, so let go of the bait. These products aren't why Victoria Principal is beautiful.

Joining her "club" is no bargain either. Every 90 days a club member receives the original "Value Order" she purchased (either the three-piece group for $49.95 or the six-piece group for $79.95), and then every fifth shipment is free. That means that in a year's time, your bill for skin care alone will be somewhere between $219.80 to $347.80, including shipping and handling. Extra products, which are discounted between 20 percent and 50 percent when you belong to the club, could bring your yearly total to more than $500.

Having gotten all this anger about infomercials off my chest, I should mention that several of these products aren't bad, and a few are actually quite nice, specifically for someone with normal to dry skin. Someone with oily, sensitive, or blemished skin could have problems with this skin care routine. Another benefit is that none of these products are tested on animals. But my opinion about the price remains. Plus, no one needs six to ten products (especially expensive ones) to take care of her face and body. Did I forget to state that the claims are also exaggerated?

The following is a review of the Victoria Principal products; all prices listed are retail. If you do decide to use these products, the club is a good idea, because you will need to reorder frequently as most products come in only 0.25- to 4-ounce sizes. Four ounces of any cleanser won't last for more than a month.

Gentle Deep Cleanser (*$16 for 4 ounces*) is best for someone with normal to dry skin. It cleans well, but leaves a slight greasy feel after it is rinsed, and it can burn over the eye area. The directions suggest a washcloth, which would help the greasy feel, but I never recommend using a washcloth because it abrades the skin and pulls at it. It does clean well, but is probably best only for someone with normal to oily skin.

Time Release Moisture (*$35 for 2 ounces*) contains some type of ingredient that sounds like a liposome, but I am not familiar with it, so I can't say how truly time-release it is, but it should work. The ingredients are fairly standard: water, thickener, shark oil, more thickeners, a form of mineral oil, water binding ingredients, more thickeners, and, down at the very bottom of the list, vitamin E, glycerin, another water binding ingredient, and preservatives. It is OK for normal to slightly dry skin, but it isn't very emollient and most of the good stuff is at the end of the ingredient list. It is supposed to be applied twice a day, but without a high SPF the claim of anti-aging action is just not true.

Eye Relief *($30 for 2 ounces)* is a light gel that has a cool, soft feel. It isn't very emollient, but it does have good water binding ingredients. This would be good for someone with normal to combination skin. The claim is that it can prevent the formation of wrinkles, which is completely untrue.

Intensive Serum *($40 for 0.25 ounce)* is an almost minuscule vial of some good water binding ingredients, however, it contains quaternium-15, which is a fairly irritating preservative. It is absurdly overpriced. Forty dollars for 0.25 ounce comes to $2,560 a pound! Now what cosmetic is possibly worth that much for mostly water and a pinch of some water binding ingredients?

Extra Nurturing Cream *($40 for 2 ounces)* is a good moisturizer for dry skin; it contains mostly water, shark oil, several thickeners, vitamin A, more thickeners, glycerin, more thickeners, water binding ingredients, more thickeners, more water binding ingredients, and preservatives.

Invisible Toning Masque *($23 for 2 ounces)* is unusual for a mask because it doesn't contain clay. Rather, it is a moisturizing mask. Containing mostly water, egg yolk, thickener, glycerin, more thickeners, castor oil, water binding ingredients, and preservatives, it closely resembles the Extra Nurturing Cream. It seems to be an unnecessary step, when so many of the other products contain the exact same ingredients.

Self-Tanning Milk *($15 for 4 ounces)*. All products of this type use the same ingredient—dihydroxyacetone—to turn the skin brown. Other than that, this is a good moisturizer with an insignificant amount of sunscreen. It also contains a small amount of salicylic acid, I suppose to help peel the skin, which could cause the skin to tan unevenly. You are supposed to slough the skin *before* you apply self-tanning products, not during.

Body Moisture *($20 for 8 ounces)* is a lightweight moisturizer containing water, several thickeners, castor oil, glycerin, more thickeners, water binding ingredients, herbal extracts (tea), vitamin E, and preservatives.

Time Release Tinted Moisture *($35 for 2 ounces)* is more like a foundation than a tint providing light to medium coverage. The color selection is limited, with only four colors to choose from: Sheer Peach, which is actually quite neutral, but would only be good for a medium skin tone; Sheer Rose, which turns very orange on most skin types; Sheer Gold, which has a good tan color quality for medium to dark skin tones, but may appear sallow on some skin types; and Sheer Bronze, which I did not receive a sample of. With an SPF of 8, it can't protect from the sun and thereby does not live up to its claim of anti-aging action.

Gentle Exfoliating Scrub *($20 for 4 ounces)* isn't exactly gentle. The third ingredient is polyacrylamide, which is considered to be highly irritating and caustic on the skin. Another ingredient is a form of acrylate, which is very irritating. It also contains salicylic acid, which can peel the skin. There are too many irritating ingredients for this to help any skin type and too many for a so-called gentle product.

Purpose by Johnson & Johnson

Gentle Cleansing Soap *($3.75 for 6 ounces)* is just a standard bar soap with a little glycerin added, but that won't counteract the drying effect of the soap. It can irritate and dry the skin and possibly burn the eyes.

Gentle Cleansing Wash *($5.75 for 6 ounces)* isn't all that gentle. It is a standard detergent cleanser that can dry out the skin. It could be good for someone with oily skin, but it contains quaternium-15, a very irritating preservative.

Rachel Perry

Health food stores have been selling Rachel Perry products for years. One of the original "natural" lines, it is now also available at some large drugstore chains. In spite of its unexciting status in comparison to the highbrow Aveda line, Rachel Perry products contain many of the same "natural" ingredients. For the consumer on a budget interested in the ballyhoo surrounding botanical skin care products, this line could satisfy that curiosity, prove quite interesting, and not hurt your pocketbook or skin. That isn't to say that the infusions of herbs and essential oils will do anything spectacular for your skin, but there are enough consumers out there who want to find out for themselves and here is an inexpensive alternative.

Citrus-Aloe Cleanser and Face Wash *($7.88 for 4 ounces)* contains a tea of aloe vera, nettles, sage, chamomile, linden, cucumber, arnica, marsh mallow, and rose hips (all can be soothing to the skin); thickeners; apricot oil; more thickeners; and more oils. The oils in this product make this more a wipe-off product than a face wash. It will leave a greasy residue on the skin.

Sea Kelp-Herbal Facial Scrub *($7.88 for 2.5 ounces)* contains mostly water, cornmeal, glycerin, slip agent, rye flour, mineral oil, titanium dioxide, almond meal, sea kelp and sea salt, some herbs, and preservatives. This is a pretty thick mess to use as a scrub. You would be better off using plain cornmeal or sea salt all by itself as a scrub. It would be cheaper and better for the skin. There is no benefit from using sea kelp on the skin.

Violet Rose Skin Toner *($7.19 for 8 ounces)* contains mostly a tea of aloe vera, chamomile, rose hips, comfrey, calendula, and juniper; water binding agents; soothing agent; and preservatives. This would be good irritant-free toner for most skin types.

Elastin and Collagen Firming Treatment *($10.88 for 2 ounces)* contains mostly a tea of horsetail, comfrey, chamomile, ginseng, marsh mallow, linden, and yarrow (all can be soothing to the skin); witch hazel extract (can be a skin irritant); collagen; elastin; thickeners; water binding agent; thickener; and fragrance. This won't firm anything, but it is a good moisturizer for someone with normal to slightly dry skin.

Bee Pollen-Jojoba Maximum Moisture Cream *($9.38 for 2 ounces)* contains a long list of herbs similar to those above, and, of course, bee pollen. If you want to believe bee pollen can do something for your skin, that's fine, but there is no independent research that supports its use for skin care. The next ingredients are oil; thickeners; jojoba oil; vitamins A, D, and E; and preservatives. One of the preservatives is quaternium-15, which is considered one of the more irritating preservatives used in cosmetics. Other than that this would be a good moisturizer for most skin types.

Ginseng and Collagen Wrinkle Treatment *($10.88 for 2 ounces)* contains a long list of herbs similar to those above: safflower oil; several thickeners; collagen; vitamins A, B, C, D, and E; more oils; and preservatives. The vitamins are way down in the ingredient list, but they still can provide some antioxidant benefit. This would be a good moisturizer for dry skin, but it won't change wrinkles as the name implies.

Hi Potency "E" Special Treatment Line Control *($10.88 for 2 ounces)* contains mostly water, vitamin E (16,000 I.U.), thickeners, safflower oil, shea butter, glycerin, apricot and sesame oil, aloe vera, vitamin A, more vitamin E, royal bee jelly, and preservatives. One of the preservatives is quaternium-15, which is considered one of the more irritating preservatives used in cosmetics. Vitamins A and E are good antioxidants and can prevent dehydration, but they do not nourish the skin. This stuff won't control lines, but it is a very good moisturizer for dry skin.

Clay and Ginseng Texturizing Mask *($7.88 for 2 ounces)* contains mostly water; clay (supposedly French clay, but clay is clay no matter what country it comes from); talc; more clay; castor oil; clay; titanium dioxide; glycerin; ginseng; vitamin E oil; extracts of mint, eucalyptus, and mint (which can all be irritating to the skin); and preservatives. This is just a standard clay mask, and the plant extracts can prove to be too irritating, particularly when combined with the drying effect of the clay.

Revlon

Revlon's standard lines—Eterna '27', Natural Collagen Complex, and Moon Drops—have recently been joined by a line of products called Revlon Results. Before I discuss this product line, let me relate a story that might sound familiar. Back in 1987, Retin-A was being heralded by the media as a possible wrinkle cream for sun-damaged skin. Shortly, and I mean shortly, after that, an unbelievable number of cosmetics companies created fake Retin-A copycat products. "Retinol," "Vitamin A therapy," and "Works just like Retin-A, only more gentle" proclaimed the product labels. Could any of these substitute for Retin-A? No, absolutely not, but that never stops the cosmetics industry, and there was little the FDA could do about it.

Now, with alpha hydroxy acids making cosmetic news, Revlon is the first company to come out with an AHA look-alike that has no AHA in it. Revlon Results is a product line that contains an ingredient complex called Alpha Recap. It is supposed to exfoliate the skin like AHA but more gently, because it is not an acid. There are a few problems with this kind of marketing. First, the only reason we know AHA can do what it can do is because it was first tested as a prescription drug and therefore we have quantitative test results that let us know how it works. AHA never became exclusively a drug; it is a cosmetic ingredient. Alpha Recap is simply a cosmetic ingredient, and because of that status Revlon is not required to back up any of its claims with proof. You may be impressed by the patent and trademark information, which make Alpha Recap sound very exclusive, but only the name is being protected. The trademark has nothing to do with the ingredients. My advice, based on the ingredient list, is to not expect Revlon Results to behave in any way like AHA. That doesn't mean these aren't good moisturizers, but they are misleading if what you are expecting is an AHA product.

Eterna '27' All Day Moisture Lotion *($13.25 for 2 ounces)* is a very emollient, good moisturizer for dry skin; it contains mostly water, standard water binding agent, thickener, olive oil, a long list of thickeners, a nominal amount of amino acids, and preservatives.

Eterna '27' All Day Moisture Cream *($13.25 for 1 ounce)* is very similar to the lotion above. The major difference is that it contains more thickeners. It would be good for dry skin.

Eterna '27' with Exclusive Progenitin *($15 for 2 ounces)* is going to sound strange, but just remember, I'm only describing this product, I didn't formulate it. The active ingredient in this product is called pregnenolone acetate. It is derived from the urine of pregnant women and is considered to be an anti-inflammatory agent. Therefore, this moisturizer is actually a very mild topical cortisone-type cream. In my opinion, unless your dry skin is a result of a slight dermatitis, this cream is unnecessary. In any case, there are cheaper topical cortisone creams on the market. Beyond the price, this is a very emollient cream for dry skin only; it contains mostly water, mineral oil, beeswax, petrolatum, standard water binding agent, thickener, almond oil, avocado and sesame oil, and preservatives.

Eterna '27' Skin Recharger *($6.25 for 2 ounces)* is released via propellant. It shoots out of a spray bottle like bug spray and has a similar initial odor due to the isobutane. It is a good moisturizer if you can get past the smell and the way it is dispensed. It contains standard water binding agents, thickener, water binding agents, amino acids, thickeners, plant extract, protein, collagen, fragrance, and preservatives.

Natural Collagen Complex SPF 15 *($9.87 for 3.85 ounces)* is a lightweight moisturizer with a good SPF; it contains mostly thickeners and some good water binding agents. It also contains collagen, which is a good water binding agent (nothing more), and some algae extract, which sounds more exotic than it is beneficial.

Natural Collagen Complex SPF 6 *($9.87 for 3 ounces)* is similar to the SPF 15 except it is more emollient due to the inclusion of mineral oil and petrolatum. This would be good for someone with dry skin, but the SPF isn't high enough to protect adequately from the sun.

Natural Collagen Complex Protective Eye Cream Vitamin E SPF 4 *($8.89 for 0.5 ounce)* is a nonchemical sunscreen that would be better if it had a higher SPF. It is very emollient and would be good for someone with dry skin, but it doesn't contain enough vitamin E to warrant a plug in the name.

Revlon Results Day-Light Replenisher SPF 8 *($9.49 for 1.75 ounces)* contains mostly water, standard water binding agents, thickeners, petrolatum, more thickeners, water binding agents, vitamin E, and preservatives. This is a good moisturizer with a small amount of sunscreen that is not adequate to protect from the sun.

Revlon Results Daily Requirement Moisture Cream SPF 8 *($9.49 for 1.75 ounces)* is almost identical to the Day-Light Replenisher and the same critique applies.

Revlon Results Day-Light Moisturizer SPF 8 *($9.49 for 1.75 ounces)* contains mostly water, thickeners, standard water binding agents, more thickeners, vitamin E, water binding agents, more thickeners, and preservatives. This is a good moisturizer.

Revlon Results Rest & Renewal Night Cream Concentrate *($14.49 for 2 ounces)* is almost identical to the Day-Light Moisturizer, minus the sunscreen and with the addition of mineral oil. The same critique applies.

Brighten-Up Eye Cream *($12.99 for 0.75 ounce)* is almost identical to the Rest & Renewal Cream, minus the mineral oil and with the addition of petrolatum, which makes it somewhat heavier. It is still a good moisturizer for extra-dry skin around the eyes.

Shiseido

This is a huge skin care line, to say the least, and it is one of the more confusing I've encountered. There are several skin care divisions within the line that have absurdly similar names. For example, Facial Cleansing Foam is one product from one of the categories, Cleansing Foam Concentrate is another, and Cleansing Foam is yet another. Surely there are enough words to come up with different names that would help separate the products, but that name game may be more irksome for me than for the consumer. Anyway, the reality is that the cleansers, moisturizers, and toners aren't really all that different. Some of the product divisions seem to be more a marketing consideration to convince a woman that her specific skin care needs are being met than anything to do with content. The Pureness group of products is supposed to be for oily skin; Vital Perfection is for normal/combination skin; Facial Concentrate is for dry/mature skin; and Facial Skin Care is for normal/dry skin. There is also a group of specialty products for those who think their skin care needs aren't being met by all the other items.

I have to admit that at the counter the products are organized nicely in separate cases according to the different skin types, but as is true with every product grouping of this type, oily skin is stuck with products that dry and irritate the skin and dry skin is lumped in with mature skin (as if all mature skin is dry). It is always best to look at products individually and not in groups. That way you won't inadvertently buy an irritating product or one that is too greasy.

Facial Concentrates Facial Cleansing Foam *($27 for 5.5 ounces)* is a standard detergent cleanser that can have a drying effect on the skin.

Facial Concentrates Facial Softening Lotion *($34 for 5 ounces)* is a toner that is mostly water, propylene glycol, and alcohol. Alcohol is never great for the skin and definitely can't soften it.

Facial Concentrates Facial Moisturizing Lotion *($35 for 3.3 ounces)* is a good moisturizer for dry skin; it contains mostly water, shark oil, standard water binding agents, petrolatum, thickeners, jojoba oil, more thickeners, and preservatives. It does contain some water binding agents and vitamin E, but they are too far down on the ingredient list to count.

Facial Concentrates Facial Eye Wrinkle Cream Concentrate *($40 for 0.5 ounce)* is a very rich, thick cream that contains mostly water, squalene (shark oil), mineral oil, petrolatum, and sodium PCA. It won't change the wrinkles around your eye, but it will improve your dry skin.

Facial Concentrates Facial Nourishing Cream *($50 for 1 ounce)* contains mostly shark oil, glycerin, water, petrolatum, jojoba oil, thickeners, preservatives, fragrance, and preservatives. This is a good moisturizer for someone with very dry skin.

Facial Concentrates Throat Firming Cream Concentrate *($33 for 1.7 ounces)* won't firm anyones's neck, but you don't really need me to tell you that anymore, do you? This is an OK moisturizer that contains mostly water, standard water binding agents, shark oil, jojoba oil, several thickeners, palm oil, more thickeners, and preservatives. It does contain vitamin E and some plant extracts, but besides being useless for firming the skin, they are at the end of the ingredient list and basically trivial.

Facial Concentrates Essential Concentrate *($46 for 1 ounce)* contains mostly water, standard water binding agents, alcohol, slip agents, seaweed, and preservatives. Putting alcohol on dry skin is foolish and not recommended, and at these prices it is criminal.

Facial Concentrates Facial Moisture Mask *($36 for 4.5 ounces)* contains some oil and water binding agents, but it also contains some very drying ingredients as well. I wouldn't consider this a great mask.

Pureness Washing Grains *($22 for 3.5 ounces)* is a detergent cleanser with scrub particles. It also contains castor oil and beeswax, which can leave a film on the skin.

Pureness Clarifying Toner *($14 for 2.5 ounces)* is a standard alcohol-based toner that also contains clay, sulphur, and salicylic acid. All of these ingredients are potentially very irritating and drying on the skin.

Pureness Oil Control Treatment Compact *($17.50 for 3.5 ounces)* contains mostly talc, shark oil, thickeners, and preservatives. Shark oil is not great for someone with oily skin. There is absolutely nothing in this product that will control oil.

Pureness Oil Free Moisture Essence *($18 for 1.69 ounces)* contains water, alcohol, standard water binding agents, thickeners, preservatives, and salicylic acid. This isn't really oil-free; one of the thickeners is a form of castor oil. The other ingredients are too drying and irritating to consider this any kind of a moisturizer.

Pureness Exfoliating Masque *($17 for 2.8 ounces)* is a standard peel-off mask that contains alcohol, thickeners, salicylic acid, and preservatives. The alcohol and salicylic acid are very drying and irritating.

Pureness Spot Cream *($14 for 0.5 ounce)* contains sulphur, clay, talc, and alcohol. Just like all acne lines, this group of products is based on the premise that sulphur, clay, and alcohol can do something for acne or oily skin. They can't, but they can make it irritated, dry, and potentially more oily.

Pureness Oil Blotting Paper *($9.50 for 100 sheets)* is a thin sheet of paper dusted with a tiny amount of clay and preservatives. I find no difference between using this and blotting a facial tissue over the face and then dusting with a translucent powder.

Facial Skincare Cleansing Foam *($20 for 4.5 ounces)* is a standard detergent facial cleanser that can be very drying.

Facial Skincare Facial Astringent Lotion *($26.50 for 5 ounces)* is like most astringents that contain mostly water and alcohol, and is too irritating for most skin types.

Facial Skincare Facial Astringent Lotion (Mild) *($26.50 for 5 ounces)* is almost identical to the one above, which makes it anything but mild. Alcohol dries and irritates the skin, period.

Facial Skincare Facial Soothing Lotion *($26.50 for 5 ounces)* is designed for oily skin and it can indeed absorb oil, but I would not necessarily call it soothing. The ingredients are water, butylene glycol, and two types of clay.

Facial Skincare Facial Moisturizing Lotion (Rich) *($27.50 for 3.3 ounces)* contains mostly water, shark oil, standard water binding agent, jojoba oil, petrolatum, thickeners, fragrance, and preservatives. This is a good emollient moisturizer for dry skin.

Facial Skincare Facial Nourishing Cream *($38 for 1 ounce)* is very similar to the Moisturizing Lotion (Rich) above, and the same critique applies.

Facial Skin Care Pre-Makeup Cream *($23 for 1 ounce)* contains mostly water, standard water binding agent, a long list of thickeners, jojoba oil, shark oil, petrolatum, palm oil, more thickeners, and preservatives. This is a good moisturizer for dry skin, but there is nothing unique about this that makes it better for wearing under makeup, particularly when it doesn't contain a sunscreen.

Facial Skincare Facial Nourishing Stick *($24 for 0.21 ounce)* contains mostly mineral oil, shark oil, wax thickeners, water, more thickeners, water binding agents, jojoba oil, vitamin E, water binding agent, and preservatives. This is a good emollient for dry skin, but it is absurdly overpriced. When you consider the cost is about $120 per ounce, this is outrageous.

Facial Skincare Facial Masque Peel-Off *($26 for 2.8 ounces)* is an ordinary peel-off mask that contains alcohol and little else. It would be drying for the skin, but it can exfoliate the skin.

Facial Skincare Facial Masque Rinse-Off *($26 for 4.2 ounces)* is a standard clay mask that contains no other irritants. It does contain mineral oil, which would make it less drying than other clay masks.

Vital Perfection Cleansing Cream *($22 for 3.9 ounces)* is a typical mineral oil- and petrolatum-based wipe-off cleanser that leaves a greasy residue on the skin.

Vital Perfection Cleansing Foam *($22 for 4.5 ounces)* is a water-soluble cleanser containing several standard detergent cleansers that can probably dry out the skin.

Vital Perfection Conditioning Cleansing Soap *($20 for 5.2 ounces)* is a standard bar soap with detergent cleansers. There is nothing conditioning about this soap; it can be very drying and possibly burn the eyes.

Vital Perfection Cleansing Gel *($23 for 4.2 ounces)* is supposed to be a water-soluble cleanser, but it leaves a greasy film on the face and doesn't take off makeup without the aid of a washcloth.

Vital Perfection T-Zone Balancing Toner *($25 for 2.5 ounces)* is an alcohol-based toner that also contains some clay, preservatives, and menthol. This toner won't balance anything, but it can dry out the skin and irritate it.

Vital Balancing Softener *($30 for 5 ounces)* is an OK irritant-free toner. It does contain magnesium and calcium chloride, which could be irritating to some skin types.

Vital Perfection Moisture Active Emulsion *($32 for 2.3 ounces)* contains mostly water, shark oil, petrolatum, thickener, standard water binding agents, thickeners, a small amount of sunscreen, and preservatives. This is a good emollient moisturizer for dry skin (not combination skin), but there isn't enough sunscreen to adequately protect from the sun.

Vital Perfection Active Lotion *($32 for 2.3 ounces)* contains mostly water, standard water binding agents, alcohol, thickeners, nut oil, shark oil, a small amount of sunscreen, and preservatives. This is a poor sunscreen and moisturizer. Why anyone would put alcohol in a moisture lotion is beyond me.

Vital Protection Daily Eye Primer *($30 for 0.5 ounce)* contains mostly water, standard water binding agents, mineral oil, thickeners, nut oil, more thickeners, and preservatives. This is a fairly ordinary mineral oil-based moisturizer that is overly expensive for what you get.

Vital Perfection Hydro-Intensive Mask *($28 for 1.4 ounces)* contains mostly water, standard water binding agents, alcohol, thickeners, nut oil, more thickeners, and preservatives. There is nothing intensive about this mask and the alcohol can be drying.

Vital Perfection Rinse-Off Clarifying Mask *($25 for 2.7 ounces)* is a standard clay mask that contains mostly water, clay, alcohol, talc, thickeners, standard water binding agents, and preservatives. The alcohol makes this basic clay mask more irritating than it needs to be. This won't clarify the skin, but it can cause irritation.

Bio Performance Super Revitalize Creme *($60 for 1.4 ounces)*. A four-page, full-color glossy brochure, including graphs and charts, explained why this product would do more for your skin "than ever dreamed possible." Despite this presentation, it is a good lightweight moisturizer that contains mostly water, standard water binding agents, thickeners, shark oil, petrolatum, thickeners, preservatives, fragrance, and more preservatives. It also contains several water binding agents, but these come well after the preservative and are therefore inconsequential.

Bio Performance Synchro Serum *($75 for 0.03 ounce of Powder and 0.5 ounce of Essence)*. Interpreting the brochure for this product requires a degree in chemistry. The before-and-after pictures, although convincing, are misleading, because the information is so limited and hokey. There are two vials in this package that you're supposed to combine. The Powder contains a thickener, protein, amino acids, water binding agents, and preservatives.

The Essence contains water, standard water binding agents, alcohol, slip agents, and preservatives. Mixed together, these two compounds do make an OK moisturizer, but nothing more, and the alcohol can be drying.

Revitalizing Cream *($125 for 1.4 ounces)* is hopelessly ordinary for this kind of absurd price. It contains mostly water, shark oil, petrolatum, glycerin, mineral oil, water binding agent, thickeners, amino acid, preservatives, fragrance, and preservative. It does contain placenta extract and vitamin E, but they come well after the preservatives and are meaningless in both amount and what they can do for the skin anyway.

B.H-24-Day/Night Essence *($65 for 1 ounce)* are two very small bottles of liquid that are supposed to be worn under your regular moisturizer. The Day Essence contains mostly water, standard water binding agents, alcohol, thickeners, collagen, PABA (a sunscreen that is considered a strong irritant and is rarely used anymore), amino acid, water binding agents, vitamin E, and preservatives. The Night Essence essentially has the same formulation minus the PABA. The alcohol is an irritant in both cases. Basically, this is an overpriced toner, and if the moisturizer you are using is good you shouldn't need a second undercoat. If you have dry skin you shouldn't be using a moisturizer with alcohol.

Sudden Youth

We've all seen before-and-after pictures that are remarkably impressive. As a professional makeup artist, I know how to make that kind of effect happen. The Sudden Youth infomercials take advantage of every known makeup and photographic trick in the book to make it look like their products can do what they simply can't do. Women "anonymously" pulled from the biased audience (remember, these are paid commercials; the audience is hand-picked and told what to say and how to act) rave about the results, but they're not telling you the whole story. If you look closely, the lighting, facial position, backdrop, and makeup in the "before" photograph are different from the "after" photograph. Sudden Youth would like you to believe that their products create the difference, but that is not the whole truth. When you look at the ingredient lists, you find that these products are not unusual in any way. Their ingredients are not unique or sufficiently different from any other face-lift-type product on the market to warrant the hoopla. The following review is of the five skin-care products *($85.85)* sold by Sudden Youth directly from their infomercial.

Pearlized Facial Wash *(8 ounces)* contains aloe, water, detergent, thickeners, safflower oil, more thickeners, more oils, and preservatives. Because of the oils it is not all that water-soluble and it can leave a greasy residue on the face, but it will take off makeup. The detergent used is a typical cleansing agent found in most water-soluble cleansers.

Facial Moisture Lotion *(8 ounces)* contains aloe, water, thickeners, several vegetable oils, more thickeners, water binding ingredients, preservatives, and, at the very end of the list, vitamins C and E. This would be a good moisturizer for someone with dry skin, but it's not exceptional or anything unusual.

Essential Beauty Complex *(1 ounce)* contains almond oil, sunflower oil, peach oil, walnut oil, safflower oil, and vitamins A, D, and E. You would do just as well buying a bottle of sunflower oil or using a vitamin E capsule from your local health food store.

Facial Recovery Activator *(4 ounces)* is supposed to be mixed with the Facial Recovery Contour Blend below to create a mask. The Activator contains aloe, water, stabilizer, and quarternium-15, considered to be one of the most potentially irritating preservatives used in cosmetics.

Facial Recovery Contour Blend *(2 ounces)* contains cornstarch, egg white, thickener, collagen, and some herbs. Cornstarch and egg white mixed with aloe and water will not change a wrinkle on your face. These ingredients are worthless for changing the skin in any positive way. You could make the same thing yourself by mixing a little egg white with cornstarch and applying it to the face. But why bother—it won't do anything for the skin other than stiffen it for an hour or two.

Ultima II

CHR Extraordinary Lotion Cleanser *($17 for 6 ounces)* is a cleanser that does not rinse off without the help of a washcloth and can leave a greasy film on the face.

CHR Extraordinary Cream Cleanser *($17 for 4 ounces)* is a standard mineral oil-based cleanser that has to be wiped off and can leave a greasy film on the skin.

CHR Extraordinary Gentle Toner for Very Dry Skin *($17 for 6 ounces)* is an alcohol-free toner that would be soothing and emollient for dry skin. It does contain menthol, which can be an irritant for sensitive skin types.

CHR Extraordinary Lotion *($65 for 2 ounces)* contains mostly water, thickeners, collagen, protein, water binding agents, almond oil, rice oil, mineral oil, thickeners, and preservatives. This is a good emollient moisturizer for dry skin, but very overpriced.

CHR Moisture Lotion Concentrate *($28 for 3 ounces)* contains mostly water, standard water binding agent, thickeners, collagen, protein, more thickeners, and preservatives. It would be good for dry skin, but don't expect the collagen and protein to change anything about your skin.

The Cleanser for Dry Skin *($12.50 for 5.8 ounces)* is a standard mineral oil-based cleanser that needs to be wiped off. It can leave a greasy film on the face.

The Cleanser for Normal/Combination Skin *($12.50 for 5.8 ounces)* is a standard detergent cleanser that also contains some glycerin. The glycerin can be soothing, but for most skin types it may not counteract the irritation caused by the detergent cleansing agent.

The Soap for Oily Skin *($9.50 for 5.25 ounces)* is a standard bar soap that also contains lemon and grapefruit extract, which along with the soap can irritate and burn the skin and eyes.

The Remover *($11 for 3.6 ounces)* is an OK eye makeup remover that can be slightly irritating to the eye area. It contains mineral oil, but still has a nongreasy feel.

The Toner for Oily Skin *($12.50 for 7.8 ounces)* contains alcohol and eucalyptus oil; both are very irritating for the skin and can make oily skin oilier.

The Toner for Dry Skin *($12.50 for 7.8 ounces)* contains witch hazel, eucalyptus oil, and sodium phosphate, which can all be very irritating and drying for most skin types, but particularly dry skin.

The Toner for Normal/Combination Skin *($12.50 for 7.8 ounces)* is similar to the dry skin toner with the addition of menthol, which is also a skin irritant. None of these toners are recommeneded.

The Moisturizer *($10 for 1.8 ounces)* contains mostly water, standard water binding agents, thickeners, petrolatum, several water binding agents, vitamin E, shark oil, and preservatives. This would be a good moisturizer for someone with dry skin.

The Moisturizer for Normal/Combination Skin *($10 for 1.8 ounces)* contains mostly water, thickeners, standard water binding agents, thickeners, sunscreen (SPF 8, not enough to adequately protect from the sun), water binding agents, eucalyptus oil, and preservatives. Someone with combination skin is going to find this too emollient, and the eucalyptus oil can irritate the skin.

The Oil-Free Moisturizer for Oily Skin *($10 for 1.8 ounces)* contains mostly water, standard water binding agent, talc, clay, thickeners, water binding agents, thickeners, a small amount of sunscreen, and preservatives. This is a confused moisturizer; all of these water binding agents are useless when you include water absorbing agents like talc and clay.

Under Makeup Moisture Cream *($22 for 2 ounces)* is a very emollient moisturizer for dry skin, but the second ingredient is isopropyl myristate, which can cause blackheads.

ProCollagen *($40 for 2 ounces)* contains a small amount of sunscreen and water, standard water binding agents, collagen, mineral oil, more collagen, water binding agents, thickeners, and preservatives. Collagen is a good water binding agent, but not much else; the fact that this product contains a lot of collagen doesn't make it better for the skin.

ProCollagen Face and Throat *($40 for 2 ounces)* is almost identical to the ProCollagen above, and the same critique applies.

ProCollagen For Eyes *($26 for 0.9 ounce)* is almost identical to the ProCollagen above, and the same critique applies.

Megadose *($40 for 1.65 ounces)* contains mostly water thickener, mineral oil, standard water binding agents, thickeners, safflower oil, more thickeners, water binding agents, and preservatives. This is a good moisturizer for dry skin, but nothing more. It is not any better than or really different from any of the other moisturizers in this line.

Energizer *($30 for 1.7 ounces)* is a good moisturizer, but it is supposed to balance and recharge the skin. It contains mostly water, standard water binding agents, thickeners, algae extract, more thickeners, water binding agents, more thickeners, almond oil, vitamin E, plant extracts, and preservatives. These are standard cosmetic ingredients, and this moisturizer can't do any more than any other moisturizer. It also contains a small amount of eucalyptus oil, which can irritate the skin.

Mineral Mask 3-Minute Purifying Clay Mask *($12.50 for 4 ounces)* is a standard clay mask that also contains peppermint oil, menthol, and eucalyptus oil, all of which can cause skin irritation.

5-Minute Rehydrating Moisture Mask *($12.50 for 4 ounces)* contains mostly water, thickeners, standard water binding agents, more thickeners, water binding agents, and preservatives. This is an OK mask, but it won't replenish your skin any better than your moisturizer will.

30-Second Refining Scrub Mask *($12.50 for 4 ounces)* is a good lightweight scrub that contains a small amount of eucalyptus oil, which can irritate the skin.

Vaseline Intensive Care

UV Daily Defense Lotion for Body and Hands *($2.67 for 6 ounces)* has an SPF of 4, which isn't enough to defend the skin against the sun.

Dry Skin Formula *($2.67 for 6 ounces)* contains mostly water, glycerin, thickeners, mineral oil, more thickeners, lanolin, and preservatives. This is a good moisturizer for dry skin if there are not allergies to lanolin.

Extra Strength *($2.67 for 6 ounces)* is almost identical to the Dry Skin Formula and the same critique applies.

Aloe & Lanolin *($2.67 for 6 ounces)* is almost identical to the Dry Skin Formula except for the addition of aloe. If you want a good emollient for dry skin, this is just fine.

Overnight Moisture Treatment Cream *($2.67 for 6 ounces)* contains mostly water, standard water binding agents, petrolatum, and preservatives. This is an OK moisturizer.

Sensitive Skin with Vitamin E *($2.67 for 6 ounces)* contains mostly water, glycerin, thickeners, mineral oil, petrolaum, more thickeners, lanolin, and preservatives. This product contains menthol and dmdm hydantoin (a preservative), both of which can be skin irritants. I would not recommend this product for someone with sensitive skin.

Victoria Jackson

The handful of skin care products in the Victoria Jackson line are supposed to be suitable for all skin types. It's an interesting and unusual concept for a cosmetics company, and one that I find hard to accept. Skin care for someone with oily skin cannot be the same as for someone with extremely dry or even normal skin. Still, I liked some of these products very much, and the price range (if you buy more than $20 worth of products at a time) is quite reasonable.

Note: The first price listed is for the individual product; the second price applies when you order more than $20 worth of products at one time.

Facial Cleanser *($12.50/$7.25 for 4 ounces)*. You are meant to wipe off your makeup using this watery cleanser applied to a cotton ball, and then rinse off any residue. The main ingredients are water, a form of coconut oil (considered to be a good, nongreasy cleansing agent), collagen, hyaluronic acid, and sodium PCA; the water binding agents are unnecessary in a cleanser because they are rinsed off. It actually feels quite light on the skin, and the ingredients are very moisturizing, but I'm still not a proponent of wiping off makeup.

Toning Mist *($13.50/$7.75 for 4 ounces)* would be a great toner for all skin types, but like many of these products it contains quaternium-15, a preservative that can be a strong skin irritant.

Moisturizer *($19.50/$11.75 for 2 ounces)* contains mostly water, standard water binding agents, thickeners, water binding agents, collagen, vitamins E and A, and preservatives. This would be a very good moisturizer for dry skin except it contains quaternium-15, a preservative that can be a strong skin irritant.

Skin Renewal System *($24.95 for 1.4 ounces of Eye Cream and 1.25 ounces of Night Cream)* is a rather uniquely packaged moisturizer. The Night Cream is in the bottom half of the jar and the Eye Cream is in the top half. Very cute. However, the ingredients are not all that different, so the division seems unnecessary. This is a good moisturizer, but the regular moisturizer has a more impressive ingredient list.

Eye Repair Gel *($18.50/$10.50 for 0.5 ounce)* contains mostly water, several water binding agents, and preservatives. This would be a good lightweight moisturizer for around the eyes except that one of the preservatives is quaternium-15, which can be a strong skin irritant.

Firming Gel Masque *($16.50/$9.95 for 4 ounces)* won't firm anything, and the second ingredient is a strong skin irritant. If your skin looks tighter after you take this mask off it's due to the irritation. It also contains quaternium-15, a preservative that can be a strong skin irritant.

Yves St. Laurent

Foaming Cleansing Gel *($24 for 6.6 ounces)* is a fairly good water-soluble cleanser that rinses well and takes off all the makeup without irritating the skin. Unfortunately, it has a tendency to burn the eyes, which makes it an unreliable product to recommend.

Instant Cleansing Milk *($24 for 6.6 ounces)* doesn't really remove makeup all that well and is not very water-soluble without the aid of a washcloth.

Soothing Creme Cleanser *($24 for 6.6 ounces)* is a standard mineral oil-based cleanser. It can leave a greasy film on the skin and requires a washcloth to really get off all the makeup, which is not very soothing.

Extra-Gentle Tonic Alcohol-Free *($24 for 6.6 ounces)* contains standard water binding agents, some plant extracts, and preservatives. It is over-priced, and I am skeptical about it being extra gentle when the fragrance is so high up in the ingredient list.

Mild Clarifying Tonic *($24 for 6.6 ounces)* is an OK toner that contains sodium phosphate, which can be a possible skin irritant. This isn't all that mild, but it could be an option for someone with normal to oily skin.

Oil-Control Tonic *($24 for 6.6 ounces)* is a standard alcohol-based toner that won't control oil, but will irritate the skin.

Hydro-Intensive Day Creme *($50 for 1.6 ounces)* contains mostly water, thickeners, standard water binding agents, water binding agent, petrolatum, vitamin E, more thickeners, mineral oil, and preservatives. This is a fairly ordinary moisturizer for dry skin, with a small amount of sunscreen. Many of the good moisturizing ingredients come way after the preservatives and don't amount to much.

Hydro-Light Day Creme *($50 for 1.6 ounces)* is almost identical to the Hydro-Intensive Day Creme except it excludes petrolatum and sunscreen. It is lighter than the one above and is just as ordinary.

Intensive Nighttime Revitalizer *($55 for 1 ounce)* contains mostly water, standard water binding agents, collagen, almond oil, mineral oil, plant oil, a small amount of sunscreen (which is strange to find in a night cream), fragrance, and preservatives. Vitamins A and E are in here, but too far down in the list to count. This is a good emollient moisturizer for dry skin, but nothing special or unique.

Nighttime Revitalizer *($55 for 1 ounce)* is almost identical to the Intensive Nighttime Revitalizer, with just a few minor changes, and the same critique applies.

Soothing Eye Contour Gel *($45 for 0.5 ounce)* contains mostly water, standard water binding agent, plant extract, soothing agent, protein, thickeners, aloe vera, and preservatives. There are some other interesting water binding ingredients in here, but they come well after the preservatives, which makes them useless. Other than that, this is a good lightweight moisturizer for the eye area, but nothing unique or special.

Time Interceptor Fortifying Complex *($66 for 1 ounce)* won't intercept anything. It contains water, standard slip agents, mineral oil, soothing agent, preservatives (very high up in the ingredient list), amino acid, more preservatives, and fragrance. There are some other interesting water binding ingredients in here, but they come well after the preservatives, which makes them worthless.

Hydro-Active Moisture Masque *($35 for 1.6 ounces)* contains mostly water, mineral oil, thickeners, plant oil, thickeners, vitamin E, preservatives, more thickeners, and preservatives. This is a good, somewhat ordinary moisturizer/mask for dry skin, but it won't alter the skin or change it in any way.

Instant Clarifying Masque *($35 for 2.5 ounces)* contains mostly water, glycerin, thickeners, soothing agent, preservatives, fragrance, plant extracts, and more preservatives. There is nothing clarifying about this mask. The ingredients are rather ordinary and the exotic plants come well after the preservatives, making the amount totally insignificant.

The Products You and I Liked the Most

COSMETICS COUNTER UPDATE OPINION POLL

This past summer I inserted a questionnaire regarding women's experiences with cosmetics in about 1,500 copies of my newsletter. The *Cosmetics Counter Update* 1993 Opinion Poll included a list of questions regarding which cosmetic products were liked the best and which were liked the least. More than 600 women took the time to express their feelings, opinions, and thoughts on the subject of makeup and skin care. I want to express my deepest appreciation to all of you who responded. Taking the time to add your voice to the cause of putting some objectivity into shopping for cosmetics was extremely helpful. Your comments were enlightening and immensely constructive. We didn't always agree, but that wasn't the purpose of the survey. It was to get feedback from a diverse group of women who were interested in delving beneath the hype and into the reality of what does and doesn't work in the world of cosmetics.

I know it might seem strange to some of you that I have added the results of a survey that at times pointedly disagreed with my research and evaluations. There were those who said they liked Clinique's astringents, yet I think they are the most drying and irritating on the market. Some respondents said they thought Revlon was a bad line of products because they had had an allergic reaction to one of their foundations ten years ago. Of course, an allergic reaction to one product doesn't speak to the quality of a line or even the quality of that product. If you were allergic to roses, would you condemn the value of roses for others?

Many women base their decisions on different criteria than I do. A lot of women liked eyeshadows and blushes from various lines that I would consider too shiny to wear, or eye pencils that were too greasy, or toners and cleansers that were too drying. When a woman complained that her mascara smeared there was no way for me to tell what was causing the problem. If someone wears heavy eye creams or uses a greasy foundation, almost every mascara she chooses will smear. When a cleanser received a poor rating, I couldn't tell if that was due to the product itself or if it failed to live up to what the women expected from the product. Sometimes one woman's clean feeling is another woman's dried out and irritated.

I am pleased to say that the preponderance of the feedback from the surveys agreed with what I found to be true about most cosmetics. Still, I felt it was important to share a wide range of opinions from women who use cosmetics. Use the information as a guide to compare to my evaluations and what you discover when you test a product.

Beauty Note: Keep in mind that the women who participated in this survey have read much of what I have written about cosmetics, so they are not exactly a random group. These women are influenced by my information and not just the cosmetics industry. Statistically speaking, the population who responded to the survey is definitely skewed. A woman who was only influenced by the cosmetics industry's information (advertising, product labels, brochures, fashion magazines, and salespeople) might have responded differently. Of course, I believe the skew is more helpful to getting reasonable data. The women who answered my survey have some amount of investment in becoming more rational and sensible consumers when it comes to cosmetics because they have spent money on my books and/or newsletter. You need to know the bias of the respondents, however, I believe that in many ways the information is more reliable.

ABOUT THE RESULTS

I categorized the answers by products you liked and products you disliked. Only products that received more than two positive or negative comments were included. That way I could be sure the comment was not circumstantial but more broad-based. I used only those comments that most reflected the general feeling about a specific product. I did not include complaints about allergic reactions unless I received four or more complaints.

One theme that ran throughout over 80 percent of the questionnaires was the decision to shop different makeup lines rather than using one makeup line for all needs. I was thrilled to discover that women (at least the women who read my books and newsletter) are not as susceptible to line loyalty as they once were. Buying expensive foundation and eyeshadows isn't so bad when the lipstick, eye pencil, blush, mascara, and moisturizer are inexpensive.

Please note that the one weakness of this compilation is that there were a good number of respondents who said, for example, that they liked or disliked Revlon mascara or Estee Lauder foundation. Without a specific name, it was impossible to know which particular product they meant. The intent of organizing this list is to home in on the individual deficiency in each line.

THE PRODUCTS YOU LIKED THE MOST

After reading each survey, I compiled the overall positive responses for each product category. The numbers in parentheses reflect the total number of responses for that product.

Cleansers

BeautiControl Cleansing Wash Lotion (3)
Cetaphil (obviously; took high marks because most of the respondents have previously read my books; good in winter; doesn't irritate eyes; I wish it wasn't tested on animals!) (108)
Chanel Cleansing Milk (2)
Clarins Facial Foaming Cleanser (2)
Clarins Oil Control Cleansing Gel (2)
Clinique Mild Cleansing Bar (4)
Dove Liquid Beauty Wash (3)
Dove Unscented Bar (5)
Estee Lauder Face Wash (2)
Lancome Bi-Ficils Eye Makeup Remover (fabulous) (5)
Moisturel Sensitive Skin Cleanser (7)
Neutrogena Liquid Cleansing Formula (8)
Pond's Foaming Cleanser & Toner In One (6)
Purpose Soap (6)

Exfoliants

Baking soda (9)
Clinique Gentle Exfoliant (2)
L'Oreal Plenitude Gentle Exfoliating Scrub (2)

Toners

Clarion Toner (2)
Clinique Alcohol-Free Toner (2)
Clinique Clarifying Lotions (5)
Estee Lauder Skin Perfecting Lotion (2)
Hydrogen peroxide 3% (gets rid of blackheads; one woman mixes it with water) (24)
Lancome Alcohol-Free Toner (2)
Lancome Clarifiance Alcohol-Free Natural Astringent (9)
L'Oreal Plenitude Floral Toner for Normal to Dry Skin (14)
Mary Kay Toner (4)
Neutrogena Alcohol-Free Toner (2)
Physicians Formula Gentle Refreshing Toner (5)

Moisturizers

Candermyl Cream (6)
Chanel Lotion #1 (even though ridiculously overpriced) (2)
Clarins Oil-Control Moisturizing Lotion (2)
Clinique Turn Around Cream (3)
Complex 15 Moisturizer (3)
Elizabeth Arden Ceramide Time Complex Moisture Cream (2)
Estee Lauder Equalizer Oil-Free Hydrogel (3)
Estee Lauder Eye Cream (2)
Eucerin Lotion (2)
Lancome Niosome (2)
Lancome Renergie Anti-Wrinkle Cream (expensive, but a little goes a long way) (2)
Lancome Trans Hydrix Moisturizer (2)
L'Oreal Plenitude Moisturizer with Liposomes (5)
L'Oreal Plenitude Oil Free Daily Moisture Lotion SPF 12 (3)
Lubriderm Lotion (14)
Mary Kay Balancing Moisturizer (3)
Mary Kay Nighttime Recovery System (2)
Moisturel Skin Protectant (6)
Neutrogena Eye Cream (4)

Neutrogena Moisturizer (4)

Nivea Visage Moisture Lotion (4)

Nivea Visage Moisturizing Lotion with Vitamin E (penetrates skin well; an incredible moisturizer for dry skin) (7)

Nutraderm (12)

Oil of Olay Daily UV Protectant Beauty Fluid (SPF 15) (3)

Oil of Olay Sensitive Skin Beauty Fluid (4)

Prescriptives All You Need Moisturizer (5)

Purpose Moisturizer (4)

Yves St. Laurent Eye Gel (7)

Sunscreen/Moisturizers

Avon Sunseekers SPF 30 (2)

Bain de Soleil All-Day Waterproof Sport Lotion SPF 15 (2)

Banana Boat Faces Sunscreen (unscented) (3)

Clinique City Block SPF 13 (the best for my sensitive face) (12)

Clinique 15 SPF Face-Zone Sun Block (2)

Coppertone Sport Sweatproof/Waterproof Dry Lotion Sunblock (2)

Lubriderm Lotion UV SPF 15 (13)

Neutrogena Chemical Free Sunblock SPF 17 (5)

Neutrogena Moisturizer SPF 15 (13)

Oil of Olay Daily UV Protectant Beauty Fluid SPF 15 (9)

Physicians Formula Vital Defense Moisture Lotion SPF 15 (7)

AHA Products

Alpha Hydrox Lotion (just as good as Fruition; works miracles; love it!) (36)

Aqua Glycolic Lotion—Herald Pharmacal (3)

Avon Anew (want the benefits but would like a lighter product; best AHA product I have found) (4)

Estee Lauder Fruition (3)

M.D. Formulations Smoothing Complex (5)

NeoStrata AHA Gel for Age Spots (3)

NeoStrata AHA Smoothing Lotion (19)

Acne Products

There was no consensus on acne products.

Facial Masks

There was no consensus on facial masks.

Foundations

Almay Liquid to Powder Makeup (similar to Borghese's) (3)

Borghese Liquid to Powder Makeup (perfection) (6)

Clinique Balanced Makeup (goes on easily and stays put) (13)

Clinique Continuous Coverage (2)

Clinique Sensitive Skin Makeup SPF 15 (4)

Clinique Stay True Oil-Free Foundation (great for oily skin) (12)

Estee Lauder Demi Matte Foundation (easily applied; nonirritating) (3)

Estee Lauder Lucidity Light Diffusing Makeup (3)

Lancome Dual Finish Makeup (lasts all day) (2)

Lancome Maquicontrole Foundation (good coverage; keeps my face from looking like an oil slick) (14)

L'Oreal Hydra Perfect Foundation SPF 10 (very natural looking) (5)

L'Oreal Lightnesse Makeup (2)

L'Oreal Mattique (natural look and didn't give a caked look; good shades; good price) (2)

L'Oreal Visuelle Foundation (light, smooth coverage) (3)

M.A.C. (3)

Mary Kay Oil-Free Foundation (3)

Max Factor New Definition Makeup Base (good for the price) (2)

Prescriptives Oil-Free Foundation SPF 15 (sunscreen is great; great texture; beautiful finish) (6)

Revlon Double Play Foundation (6)

Revlon New Complexion (2)

Revlon Springwater Foundation (good shades; good price) (7)

Ultima II Beautiful Nutrient Makeup (2)

Ultima II Oil Control Formula Foundation (2)

Concealers

There was no consensus on concealers.

Powders

Clinique Pressed Powder (3)

Clinique Superpowder Double Face Powder (3)

Coty Airspun Face Powder (2)

Coty Loose Face Powder (2)

Estee Lauder Demi Matte Loose Powder (2)

Lancome Pressed Powder (5)

Merle Norman Pressed Powder (2)

Revlon Springwater Pressed Powder (2)

Eyeshadows

Clinique Eyeshadows (2)
Estee Lauder Eyeshadows (smooth; silky; good colors) (2)
Lancome Eyeshadows (last all day) (4)
M.A.C. Eyeshadows (excellent price) (13)
Mary Kay Matte Eyeshadows (4)
Max Factor Matte Eyeshadows (lasts hours without creasing) (4)
Maybelline Matte Eyeshadows (5)
Merle Norman Matte Eyeshadows (4)
Physicians Formula Matte Eyeshadows (4)
Prescriptives Eyeshadows (6)
Revlon Matte Eyeshadows (good texture; easy to apply; neutral colors) (15)
Ultima II Eyeshadows (amazing! super soft!) (10)

Blushes

Almay Cheek Color Blushes (soft and beautiful; looks natural) (3)
Borghese (easy to apply; blends well) (2)
Borghese Liquid to Powder Blush (nothing quite like it) (1)
Chanel Blushes (only the nonshiny ones) (3)
Christian Dior (didn't smear; natural; no sparkles; velvety) (3)
Clinique Beyond Blusher (7)
Clinique Oil-Free Blush (3)
Clinique Powder Blush (good color choice and it stays on) (2)
Clinique Soft Powder Blush (hard to overdo) (5)
Color Me Beautiful Blushes (2)
Cover Girl Blush-Natural Glow (natural color) (4)
Estee Lauder Signature Blush (3)
Lancome Blush (they're all great) (12)
Maybelline Brush Blush (very blendable) (2)
Merle Norman Blusher (3)
Origins Blushes (2)
Prescriptives Blushes (5)
Revlon Naturally Glamorous Blush (4)
Revlon Powder Creme Blush (5)
Revlon Springwater Blush (2)
Shiseido Blush (soft; natural-looking) (2)
Ultima II Nakeds Blush (3)
Victoria Jackson Blushers (inexpensive; soft colors) (2)

Lipsticks

Almay Color Protective Lipstick (good staying power without much bleeding; stays on all day) (4)

Aveda Lipstick (not a creamy application but doesn't change color; wears well; smells good; doesn't dry out lips) (3)

Avon Lipsticks (3)

BeautiControl Lipsticks (2)

Borghese Spa Lipstick (long-lasting) (2)

Chanel Lipsticks (2)

Clarion Lipsticks (inexpensive and they last) (3)

Clinique Lipsticks (superb texture and colors; smooth; stays on) (8)

Clinique Semi-Lipstick (4)

Clinique Super Lipstick (2)

Color Me Beautiful Lipsticks (3)

Coty Lipstick (really lasts; stays on) (4)

Coty Stop It (it really works) (3)

Elizabeth Arden Lip Spa (colors last; feels good; colors don't change on me) (3)

Estee Lauder All-Day Lipstick (stays on a long time) (8)

Estee Lauder Perfect Lipstick (5)

Lancome Lipsticks (creamy; beautiful colors; little fragrance) (4)

L'Oreal Lipsticks (3)

M.A.C. (creamy; very long-lasting; great colors; stays on forever) (12)

Mary Kay Lipstick (goes on smoothly) (3)

Max Factor Lasting Color Lipstick (amazing staying ability) (2)

Maybelline Lipsticks (not too dry) (2)

Prescriptives Classic Lipsticks (moist, without greasy feeling) (2)

Revlon Lipsticks (all of them are great) (17)

Eyebrow Products

There was no consensus on brow products.

Eyeliners

Cover Girl Pro-Line Eyeliner (5)

Estee Lauder Eye Pencil (doesn't pull) (4)

Lancome Le Kohl Crayon Eye Pencil (3)

Mary Kay Liners (2)

Max Factor Featherblend Kohl Liner (2)

Maybelline Expert Eyes (4)

Revlon Soft Stroke Powderliner (goes on soft; blends easily) (3)

Victoria Jackson Eyeliner (2)

Lip Liners

There was no consensus on lip liners

Mascaras

Almay One Coat Mascara (gives me eyelashes; no clumping; makes lashes look long and full) (8)

Cover Girl Extremely Gentle Mascara (the only mascara that doesn't irritate my eyes) (2)

Cover Girl Marathon Mascara (2)

Estee Lauder More Than Mascara (goes on thick and doesn't clump; expensive but very easy product to apply) (5)

Lancome Defincils (builds thick and long lashes; lengthens well; doesn't flake or smudge; nice consistency) (13)

L'Oreal Accentuous Mascara (7)

L'Oreal Formula Riche (as good as Chanel's for a third of the price; doesn't smudge or clump) (7)

L'Oreal Lash Out (best coverage; no flaking or smudging; the best no money can buy) (12)

L'Oreal Voluminous (the thickest lashes ever; never smudges and always looks full) (14)

M.A.C. Mascara (thickens lashes) (1)

Max Factor 2000 (13)

Maybelline Great Lash Mascara (comes off easily; lengthens) (5)

Maybelline Illegal Lengths (5)

Maybelline No Problem Mascara (goes on evenly; doesn't clump or flake; lengthens and thickens lashes; washes off easily) (4)

Revlon Lashfull (finally a mascara that doesn't clump!) (11)

Victoria Jackson Mascara (doesn't clump or smudge) (2)

THE PRODUCTS YOU LIKED THE LEAST

Cleansers

Almay Moisture Balance Cleansing Lotion (too greasy) (2)

Basis Soap (advertised for sensitive skin and was still irritating) (3)

Borghese Eye Makeup Remover (stings) (2)

Clinique Soap (too drying; too harsh) (3)

Johnson & Johnson's Clean & Clear (loved it before J&J changed it) (3)

Lancome's Gelatee (greasy; doesn't rinse off; doesn't remove makeup) (2)

L'Oreal Eye Makeup Remover (doesn't clean and leaves residue behind; stings) (2)

Neutrogena Facial Soap Original Formula (drying) (2)
Neutrogena Liquid Facial Cleansing Formula (too drying; burned eyes; smelled like shampoo) (7)
Noxzema (too drying) (9)
Oil of Olay Face Wash (didn't rinse well) (2)

Exfoliants

There was no consensus on exfoliants.

Toners

Clinique Clarifying Lotions (way too strong) (11)
Lancome Ablutia and Toner (too costly for no apparent benefits) (3)

Moisturizers

Avon Anew Moisturizer (disagree with Paula: very heavy and greasy) (2)
Avon Daily Revival Oil-Free Moisture Lotion (2)
Elizabeth Arden Ceramide Time Capsules for Eyes (felt like cooking oil; does not perform) (4)
Elizabeth Arden Visible Difference Eye Cream (there was no difference) (2)
Estee Lauder Advanced Night Repair (can't see benefits) (4)
Oil of Olay Moisturizer (too greasy; too much fragrance; too highly scented) (6)

Sunscreen/Moisturizers

There was no consensus on sun products, but there was a recurring request for sun products without oil, coloring, and fragrance.

AHA Products

Estee Lauder Fruition (it is the "emperor's new clothes" syndrome: people pretend it's great and it does nothing) (2)
Murad AHA products (double the price of NeoStrata or Alpha Hydrox but does the same) (2)
NeoStrata Enhanced Gel Formula (very drying and caused breakouts) (2)

Facial Masks

There was no consensus on facial masks.

Acne Products

Acne Statin (what a joke!; did not clean) (2)
All over-the-counter acne products (extremely irritating; criminal) (11)

Foundations

Almay Foundations (wears off; unnatural colors; doesn't absorb) (3)
Clinique Pore Minimizer (too cakey; too drying) (6)
Estee Lauder Fresh Air (remains sticky; poor color choice) (2)
Estee Lauder Lucidity Foundation (awful; too thick and cakey; bad col-

ors; didn't do what the product promised) (5)

Lancome Maquicontrole Foundation (made my face look and feel oily; too heavy; too dry; too pasty) (Editor's note: This could be the old formula; the new one is lighter weight) (7)

L'Oreal Mattique Foundation (streaks) (2)

Merle Norman Foundation (too heavy; too pink) (2)

Merle Norman Total Finish Compact Makeup (too thick; stinky)

Origins Foundation (poor coverage) (1)

Physicians Formula Sunshield Liquid Makeup (started turning orange a few weeks after opening it) (1)

Prescriptives Oil-Free Foundation (3)

Revlon Springwater Oil-Free Foundation (did not stay on well) (2)

Victoria Jackson Foundations (too greasy; too orange; they should include a putty knife instead of a sponge; too thick) (4)

Concealers

Almay Cover Stick (covers absolutely nil) (2)

Clarion Protection 15 Concealer (orange) (2)

Clinique's Advance Concealer (too dry) (2)

Cover Girl Moisture Wear Concealer (does not blend) (2)

Powders

There was no consensus on powders.

Eyeshadows

There was no consensus on eyeshadows, but there was a recurring complaint about any eyeshadows that were shiny.

Blushes

There was no consensus on blushes.

Lipsticks

Avon (too much fragrance; tended to cake) (3)

Clinique Lipsticks (poor color choice; too greasy and sheer) (4)

Coty Lipsticks (all caked; some dry; some greasy; all are gone after ten minutes) (2)

M.A.C. Lipsticks (matte lipsticks are too drying) (2)

Mary Kay Lipsticks (2)

Eyebrow Products

There was no consensus on eyebrow products.

Eyeliners

Clinique Eye Pencil (broke off too easily; didn't go on smoothly; pulled skin) (2)

Estee Lauder Eye Pencil (broke constantly; goes on greasy; hard to wash off) (3)

Lancome Le Kohl Crayon (very dry; impossible to sharpen) (2)

Mary Kay Eye Liner Pencils (smudge and bleed easily) (4)

Lip Liners

There was no consensus on lip liners.

Mascaras

Clinique Glossy Mascara (makes lashes thin and spiky; smudges easily) (2)

Lancome Defincils Mascara (made lashes stick together; smudged easily) (2)

L'Oreal Lash Out (flaked and clumped; smudged badly; hated the wand) (2)

M.A.C. Mascara (it clumped!) (2)

Mary Kay Mascara (clumped and smudged) (2)

Max Factor 2000 Calorie Mascara (runs; hard to get off; clumps) (2)

Maybelline Great Lash (ended up with raccoon eyes!; overrated—smudges) (17)

THE PRODUCTS I LIKED THE MOST

The recommendations below reflect summaries of the individual reviews in Chapters Seven and Eight. Be sure to read the more detailed product evaluations in each chapter before making any decisions. There are a handful of products listed below from companies I did not review in the previous chapters. I've included these products because they worked so well. I hope all of these recommendations will make shopping for makeup a more stress-free experience.

Beauty Note: Most cosmetics companies have skin care routines for specific skin types. It is my heartfelt and strong suggestion that you ignore these categories. Most of the time they will get your skin in trouble. If you have dry skin you may be using too many products that will overgrease the skin and cause a build-up, making the skin look dull. If you have oily skin you will most likely be sold products that contain strong irritants that can make oily and acned skin worse. Please consider each product individually for its quality and value to your skin, instead of its placement in a series of products.

Foundation

Perhaps there is no area of makeup more treacherous and just plain hard to get exactly right than finding the perfect foundation. The problems are many, but the most difficult to overcome are expectations, color choice, and texture. Women want a foundation that fits like a second secret skin; it should look invisible, but still provide coverage, camouflage, and look radiant. That is no short order—it is like eating a piece of cake and hoping it won't go to your hips. Foundations have their limitations, and that is hard for some women to accept. Take the endless search for an oil-free foundation that will last through the evening. If you have oily skin, that just isn't possible without serious touch-ups several times during the day. Some expectations are more than possible, but some are not.

Choosing the right foundation color is not only time-consuming, it is exceedingly frustrating. How many foundations can you test on one face before it becomes raw from wiping off the one you don't like and then trying another, and another, and another? Yet that is what it takes to narrow the choices down to the right color. The last hurdle is finding a pleasing texture that feels soft and silky but doesn't streak, cake, or look thick. Now tell me that isn't a challenge.

Be patient about finding the right foundation and remember that if there is one area to splurge on it is foundation. Taking the time to check the color and texture in daylight is essential. There is no way around this if you want to get the best foundation possible for your skin's needs.

At the drugstore, only L'Oreal consistently had testers for every foundation shade, but be careful, some of their colors are too peach or too rose to recommend. Revlon's Color Style and Maybelline's Shades of You both have wonderful testers for their entire color line, but in particular they have testers for all their foundations. I was surprised that I did not find many great foundations from in-home sales. Mary Kay received higher marks last time out, but this time the colors seemed much less reliable; either their formulas have changed or my testing methods have.

Max Factor's Satin Splendor (cream-to-powder) foundation is still great and the colors are very reliable. The same is true for Revlon's Powder Cream Makeup Base and their Springwater Oil-Free Makeup, but again you have to guess which color is best for you and that can be a problem. I also really liked Cover Girl's Liquid Powder Foundation, but more than half a dozen respondents to my cosmetic poll said they hated it. I still like it, but I'm hard put to ignore that number of comments; the choice is up to you. Perhaps those women had normal to oily skin, and this foundation is geared toward someone with dry skin.

For general excellence, high marks go to: Avon, Charles of the Ritz, Borghese, Clinique, Color Me Beautiful, Fashion Fair, Estee Lauder, Lancome (particularly since they have reformulated), L'Oreal, Maybelline's Shades of You, M.A.C., Monteil of Paris, New Essentials, Prescriptives (not including their Oil-Free Foundation, which is half glycerin and half talc), Revlon Color Style, Shiseido, Ultima II's New Nakeds, and Yves St. Laurent.

Overall best buys are: Avon, Charles of the Ritz (which has great foundations, but some of the colors are not the best), Clinique, Fashion Fair, L'Oreal, M.A.C., Maybelline, Revlon, and Ultima II's New Nakeds.

For oily skin, my favorite foundations are: Avon Oil-Free Liquid; Charles of the Ritz Perfect Finish Makeup SPF 6 for Oily Skin; Clinique Stay True Makeup and Sensitive Skin Makeup SPF 15; Elizabeth Arden Simply Mousse Makeup (can be tricky to use) and Flawless Finish Liquid Makeup Matte Finish; Erno Laszlo Oil-Free Normalizing Base; Estee Lauder Demi Matte; Fashion Fair Oil-Free Liquid Foundation and Oil-Free Souffle Foundation; Lancome Maquicontrole SPF 4; L'Oreal Mattique Illuminating Matte Makeup; M.A.C. Matte; Mary Kay Oil-Free Foundation; Maybelline Shades of You Oil-Free Liquid and Shades of You 100% Oil-Free Souffle; New Essentials Skin Balancing Foundation 100% Oil-Free; Prescriptives 100% Oil-Free Liquid Makeup SPF 15; Revlon Springwater Oil-Free Foundation and Color Style Natural Color Oil-Free Makeup; and Ultima II The Foundation Oil-Control Formula.

The best buys in oil-free foundations are: Clinique, Fashion Fair, Lancome, L'Oreal, Revlon (although there are no testers available), and Ultima II.

For normal to slightly oily or combination skin, the best choices are: Borghese Hydro Minerali Natural Finish Makeup with SPF 4; Charles of the Ritz Superior Foundation for Normal to Oily; Clinique Balanced Makeup; Guerlain Elysemat Liquid Foundation; Lancome Maqui Mat; and Prescriptives Soft Matte Foundation.

For normal to dry skin, the best choices are: Avon Enhancing Liquid for Normal to Dry Skin; Borghese Milano 2000; Chanel Teint Naturel; Christian Dior Teint Dior; Clinique Balanced Makeup; Color Me Beautiful Liquid Foundation; Erno Laszlo Phelitone Fluid for Normal to Dry; Estee Lauder Polished Performance, Sportswear Tint SPF 12, and Lucidity Light Diffusing Makeup; Flori Roberts Hydrophillic

Foundation for Normal to Dry Skin; Guerlain Opalissime Complexion Base; Lancome Maqui Eclat and Imanance Tinted Creme SPF 8; L'Oreal Hydrating Makeup SPF 10, Lightnesse Light Natural Makeup, and Visuelle Invisible Coverage Makeup; M.A.C. Satin; Mary Kay Formula-2 Day Radiance Liquid; Monteil Habitat Natural Foundation Chemical-Free SPF 4; New Essentials Skin Balancing Foundation Moisturizing SPF 8; Prescriptives Makeup 1; Shiseido Fluid Foundation; Ultima II The Foundation Moisturizing Formula; and Yves St. Laurent Line Smoothing Foundation.

For dry to seriously dry skin, the best choices are: Avon Perfecting Creme for Dry Skin; Borghese Effetto Immediato Spa Firming Makeup SPF 8 and Effetto Bellezza Targeted Treatment Makeup SPF 8; Chanel Teint Creme; Christian Dior D'Ete; Clinique Extra Help; Estee Lauder Country Mist; Flori Roberts Touche Satin Finish for Dry Skin; Lancaster Rich Foundation; Lancome Maquivelour; Mary Kay Formula 2; Prescriptives Makeup 2; Shiseido Stick Foundation; and Ultima II CHR Foundation.

There are a wide variety of liquid and compact foundations available for dry skin that are not the best. My only warning is to avoid foundations that are too heavy and greasy. Having dry skin does not mean your skin needs to be greased up. Be careful!

Alternatives to liquid foundations: Someone with normal to slightly dry or slightly oily skin (better known as combination skin, depending on how serious the dry or oily areas are) may love trying one of the cream-to-powder foundations. The best ones are Adrien Arpel Creme Powder Foundation; Borghese Lumina Compact Foundation; Chanel Teint Facettes; Lancome Creme Compact Makeup; Max Factor Satin Splendor; Revlon Powder Cream Foundation and Double Play Cream to Powder; Shiseido Creme Powder Compact; and Ultima II Brush-On Foundation.

The best buys without sacrificing quality are: Max Factor, Maybelline, Revlon, and Ultima II.

Concealer

Trying to find a good under-eye concealer is still not an easy task. A lot of concealers are too dry or greasy, or they crease into the lines under the eye. Many concealers are also either too thick, too peach, too pink, too dark, or too expensive. I found some good under-eye concealers in all price categories, but I have to say that this time my favorite concealers were at the department store. Several concealers had great colors to choose from, but the tendency for slight creasing could not be ignored, particularly for those of us with an increasing number of lines under the eye area.

The best concealers are: Monteil Hide Anything Concealer and Charles of the Ritz Hide and Chic Concealer.

Other good concealers worth checking out are: Almay Coverup Stick and Undereye Cover Cream; Borghese Absolute Concealer; Clinique Quick Corrector and Advanced Concealer (for oily skin only); Cover Girl Moisturizing Concealer; Fashion Fair Fragrance-Free Cover Stick; Lancaster Concealing Creme; L'Oreal Mattique Conceal Oil-Control Coverup; M.A.C. TV Touch; Maybelline Undetectable Creme Concealer; Monteil Hides Anything Moisturizing Concealer; Origins Concealer; Prescriptives Camouflage Cream; Revlon Color Style Natural Blend Concealer; Ultima II The Concealer; and Yves St. Laurent Radiant Touch.

Powder

If there is one major aspect of makeup that stayed the same from the last edition of *Don't Go To The Cosmetics Counter Without Me* to this one, it is powders. It still doesn't make sense to spend too much money on a finishing powder because there is so little difference between products. More than 95 percent of them are talc-based; the rest of the ingredients vary only slightly, although the advertising makes claims about light-reflecting properties and micro-encapsulated color, all of which is nonsense. When I think of the number of pressed powders priced between $16 and $30, I just shake my head at the audacity of the cosmetics companies. Unfortunately, after having recommended that you go inexpensive for this product group, it is hard to recommend with any enthusiasm the finishing powders available at the drugstore. Some of these are superior products, but there is no way to test the color ahead of time. For drugstore finishing powders I will make my suggestions based on what I think are the safest choices, but if you are inexperienced or haven't had luck with finding the best color, trying on a powder is generally the best way to make a decision, and then you are back at the cosmetics counters. But you can definitely shop the less expensive lines there.

The best finishing powders are: Almay Real Silk Pressed Powders Shine Free and Sheer Finish; Borghese (both loose and pressed); Charles of the Ritz (both loose and pressed); Clarion Silk Perfection Pressed Powder, Natural Finish Press Powder, and Oil-Free Translucent Powder; Clinique (both loose and pressed); Elizabeth Arden Flawless Finish Pressed and Loose Powder; Fashion Fair (both loose and pressed); Lancome (both loose and pressed); L'Oreal (both loose and pressed); M.A.C. (both loose and pressed); Mary Kay (pressed only); Maybelline (pressed only); Monteil Pressed Powder; Origins Translucent Powder; Prescriptives (both loose and pressed); Revlon Springwater Powder Oil-Free and Color Style Color Balancing Pressed Powder; Shiseido (pressed only); Ultima II (both loose and pressed); and Yves St. Laurent Silk Finish Pressed Powder.

The best buys without sacrificing quality are: Almay, Clarion, L'Oreal, Revlon, Maybelline, and Mary Kay.

Eyeshadow

By now I am well known for my opinion of both shiny eyeshadows and blue and green eyeshadows (or any brightly colored eyeshadow, for that matter). It was and still is my goal to find the best matte shades available, and I am thrilled to say that the cosmetics industry has caught on and there are more than enough matte shades available in all price ranges. You can shop both the drugstores and cosmetics counters and find wonderful textures and colors. There is no reason to wear shiny eyeshadows, so why not give them up forever.

Be aware that almost all of the lines I'm listing here have some shiny eyeshadows mixed in with their matte colors. Please avoid the shiny ones at all costs.

The best matte eyeshadows are: Almay Matte Classic Duo; Borghese (excellent silky texture); Clarion; Clinique; Charles of the Ritz; Cover Girl Pro Color, Natural Breeze-On, and Soft Radiant; Elizabeth Arden; Estee Lauder; Lancome; L'Oreal; M.A.C.; Marcelle; Mary Kay; Max Factor; Maybelline; Monteil; Origins; Physicians Formula; Prescriptives; Revlon; Shiseido; and Ultima II.

The best buys for matte eyeshadows are: Almay, Maybelline, Revlon, L'Oreal, and Physicians Formula; they have the most selections, but that isn't saying much. The department store cosmetics counters are where you can find the largest assortment of matte shades. The best selections are found at Charles of the Ritz, Origins, Prescriptives, and Ultima II.

There are only a few unique eye products to recommend, but they are worth a closer investigation. Clinique Beyond Shadow and Almay Liquid to Powder Eye Tints both have creamy textures that dry to a powder and have incredible staying power.

Blush

Blush is probably one of the easiest makeup components to get right. It is simply hard to buy a bad blush. Not that there aren't some real duds out there, but there are decidedly more winners than losers. The problem with blush is usually application, and that is where good brushes come into play. Using proper brushes is essential for getting blushes (and eyeshadows) to go on correctly.

Blushes received high marks if they were matte, had a soft non-grainy texture, blended on smoothly, did not absorb or dissipate with time, and had a good selection of colors. There are plenty that qualify, so it is not sensible to spend a lot of money on blushes unless you need to test the color first. Many of the blushes at the drugstore are of a superior quality and provide the same results as those at the department store. I particularly liked many of the new cream-to-powder blushes that I tried.

The best blushes are: Adrien Arpel Powdery Creme Blush; Almay Cheek Color Blush, Cream-to-Powder Blush, and Brush-On Blush; Borghese Liquid Powder Blush and regular blush (only those shades that aren't shiny); Chanel blushes (only those shades that aren't shiny); Charles of the Ritz blushes; Christian Dior Blush Final; Clarins Cream to Powder Blush (only); Clarion (all blush types); Clinique Young Face Powder Blush, Beyond Blusher, and Creamy Blush; Color Me Beautiful Blush; Cover Girl (all types, but only if you can stand the fragrance); Elizabeth Arden Luxury Cheek Color Matte (only) and Cream Powder Blush; Estee Lauder Just Blush, Soft Color Creme Blush, and Signature Powder Blush (only those that aren't shiny); Fashion Fair Blush; Frances Denny Moisture Silk Powder Blush; Guerlain Blush; Lancome Blush Majeur and Blush Subtil; L'Oreal Visuelle Powder Blush; M.A.C. Blushes; Marcelle Moisturizing Blush; Mary Kay Powder Perfect Cheek Color (powders only); Maybelline Revitalizing Color and Shades of You 100% Oil-Free Blush; Monteil Blush; New Essentials Cheek Color; Origins Blush; Physicians Formula Matte Blush; Prescriptives All Skin Face Colors and Regular Blush; Revlon Color Style Soft Color Powder Blush, Naturally Glamorous Blush-On, Powder Creme Blush, In-the-Pink Cheek Color, Sheer Face Color, and Springwater Blush; Shiseido blushes; and Ultima II Creamy Powder Blush (only those shades that aren't shiny).

The best buys without sacrificing quality are: Almay, Charles of the Ritz, Clinique, Cover Girl, L'Oreal, and Revlon.

Lipstick

By now we are all over the search for lipsticks that will last all day, right? We know that the greasier or glossier the lipstick, such as those by Clinique or Avon, the less likely it is to last, and the more matte the lipstick the longer it is likely to stick around, although powder-based lip colors—such as Ultima II Lip Sexxxy, Charles of the Ritz Powderful Lipstick, Adrien Arpel Matte Powder Creme, and Chanel Professional Lip Basics, may be too drying—and some—including M.A.C.'s matte lipsticks—can cake. However, if you don't have a problem with dry lips and you want to try a matte look, these are certainly an option worth testing.

There are a handful of creamy lipsticks with a tint added to the formula that stains the lips, including Adrien Arpel's lipsticks, Charles of the Ritz Semi Matte Lipstick, Flori Roberts Hydrophillic Lipstick, Lancome Rouge Absolu, M.A.C. Liptones, and Yves St. Laurent Rouge Intense. These do stick around longer than most, but they tend not to look all that great once the lipstick has worn away and the stain is left behind.

Remarkable lipsticks that are just creamy and last a reasonable amount of time are: Adrien Arpel Cream Lipstick; Almay Colour Protective Lipstick (matte shades only); Bonne Bell Stay True Lip Color; Chanel Rouge a Levres; Christian Dior Rouge a Levres and Rouge Accent; Color Me Beautiful Lipstick; Cover Girl Continuous Color with or without SPF 15 and Remarkable Lip Color with or without SPF 15; Estee Lauder (all types); Flori Roberts Regular and Matte Lipstick (the mattes aren't all that matte); Lancome Rouge Superb; L'Oreal Colour Supreme, Creme Riche, and L'Artiste Creme; M.A.C. Satin and Cream Lipsticks; Marcelle Lipsticks; Max Factor Moisture Rich Lipstick, New Definition, and Lasting Color Lipstick; Maybelline Moisture Whip, Long Wearing Lipstick, and Shades of You; Monteil Lipstick; Payot Lipstick; Prescriptives Classic, Demi Matte, Matte, and The Hots Lipstick; Revlon Super Lustrous Creme, Moon Drops Moisture Creme, Velvet Touch, Outrageous, and Color Style Lipsticks; Shiseido Lipsticks; Ultima II Super Luscious and Matte Lipsticks; and Yves St. Laurent Lipsticks.

The best buys and some of my absolute favorite lipsticks are: Almay, Bonne Bell, Color Me Beautiful, Cover Girl, L'Oreal, Marcelle, Max Factor, Physicians Formula, and Revlon.

How to prevent lipstick from feathering into the lines around the mouth is of interest to many women, including myself. I was thrilled when I discovered Chanel's Protective Colour Control stick. It was the first product I've used that really kept my lipstick from bleeding. Imagine my excitement when I found a product by Coty called Stop-It ($4.50) that worked just as well for one-third the price. Then I found Revlon's Color-Lock, which worked equally well for about the same price as Coty's Stop-It. (The only drawback is that Revlon's Color-Lock goes on slightly white, which will make your shade of lip color look lighter.) The only really featherproof lipstick I've tested is Estee Lauder's Featherproof Lipstick: it truly doesn't bleed. Excellent! I only wish they made more colors.

Eye and Brow Liners

Some cosmetics companies sell two different eye pencils: one for the brow and the other for lining the eye. Other cosmetics companies are more straightforward and sell only one that does both jobs. In essence that is the most practical and honest approach. There is usually little to no difference between eye and brow pencils. Most eye and brow pencils have a lot of similarities; the contrasts have little to do with where you should use the product. But whether they have a greasier or drier texture, they can all cause problems.

An eye pencil with a dry texture makes it difficult to line the eyelid after you've applied your eyeshadows. If the pencil is more on the greasy side, it will line the lid more easily, but it is also more likely to smear under the lower lashes in a very short period of time. I have always and still do prefer lining the eyes with regular eyeshadow powder and a small, thin eyeliner brush. I usually line my lower lashes with a soft brown eyeshadow and my eyelid with a black or dark brown eyeshadow. You can also wet the brush and apply the eyeshadow as you would a liquid liner in a more vivid line. In fact, even on the occasions that I line my eyes with a pencil, I go over it with an eyeshadow to make sure it has a better chance of staying all day. The difference for that look, and how long it lasts, in comparison to when you use a pencil alone, is amazing—particularly if you have oily or combination skin. If, however, the technique of lining your eyes with an eyeshadow and a tiny brush has eluded you and you still prefer pencils, you can still find many companies that have good products. You can shop the more expensive lines, but it is simply a waste of money. At all price levels, I found many more similarities among pencils than differences.

The best pencils that can be used for both the eyes and brows are: Almay's Kohl-Formula Eye Pencil (although the color selection is limited); Avon's Eye Lining Pencil; Bonne Bell's Eye Pencil; Borghese; Chanel (only those that aren't iridescent); Charles of the Ritz Classic Liners; Christian Dior Eye Pencils; Clarion Pen Silks and Lasting Effects Eye Pencil; Clinique Quick Eyes (matte colors only) and Regular Eye Pencil; Color Me Beautiful Eye Pencils; Cover Girl Eye Definer; Elizabeth Arden Slender Liner; Estee Lauder Automatic Pencil Liner for Eyes; Flori Roberts; Frances Denney; Lancaster; Lancome Le Crayon Kohl; L'Oreal; M.A.C.; Marcelle; Mary Kay Eye Defining Pencil; Max Factor Featherblend Kohliner; Maybelline Expert Eyes Pencil and Turning Point Liner; Monteil; New Essentials; Origins; Physicians Formula Gentle Eyewear Pencils; Prescriptives (great color selection); Revlon Time Liner for Eyes and Micropure Slimliner; Shiseido; Ultima II; Yves St. Laurent Automatic Pencil for Eyes; and Victoria Jackson.

The best buys without sacrificing quality are: Almay; Charles of the Ritz; L'Oreal; Mary Kay; Max Factor; Origins; Revlon (drugstore); and Victoria Jackson. I also like Shiseido's pencils very much, but they are not exactly what I would call a bargain.

Almost every cosmetics line has a selection of liquid eyeliners. They vary from a traditional tube liner to a felt-tip type liner. Although I tend not to like the look a liquid liner provides, I know that it is an option some women choose.

The best liquid liners are: Almay Skip Proof Eye Lining Pen; Elizabeth Arden; Lancome Automatic Eye Lining Felt Pen; Max Factor; and Maybelline.

When it comes just to the brows, I was very disappointed in the meager assortment of new eyebrow products. Eyebrow pencils have long been the standard product for making eyebrows appear thicker or more defined, and they still are, but greasy ones look over-madeup and dry ones are not that easy to apply.

As I mentioned above, most eyebrow pencils are identical to eyeliner pencils. Regardless of whether you choose an all-purpose pencil or a specific brow pencil, the most important consideration besides texture is color. Brow pencils generally are included due to their appropriate color range. I have excluded all pencils that are too greasy and can make the brow look "penciled." For a while, eyebrow powders were widely sold as an alternative to pencils. These brow powders were simply eyeshadows packaged under a different name. Only a handful of cosmetics companies still sell brow powders. This is not a reflection on how well they worked—eyebrow powders are an excellent, less obvious alternative to pencils, but most women seem unwilling to adopt this mode of filling in the eyebrow.

Several companies make eyebrow gels. Some gels contain color to fill, lift, and define the brows; Chanel Brow Shaper, Borghese Brow Milano, and Lancome Tinted Brow Groomer are in this category. There are no inexpensive counterparts except for the clear gels, such as Max Factor Brow Tamer, Color Me Beautiful Clear Brow Fixative, and Shiseido Eyebrow Shapeliner. (A good substitute for clear gel is putting hair spray on a toothbrush and brushing it through the brow.) For the most part, the brow gels with natural brow color choices are great. I strongly recommend them as another way to make eyebrows look fuller but not artificial. If you can learn how to use the eyebrow gels, they can be a great alternative to pencils.

The best pencils specified for the brows, regardless of price, are: Adrien Arpel; Almay; Chanel; Borghese; Charles of the Ritz; Christian Dior (although the color selection is limited); Lancome Le Crayon Brow; Mary Kay Eye Brow Pencil; Shiseido; and Yves St. Laurent.

The best eyebrow powders (which I prefer to brow pencils) are: Elizabeth Arden Brow Powders; Estee Lauder Eye Brow Color; Max Factor Brush & Brow; and Revlon Natural Brow Color.

Lip Liners

There is no reason to spend more than a few dollars on lip liners. I can say without any hesitation that lip pencils priced over $6 are a waste of money. There is little to no difference between a high-priced pencil and a less expensive one. You can spend $22 on Estee Lauder's very attractive retractable lip pencil in the metallic blue case or you can spend $3 on Almay's or Revlon's (drugstore) lip pencils and get the same look. The decision is up to you. The only real difference between pencils is that a few are more greasy than others. I recommend staying away from the greasy variety because they can smear and may not last as long as ones that are a bit drier. Rather then listing every cosmetic line I've reviewed, I can easily say that all of them have great lip liners; some have more color choices than others, but that is the only real difference. Go for it. Buy an inexpensive lip pencil from Cover Girl or Revlon—no one but you will know.

Beauty Note: Lip pencils do not stop lipstick from bleeding. They can slow it down a little, but that's about it. Lip liner shapes the mouth before you apply lipstick. I would also like to put in a vote for ignoring the fashion of outlining the lips in a darker color and then filling in with a lighter shade. Besides looking strangely obvious, it tends to have a ghoulish appearance when the lip liner is done in brown. Separate from that, personally, I rarely have time for lip liner and I like the shape of my mouth, so I skip to the chase and use any of the antifeathering products I mentioned above with my lipstick color. It looks just as good, and I'm the only one who ever knows I've forgotten to line my lips.

Mascara

I am still surprised by how many good mascaras there are at both drugstores and department stores; in fact, I think they've improved all around. All price ranges include excellent mascaras. Obviously, I think it is foolish to buy the most expensive when reasonably priced mascaras are equally as good. Given that this is one product you can't readily test at the counters for reliability, try a few of the inexpensive ones I'm suggesting and see what works for you. It really is the most sensible and beautiful decision.

The best mascaras are: Almay One Coat Mascara and Triple Thick; Borghese Maximum Mascara for Sensitive Eyes; Chanel Luxury Creme Mascara; Charles of the Ritz Perfect Finish Lash and High Density Lash; Christian Dior Thickening Lash Mascara; Cover Girl Remarkable Washable Mascara and Long N' Lush; Elizabeth Arden Twice as Thick, Twice as Long, and Two Brush Mascara; Estee Lauder More Than Mascara; Lancome Defincils and Immencils; L'Oreal Formula Riche, Lash Out, and Accentuous Mascara; Marcelle Ultimate Lash Mascara; Max Factor 2000 Calorie and Stretch Mascara; Maybelline No Problem Mascara and Illegal Lengths; Origins Fringe Benefits; Payot Mascara; and Revlon Impulse Long Distance, Impulse Quick and Thick, Lengthwise, and Lashfull.

The best buys and some of my favorite mascaras are: Almay; L'Oreal; Max Factor; Maybelline; Revlon; and Marcelle.

The best waterproof mascaras which happen to also be the best buys are: Almay Wetproof Mascara, Maybelline Great Lash Waterproof Mascara, and Revlon Lashful Waterproof Mascara. Keep in mind that I only recommend these for swimming because daily use isn't good for the lashes.

Brushes

More so than ever before, there are more professional-size brushes available at the department stores in relatively reasonable price ranges. Cosmetics lines such as at M.A.C., The Body Shop, and Merle Norman, plus brush lines such as Joan Simmons, Expressions (Canada only), and Albert Goldman, all sell a great assortment of brushes. Estee Lauder sells a good set of professional brushes, but they are so overpriced and so unexceptional as to be impossible to recommend. Take the time to check out the brushes from any of these sources—they will make a huge difference in the way you apply your makeup. As an alternative, consider shopping for eyeshadow and blush brushes at an art supply store. They have a vast selection of brushes in all price ranges and textures that are particularly great for sensitive lids.

Cleanser

Perhaps I was too emphatic years back when I began nagging about the need for water-soluble cleansers. Those were the days when the only thing available to clean the face were wipe-off cleansers and bar soaps that were all drying regardless of the claim on the bar. Now there are more water-soluble cleansers available than I ever thought possible. Not all of them are really water-soluble and many are too drying, but several remove all the makeup without causing irritation or dryness, do not burn the eyes, and leave no greasy residue, and still come close to being very gentle on the skin. It is also essential that all water-soluble cleansers be removed easily by splashing and not by being wiped off with a damp washcloth. Using a washcloth might prevent the water from dripping all around the sink after you're done splashing, but washcloths can cause irritation and that's not great for the skin.

One of the things most water-soluble cleansers shared in common, regardless of price, was the basic ingredient list. Cleansers designed for dry skin contained oils and left a greasy residue behind, while those designed for normal to oily skin contained more than one standard detergent cleanser that dried out the skin. Using a drying cleanser inevitably will require the use of a moisturizer. Moisturizers are almost always a problem for someone with oily or combination skin. Besides, this cycle of drying out oily or combination skin and then following up with a moisturizer is the fastest way I know to cause more skin problems. Using oily cleansers on dry skin and then following up with a moisturizer can cause the skin to look dull and prevent cell turnover by building up too much grease on the face.

I should mention that I am still a die-hard user of Cetaphil Lotion for a cleanser. This truly water-soluble cleanser is reasonably priced and excellent for normal to dry/sensitive skin. As often as I try other products, which I do frequently, I return to this reliable basic. I often think I'm on the verge of finding something better, but I always go back. None is really better for normal/dry/sensitive skin, particularly when you take price into consideration; a 16-ounce container costs about $10. Not bad when the average cleanser costs anywhere between $4 and $25 for 4 ounces. At $4 for 4 ounces, that makes a product about $16 a pound; that isn't such a deal. Cetaphil is definitely worth a try if your skin falls into the normal to dry category; oily skin types will want to consider other alternatives I've listed below.

Beauty Note: You will notice that several products are recommended by the company as being best for normal or oily skin types while I list them as being more appropriate for someone with dry or normal skin. After considering many aspects of a product, particularly the ingredient list, I make a suggestion on what skin type I think the product will work for, and that doesn't always agree with the cosmetics companies' view.

The best water-soluble cleansers for normal to oily skin types were: Almay Sensitive Skin Foaming Cleanser; Alpha Hydrox Foaming Face Wash; Aveda Purifying Gel Cleanser; Beauty Without Cruelty Gentle Herbal Face Wash; Borghese Gel Delicato; Chanel Foaming Gel Cleanser; Clarins Gentle Foaming Cleanser; Clarion Clear Skin Refresher and Complexion Bath; Clinique Wash-Away Gel Cleanser, Color Me Beautiful Very Effective Cleansing Gel; Cover Girl Clearly Different Deep Cleansing Face Wash and Noxzema Plus Skin Cream; Elizabeth Arden One Great Soap (extremely oily skin only); Flori Roberts Optima Gel Cleanser; Frances Denney Cleanser; Lancome Clarifiance Oil-Free Gel Cleanser; Marcelle Aquarelle Oil-Free Purifying Cleanser for Oily Skin; Moisturel Sensitive Skin Cleanser; Neutrogena Facial Cleansing Formula; and Ponds Foaming Cleanser & Toner In One.

For normal to dry/sensitive skin the best cleansers are: Almay Moisture Balance Cleansing Lotion for Normal Skin; Charles of the Ritz Revenescence Liquid; Cetaphil Lotion; Cher's Aquassentials Facial Cleanser (an exact copy of Cetaphil Lotion); Cover Girl Moisture-Gentle Cleansing Beauty Wash; Francis Denney Clean Sweep; Monteil Ice Fundamental Soft Rinse-Off Cleanser; Neutrogena Non-Drying

Cleansing Lotion; Nu Skin Cleansing Lotion; and Prescriptives Gentle Wash Lotion Cleanser.

Exfoliants

This used to be an easy area of discussion. It is well established among most beauty experts, as well as dermatologists and plastic surgeons, that exfoliating the skin is a wonderful way to take care of both oily and dry skin. A few years back, before Retin-A, there weren't many options when it came to getting dead skin cells off the face. During most of the 1970s and '80s the only choices were scrubs such as honey and almonds, cleansers with scrub particles, and facial masks. Most of these took a toll on the face and irritation was a typical problem. Then, to make matters worse, there was the question of how often should you exfoliate and what other products should you use. A scrub followed by a toner that contains irritants could really burn the skin. To solve the general obstacle of irritation, I suggested mixing Cetaphil Lotion with baking soda as a way to create your own effective, gentle, and inexpensive scrub (and I never recommend any toners that contain irritants). That is still my earnest recommendation; if you are going to use a physical scrub, this is still one of the best combinations I've found. Other scrubs with their detergent wax bases just can't compare (not to mention the extraordinarily reasonable price of baking soda and Cetaphil Lotion). But now the topic has gotten more complicated with the addition of alpha hydroxy acid products, which offer a chemical way to exfoliate the skin instead of a physical agent like a scrub.

If you are going to choose an AHA product, particularly one from my list of recommendations in the following section, then the question becomes do you still need to use a physical scrub. It's an excellent question, but the answer isn't all that easy. You will have to judge for yourself. Most women with normal to dry/sensitive skin should probably use their AHA product and no other exfoliant. Someone with normal to oily skin should probably still be using a scrub but only two or three times a week. Stick with the Cetaphil Lotion and baking soda for the most gentle results and listen closely to your skin; irritation is never the goal.

Toner

I have been preaching for years (am I dating myself?) about the need to use only nonirritating, alcohol-free toners, and to some extent I am pleased to say that the cosmetics industry has finally listened. But keep in mind that alcohol-free does not mean irritant-free.

Unfortunately, many cosmetics lines still stick other irritating ingredients in their toners. I've list the offending ingredients in Chapters Two and Eight, but I want to remind you how much trouble toners can cause the skin if they are not truly gentle.

Toners and all the products that fall into this category (refining lotions, clarifying lotions, soothing tonics, stimulating lotions, fresheners, and astringents) are an extra cleansing step, and sometimes they can be soothing, moisturizing, and, if you use the strong stuff, exfoliating. I evaluated these products strictly on how soothing and clean they felt on the face without drying the skin or leaving a greasy residue. It is not best that toners exfoliate the skin because then they almost always contain extra irritants that can do more damage than the skin can handle.

Does it make sense to spend a lot of money on a toner that doesn't contain irritating ingredients? No, I found excellent toners that had very gentle ingredients and were relatively inexpensive. Because many women enjoy using these products, and because of the soothing, fresh feeling many irritant-free toners can provide, I feel they can be beneficial for many skin types.

The best toners are: Adrien Arpel Herbal Astringent; Aveda Skin Firming/Toning Agent; The Body Shop Honey Water; Borghese Spa-Soothing Tonic for Sensitive Skin, Tonico Minerale; Chanel Firming Freshener; Cher's Aquassentials Facial Toner; Christian Dior Hydra Dior Skin Freshener for Dry Skin and Equite Alcohol-Free Softening Toner; Clarins Toning Lotion for Combination or Oily Skin and Toning Lotion for Dry to Normal Skin; Color Me Beautiful Hydrating Tonic; Elizabeth Arden Soothing Care Calming Skin Freshener; Erno Laszlo Hydraphel Skin Supplement; Estee Lauder Gentle Protection Tonic and Re-Nutriv Gentle Skin Toner; Forever Spring Ambrosia Skin Refresher; Frances Denney Nourishing Lotion and Protecting Lotion; Lancaster Suractif Preparation Lotion; La Prairie Age Management Balancer, Cellular Refining Lotion, and Cellular Purifying Lotion; L'Oreal Hydrating Floral Tonic; M.A.C. PA-3 Phyto-Astringent Purifying Toner; Mary Kay Gentle Action Freshener; Monteil Super Soft Rinse-Off Cleanser and Tonique Delicat for Dry/Sensitive Skin; Moon Drops Comforting Toner Sensitive/Delicate and Moon Drops Softening Toner Normal to Dry; Neutrogena Alcohol-Free Toner; New Essentials Refreshing Skin Tonic; Nivea Visage Alcohol Free Moisturizing Facial Toner; Nu Skin NaPCA Moisture Mist; Origins Drenching Solution, Comforting Solution, and

Managing Solution; Physicians Formula Gentle Refreshing Toner; Rachel Perry Violet Rose Skin Toner; Ultima II CHR Extraordinary Gentle Clarifier; and Yves St. Laurent Extra-Gentle Tonic Alcohol-Free.

Moisturizer

In all the letters I get, the most-asked questions are what is the best moisturizer and whether any product will really do something about wrinkles. There aren't any wrinkle creams (except sunscreens), but there are good moisturizers out there, and a lot of them. I'm including in this category all lotions, creams, even wrinkle creams, specialty creams, day creams, replenishers, liposome creams, anti-thises, and nourishing thats; all do the same thing—moisturize the skin—and they do a good job. The repetitive ingredients found in product line after product line just don't warrant the outlandish claims and ridiculous prices or your attention.

Surprisingly enough, when I ignored the claims and price tags, I liked most of the moisturizers I reviewed. Many contain ingredients that make them good moisturizers. Only a handful of moisturizers contained ingredients that I thought were potentially harmful to the skin or would dry it out and cause irritation. Other than that, there are really some remarkable emollient moisturizers on the market, in all price categories, containing great ingredients that can take care of varying degrees of dry skin.

When it comes to moisturizers, the problem for most women is finding a moisturizer that is right for their skin type. Some moisturizers contain extremely rich ingredients such as lanolin, vegetable oil, mineral oil, petrolatum, shea butter, cocoa butter, or protein, which are best for those women with very dry skin. Then there are various forms of lighter weight moisturizers that contain only one or two oils; these are best for skin that is normal to dry. If you do not have extremely dry skin, stay away from moisturizers that are loaded with the ingredients I mentioned above. If you have slightly or occasionally dry skin, you are better off with those moisturizers that contain only one or two oils. Finding the appropriate type of moisturizer for your skin will be easier if you review the ingredients I've listed for skin types in Chapter Two.

All dry skin can benefit to some degree from moisturizing ingredients such as sodium PCA, hyaluronic acid, collagen, elastin, retinyl palmitate, and vitamins E, A, and C. The other "specialty" ingredients such as cow extract, spleen extract, tissue extract, placental extract, serum protein, mineral salts, and flower or plant extracts can be completely ignored or avoided altogether.

If you are wondering about day creams versus night creams, my recommendation is to ignore those categories of products and go by what your skin needs. If your skin is extremely dry, products rich in oils and lanolin may be necessary for your skin morning and night, but the morning one needs an SPF of 15. If you have skin that is dry, but not excessively so, you may want to use a light moisturizing lotion that contains one or two oils in the morning (and an SPF of 15) and a more emollient cream at night. If you have slightly dry skin, a lightweight moisturizer or a moisturizing gel should be perfect for both morning and night. We won't even get into eye or throat creams, because you already know how unnecessary they are, right? The moisturizer you use on your face will work around your eyes. Try to disregard the scare tactics you hear at the cosmetics counters, and ignore the brochures that carry on about special formulations designed exclusively for the eye area. These claims are not substantiated by the ingredients in the products, which are practically identical to creams supposedly designed just for the face.

My strong suggestion for those women with oily skin is, please, don't get sucked into believing that all skin types, even oily skin types, require a moisturizer to prevent the skin from wrinkling or to combat surface dehydration. Unless we are talking about a sunscreen with an SPF of 15 or greater, there are no moisturizers on the market that will do more for your skin than your own oil can do without adding to the mess. Sorry, I wish it weren't so, but it is. The oil on your face is your own built-in moisturizer, and if you are not using drying and irritating skin care products you should not need a moisturizer. Also, and most important, "oil-free" doesn't mean the product won't feel slick, greasy, or oily on the skin. Many ingredients that don't sound like "oil" have a very slick, oily texture. (Oily skin types should wear an oil-free foundation that contains a high SPF number to protect their skin from the sun.)

What you all want to know is whether or not it really makes sense to spend a lot of money on moisturizers. Is a $50 product really that much better than one that costs $10? If you've read this whole book, you know the answer. For those of you who didn't read the first half of the book and just cut to chase, the answer is: The best moisturizers on the market for dry skin are to be found in almost every skin care line, so spending a lot of money does not make sense! As you read the following suggestions, understand that when I say best I mean best. A "best" moisturizer made by Almay or Avon is rated the same "best" as one by Chanel or Borghese. Please read the particular information under each skin care line in Chapter Eight to evaluate the particular product you are considering, get used to reading skin care ingredients, and ignore words like "lifts," "firms," or "energizes."

The best moisturizers for normal to dry skin regardless of price (and regardless of my disgust at the price and claims) are: Adrien Arpel Morning After Moisturizer SPF 20 (daytime only) and Underglow Line Minimizing Moisturizer; Almay Stress Cream, Anti-Irritant, Replenishing Lotion, Moisture Renew Cream for Dry Skin, and Moisture Renew Lotion for Dry Skin; Avon Daily Revival Eye Care Creme; Beauty Without Cruelty Oil-Free Hydrator with NaPCA and Oil-Free Moisturizer; The Body Shop Blue Corn Lotion and Unfragranced Lotion; Borghese Daily Skin Energy Source, Spa Lift for Face SPF 8, Spa Lift For Eyes, and Reenergizing Night Creme; Chanel Firming Eye Cream and Night Lift Cream; Charles of the Ritz Timeless Essence Night Recovery Cream; Cher's Aquassentials Continuous Release Moisturizer; Christian Dior Resultante Revitalizing Wrinkle Cream and Capture Complexe Liposomes for the Face; Clarins Gentle Night Cream for Sensitive Skin, Gentle Day Cream for Sensitive Skin, Multi-Active Day Cream, and Treatment Cream for All Skin Types; Clarion Double Defense Moisturizer; Clinique Dramatically Different Moisturizing Lotion, Sub-Skin Cream, Daily Eye Benefits, Moisture Surge Treatment Formula, and Skin Texture Lotion; Color Me Beautiful Fortifying Eye Cream, Lightweight Moisture Lotion, Oil-Free Regulating Fluid, and Regulating Night Therapy; Eb5 Facial Cream; Elizabeth Arden Ceramide Time Complex Cream, Imunage UV Defense Cream SPF 15, Imunage UV Defense Lotion SPF 15, Millenium Night Renewal Creme, and Millenium Eye Renewal Cream; Erno Laszlo pHelityl Lotion, Total Skin Revitalizer, Total Skin Revitalizer for Eyes, Total Skin Revitalizer for Night, pHelitone Firming Eye Gel, Hydraphel Emulsion, and Daily Moisture Protection Lotion SPF 15; Estee Lauder Skin Defender Sensitive Skin Protector, Advanced Night Repair, Advanced Suncare SPF 15 No Chemical Sunscreen, Eyezone Repair Gel, Time Zone Moisture Recharging Complex, Future Perfect Micro-Targeted Skin Gel, Skin Perfecting Creme, Re-Nutriv Creme Lightweight, and Non-Oily Skin

Supplement; Eucerin Daily Facial Lotion SPF 20; Flori Roberts Hydrophillic Moisture Complex; Forever Spring Ginseng Cream; Frances Denney Ultimate Repair, Eye Cream Concentrate, Moisture Infusion, Urgent Nourisher, and Oil Balancer; Freeman Beautiful Skin Chamomile & Allantoin Lite Moisturizer; Guerlain Evolution Sublicreme No. 1, Evolution Sublicreme No. 2, and Issima Anti-Wrinkle Eye Contour Fluid; Lancaster's Suractif Skin Retexturizer and Suractif Facial Treatment; Lancome's Niosome Daytime Skin Treatment and Vivifiance Hydrating Eye Gel; La Prairie Cellular Balancing Complex; L'Oreal's Oil-Free Protective Daily Moisture Lotion SPF 12, Oil-Free Active Daily Moisture, Protective Daily Moisture Lotion SPF 12, Advanced Wrinkle Defense Cream, and Eye Defense; M.A.C. CR-2 Cellular Recovery Night Emulsion; Marcelle Eye Contour Gel; Mary Kay Balancing Moisturizer; Monteil Ice Fundamental Emulsion and Firmant Des Rides; New Essentials Refreshing Eye Gel, Daily Hydrating Cream, Daily Hydrating Lotion, Hydrating Eye Cream, Daily Purifying Lotion, Moisture Maximizer, and Vitalizing Night Cream; Neutrogena Intensified Day Moisture SPF 15 and Neutrogena Chemical-Free Sunblocker SPF 17; Nivea Visage No Oil, All Moisture Hydrogel, Daily Facial Moisture Lotion SPF 15, Liposome Eye Contour Gel, and Restorative Night Cream; Nu Skin Intensive Eye Complex, Rejuvenating Cream, NaPCA Moisturizer, and Celltrex; Oil of Olay Daily UV Protectant Cream SPF 15 (fragrance free) and Daily UV Protectant Lotion SPF 15; Origins Steady Drencher, Constant Comforter, Fringe Benefits, Starting Over, Urgent Moisture, and Let The Sunshine SPF 14 No Chemical Sunscreen; Pond's Nourishing Moisturizer Lotion Oil-Free, Nourishing Moisturizer Lotion Oil-Free with SPF 15, Overnight Nourishing Complex Cream, and Dramatic Results Skin Smoothing Capsules with Nutrium; Rachel Perry Elastin and Collagen Firming Treatment, Ginseng and Collagen Wrinkle Treatment; Prescriptives Flight Cream, Line Preventor, Extra Firm Skin Care Concentrate, Simply Moisture, Multi-Moisture Pure Hydrating Cream, and Eyewear; Principal Secrets Eye Relief, and Extra Nurturing Cream; Revlon Natural Collagen Complex SPF 15; Shiseido Bio Performance Super Revitalize Creme; Ultima II CHR Extraordinary Lotion, CHR Moisture Lotion Concentrate, The Moisturizer, ProCollagen, Megadose, and Energizing Skin Recharging; and Yves St. Laurent Intensive Nighttime Revitalizer, Nighttime Revitalizer, and Soothing Eye Contour Gel.

The best moisturizers for dry skin regardless of price (and regardless of my disgust at the price and claims) are: Adrien Arpel Swiss Formula Day Cream #12 with Collagen, Vital Velvet Moisturizer, Moisturizing Blotting Lotion; Almay Moisture Balance Eye Cream for Normal Skin; Avon Daily Revival Super Moisture Creme for Dry Skin—SPF 6 and Nurtura Replenishing Cream; Basis Intensive Hydrating Oil; Beauty Without Cruelty Aloe and E Moisture Cream; The Body Shop Aloe Vera Moisture Cream, Dewberry 5 Oils Lotion, White Musk Lotion, Aloe Lotion, and Under Eye Cream; Borghese Nighttime Restorative, Charles of the Ritz Special Formula Emollient and Revenescence Cream; Cher's Aquassentials Continuous Release Eye Cream; Christian Dior Hydra-Dior Extra Rich Night Cream; Clarins Face Treatment Cream for Dry or Reddened Skin, Face Treatment Cream for Dehydrated Skin, and Treatment Cream for Very Dry, Very Devitalized Skin; Clarion Restorative Smoothing Creme, Pure Moisture, and Infinite Moisture; Clinique Advance Care Moisturizer and Very Emollient Cream; Color Me Beautiful Intensive Night Care; Elizabeth Arden Visible Difference Refining Moisturizer Creme Complex, Visible Difference Eyecare Concentrate, Millenium Day Renewal Emulsion, Skin Basics Beauty Sleep, and Special Benefit Orange Skin Cream; Erno Laszlo Active pHelityl Cream, pHelityl Cream, pHelitone Replenishing Eye Cream, and Hyrdraphel Complex; Estee Lauder Re-Nutriv Creme; Eucerin Creme; Fashion Fair Eye Cream and Moisturizing Creme; Frances Denney Multi-Layer Moisturizer, Multi-Layer Night Cream, and Cream; Eucerin Lotion for Dry Skin Care; Gueralin Evolution Specific Eye-Contour Care and Issima Midnight Secret; Jergens Advanced Therapy Lotion, Vitamin E & Lanolin; Lancome Noctosome Renewal Night Treatment, Progres Eye Creme, Progres Plus Anti-Wrinkle Creme, Nutribel Nourishing Hydrating Emulsion, Nutrix Soothing Treatment Creme, and Hydrative Continuous Hydrating Resource; La Prairie Cellular Night Cream; L'Oreal Hydra Renewal, Night Replenisher, and Wrinkle Defense Cream; Marcelle Anti-Aging Cream; Mary Kay Extra Emollient Moisturizer, Extra Emollient Night Cream, Advanced Moisture Renewal Treatment Cream, and Eye Cream Concentrate; Monteil Ice Ultimate Cream Concentrate, and Super Moist Beauty Emulsion; Neutrogena Night Cream; New Essentials Moisture Nourishing Night Cream; Physicians Formula Captyane Replenishing Eye Complex, Captyane Replenishing Gel-Cream, Elastin Collagen Moisture Lotion, and Enriched Dry Skin Concentrate; Revlon Eterna '27' All Day Moisture Lotion, Eterna and '27' All Day Moisture Cream; Shiseido Facial Concentrates Facial Moisturizing Lotion, Facial Concentrates Facial Eye Wrinkle Cream Concentrate, Facial Concentrates Facial Nourishing Cream, Facial Skincare Facial Moisturzing Lotion (Rich), Facial Skincare Facial Nourishing Cream, and Facial Skin Care Pre-Makeup Cream; and Vaseline Intensive Care Dry Skin Formula and Aloe & Lanolin.

Alpha Hydroxy Acid Products

If you are going to try this type of product, then I would encourage you to stick with those lines that are at least 8 to 15 percent AHA: NeoStrata, Murad, Aqua Glycolic, Alpha Hydrox, M.D. Formulations, and Avon's Anew (only Avon's Anew Perfecting Complex for the Hands and Body). Please stay away from any AHA products that contain alcohol, as it will irritate your skin.

Facial Masks

Although I am rarely a woman of few words, I feel quite comfortable stating that there were no facial masks on the market that I thought were particularly exceptional for the skin or worth the exceptional or even reasonable price tags. Predominantly, facial masks use clay as their main ingredients. The subsequent thickeners, standard water binding agents, and new and improved water binding agents are found in all masks, and several also included a nice litany of irritating ingredients. Obviously, I don't recommend facial masks, but some women feel that applying a mask is a great way to pamper themselves.

The least irritating facial masks are: Adrien Arpel Flower Petal and Botanical Extract Masque, and Flower Petal Mini-Facial in a Jar; Aveda Deep Cleansing Herbal Clay Masque; The Body Shop Peanut & Rosehip Face Mask; Borghese Spa Eye Energizing Mask; Chanel Maximum Moisture Mask,and Natural Exfoliating Mask; Cher's Aquassentials Revitalizing Mask; Christian Dior Hydra-Dior Cleansing Masque for Oily Skin; Clarins Gentle Facial Peeling and Absorbant Mask; Elizabeth Arden Millenium Hydra-Exfoliating Mask; Erno Laszlo Sea Mud Mask; Estee Lauder Triple Creme Hydrating Mask; Freeman Beautiful Skin Avocado & Oatmeal Facial Masque; Guerlain Issima Aquamasque; Lancaster Anti-Stress Eye Mask and Moisture Mask; Lancome Masque No. 10 Hydrating Masque; M.A.C. VM-2 Vitamin and Mineral Hydrating Mask; Mary Kay Moisture Rich Mask; Moon Drops

Three Minute Moisture Pack Skin Calming Sensitive/Delicate; New Essentials Soothing Face Mask; Nu Skin Clay Pack; Principal Secrets Invisible Toning Masque; Shiseido Facial Skincare Facial Masque Rinse-Off; Vital Perfection Moisture Active Emulsion; and Yves St. Laurent Instant Clarifying Masque and Hydro-Active Moisture Masque.

CHAPTER

T·E·N

Beauty That Respects Nature

CRUELTY-FREE MAKEUP

I received the following letter in reaction to this section in the previous edition of *Don't Go To The Cosmetics Counter Without Me*. I think it helped define the issue quite plainly.

Dear Ms. Begoun,

I was in the bookstore and about to purchase your book *Don't Go To The Cosmetics Counter Without Me* (first edition) when I realized it contained a rather serious, albeit well-meaning, error. The book ended with a chapter on the "cruelty concept" of cosmetic product testing, which you described as useless and unnecessary. You then referred the reader to groups whose primary goal is the elimination of animals from all aspects of medical research and product testing, not the safety of consumers or their children.

These groups are not reliable sources. Much of the information they distribute is badly distorted. There has been much progress in the area of reducing the number of animals needed, as well as refinements in procedures used. For example, PETA (People for the Ethical Treatment of Animals) and NAVS (National Anti-Vivisection Society) would tell you that caustic substances are routinely dripped into the eyes of rabbits [the Draize Test], whereas current standard practice is to test highly diluted solutions of products that have already passed in vitro tests for nonirritancy. The nonanimal tests are valuable prescreening tests, but do not replace all animal testing according to leading ophthalmologists and the manufacturers of the in vitro test.

Let me supply you with a more reliable source for any future revisions of your book. In 1981, Henry Spira founded the Coalition to Abolish the Draize Eye Test [the one performed on rabbits' eyes]. As a result of his efforts, the Center for Alternatives to Animal Testing was founded at Johns Hopkins University, dedicated to the development of nonanimal testing. It is their consensus that some animal testing is still necessary to ensure consumer safety.

If consumers do not wish to contribute to further animal testing, then you should recommend that they stick to old formulations of their current products to avoid the additional testing involved in the development of new ones. All ingredients have at some point been tested on animals, despite any "cruelty-free" claim on the product. No one argues the necessity of minimizing harm to animals in a humane society, but information must be provided accurately for people to make the appropriate choices for themselves.

Allison Stuart
Member, Coalition for Animals and Animal Research

Here is my response.

Dear Allison,

I appreciate your information and am willing to publish your side of the issue in the update of my book. I will be glad to utilize the sources you sent me in conjunction with other information on the subject I have researched. However, I did not state that product testing on animals was useless and unnecessary. I stated quite clearly that "*absurdly cruel* tests in the name of human safety are . . . inhumane." I also stated that I was not an expert in this arena and that the only groups I knew of working diligently to prevent cruel and merciless testing on animals were People for the Ethical Treatment of Animals (PETA), the National Anti-Vivisection Society (NAVS), the Humane Society, and a handful of other animal rights groups, and that still seems to be the way it is.

You are correct in pointing out that I did not explain that these groups are somewhat "right wing" in their approach (for example, as far as NAVS and PETA are concerned, part of their agenda is the elimination of all animal usage, including fish as a source of food), as I probably should have. But I would also have had to state that if it weren't for these so-called extremist groups creating public pressure on companies that test on animals, the wholesale slaughter and mutilation of animals without regard for their suffering or even need for the experiment would have gone on indefinitely. Research laboratories (of both cosmetics and pharmaceutical companies) weren't the ones trying to stop these nauseating tests. They are only now responding due to the pressure caused by these animal rights groups bringing their actions to the attention of the consumer.

Remember that I'm talking about cosmetics and not life-saving drugs and operations. Yet the care of these animals in any situation must be taken into consideration, and alternative tests (which are often more accurate) should be implemented absolutely whenever possible. Without getting into graphic details about what is and isn't cruel when it comes to testing, I know we may all agree on that point, but it is assuredly the animal rights groups that are implementing the pressure to change what is truly disgusting handling of animals.

I would also like to point out that your suggestion that PETA or NAVS are unreliable as sources is extremely short-sighted on your part. I quote directly from the source you mentioned in your letter, Henry Spira (who spearheaded the cause to convince Revlon, Estee Lauder, Avon, and others to stop the Draize Eye Test and use alternative nonanimal methods of testing cosmetics): "I find it encouraging that NAVS is bringing the issue of alternatives [to animal testing] to the legal profession. . . . After a decade of enormous progress in institutionalizing alternatives, in researching and developing alternatives [to animal testing], we now need to focus on implementing alternatives, on identifying and overcoming the political and legal roadblocks [excerpted from the *NAVS Bulletin*, Winter 1993]." Perhaps you are the one who should be checking your sources.

As I stated in the original version of *Don't Go To The Cosmetics Counter Without Me*, truly "natural" and "cruelty-free" products are those that have not been tested on animals. To deform and kill animal life in futile, inconclusive, and absurdly cruel tests in the name of safety is "unnatural" and inhumane. I should explain that I am not an expert on the subject of animal-free testing nor do I want to create the illusion that I am. However, I do support many knowledgeable groups that are active both politically and socially in changing common animal testing practices that they feel (and, from everything I've read about both sides of the issue, I concur) have no relevance to how a product will affect a person's skin or health. I find the research information these groups have available both disturbing and poignant. My main sources of information are: **National Anti-Vivisection Society (NAVS)**, 53 West Jackson Boulevard, Chicago, Illinois 60604, (312) 427-6065, and **People for the Ethical Treatment of Animals (PETA)**, P.O. Box 42516, Washington, D.C. 20015, (301) 770-7444. The basic philosophy of both groups is that as long as there are thousands of cruelty-free products available that are safe and effective, and as long as there are reliable means of testing without using animals, there is no excuse for the continued use of tests that torture animal life. For more details about animal-free testing alternatives, please write to these organizations.

Important note: The following lists do not reflect in any way the quality of the products the companies produce.

This first list is simply a compilation of cosmetics companies that do not test or contract with anyone to test their products on animals. I respect the responsible and humane position these businesses have chosen to follow. I applaud their lead in this controversial issue. It is through their efforts that we move closer to achieving a more caring and compassionate world. The names of the companies listed below were taken from the booklet *Personal Care with Principles,* published by the National Anti-Vivisection Society. For a complete list of such companies (not just those involved with cosmetics), I recommend that you write and request a copy of this booklet (and be sure to give a generous donation to this nonprofit organization at the same time).

The following cosmetics companies do not use animal testing:

A-Retinol

Adrien Arpel

Alexander de Markoff (Revlon)

Almay (Revlon)

Aramis (Estee Lauder)

Arbonne

Artistry by Amway

Aveda

Avon

Basis

Beauticontrol Cosmetics

Beauty Without Cruelty (England)

Beiersdorf

Bill Blass (Revlon)

The Body Shop

Bonne Bell

Borghese

Cabot Labs:

Camocare

Charles of the Ritz (Revlon)

Christian Dior

Clarins

Clinique (Estee Lauder)

Color Me Beautiful

Crabtree & Evelyn

Estee Lauder

Fashion Two Twenty

Freeman Beautiful Skin

Guerlain

HABA Laboratories

Halston (Revlon)

I Natural Cosmetics

Ida Grae Cosmetics
Jafra
Jergens
Lancaster
Lancome
L'Oreal
Lubriderm
M.A.C. Cosmetics
Mary Kay Cosmetics
Max Factor (Revlon)
Merle Norman Cosmetics
Monteil of Paris
Natural Wonder (Revlon)
Neutrogena Skincare
Nexxus Products
Nivea

Nu Skin International
Origins
Orlane
Prescriptives (Estee Lauder)
Rachel Perry
Redken Labs
Revlon
Sebastian International
Shaklee U.S.
Shiseido
St. Ives Labs
Ultima II (Revlon)
Victoria Jackson
Visage Beaute Cosmetics
Warner-Lambert Company

The following cosmetics companies continue to use animal testing:

Alberto Culver
Bain de Soleil
Breck
Bristol-Meyers
Camay
Chanel
Chesebrough-Pond's
Clairol
Clarion
Clearasil
Coty
Cover Girl
Cutex
Dermassage
Dove

Elizabeth Arden
Erno Laszlo
Helena Rubinstein
Ivory
Johnson & Johnson
Maybelline
Nina Ricci
Noxell
Oil of Olay
Pantene
Pond's
Procter & Gamble
Ralph Lauren Products
Vidal Sassoon Products
Yves St. Laurent Products

"Years younger?— Hell, I'd buy it even if it just took a couple of weeks off my life."

Overheard by a frustrated cosmetics shopper

Appendix

Consumer Relations and Customer Service Phone Numbers

Adrien Arpel	(212) 333-7700
Almay	(800) 473-8566; in Canada (919) 603-2000
Alpha Hydrox/Neoteric	(800) 552-5742
Aveda	(800) 328-0849
Avon	(800) 367-2866; in Canada (800) 265-2866
Basis (Beiersdorf)	(800) 926-4832; not sold in Canada
Beauty Without Cruelty	(707) 769-5120
The Body Shop	(800) 541-2535
Borghese	(212) 572-3100
Chanel	(212) 688-5055
Charles of the Ritz	(800) 473-8566; in Canada (919) 603-2000
Cher's Aquasentials	(800) 832-4407; in Canada (800) 228-2844
Christian Dior	(212) 759-1840
Clarins	(212) 980-1800
Clarion	(800) 862-4222; in Canada (416) 730-4225
Clinique	(212) 572-3800
Color Me Beautiful	(800) 533-5503
Coty	(212) 850-2300
Cover Girl	(800) 426-8374; in Canada (416) 730-4225
Dove	(800) 451-6679; in Canada (416) 461-9432
EB5	(503) 222-0061
Elizabeth Arden	(212) 261-1000
Erno Laszlo	(800) 793-7955
Estee Lauder	(212) 756-4801

Eucerin	(800) 233-2340; in Canada (203) 853-8008
Fashion Fair	(312) 322-9444
Flori Roberts	(800) 631-2158; in Canada (908) 905-5200
Forever Spring	(800) 523-4334; in Canada (310) 657-4402
Freeman	(310) 470-6840
Guerlain	(212) 751-1870
Jergens	(513) 421-1400
Johnson & Johnson (Purpose, Clean & Clear)	(800) 526-3967; in Canada (800) 265-8383
Lancaster	(212) 593-7400
Lancome	(212) 984-4444
La Prairie	(800) 821-5718
Lasting Kiss	(800) 388-0811; in Canada (203) 597-3951
L'Oreal	(800) 322-2036
Lubriderm	(800) 223-0182; in Canada (416) 288-2200
M.A.C.	(800) 387-6707
Mary Kay	(800) 627-9529; in Canada (800) 268-2342
Max Factor	(800) 526-8787; in Canada (416) 730-4225
Maybelline	(901) 320-4778
M.D. Formulations /Herald Pharmacal	(800) 253-9499; in Canada (408) 723-3350
Monteil of Paris	(212) 593-7400

Murad	(800) 242-1103; in Canada (310) 568-1940	*Physicians Formula*	(800) 968-3855
		Pond's	(800) 243-5804; in Canada (203) 661-2000
NeoStrata	(800) 628-9904; in Canada (215) 624-4224	*Prescriptives*	(212) 756-4801
Neutrogena	(800) 421-6857	*Principal Secret*	(800) 545-5595
New Essentials	(800) 473-8566; in Canada (919) 603-2000	*Revlon*	(800) 473-8566; in Canada (919) 603-2000
Nivea	(800) 233-2340; in Canada (203) 853-8008	*Shiseido*	(212) 752-2644
		Sudden Youth	(800) 628-6471
Nu Skin	(801) 345-1000	*Ultima II*	(800) 473-8566; in Canada (919) 603-2000
Oil of Olay	(800) 285-5170; in Canada (800) 668-0151	*Victoria Jackson*	(800) 862-5387
Origins	(212) 572-4200	*Yves St Laurent*	(212) 621-7300

Recommended Reading and Reference Material

Clinical Toxicology of Commercial Products, 6th Edition, The Williams & Wilkins Company, Baltimore, Maryland, 1976

A Consumer's Dictionary of Cosmetic Ingredients, Ruth Winter, Crown Publishers, Inc., New York, 1989

Cosmetic, Toiletry, and Fragrance Association Cosmetic Ingredient Dictionary, Library of Congress Catalog Card No. 88-071506, CTFA, Inc.

Cosmetic, Toiletry, and Fragrance Association Cosmetic Ingredient Handbook, Library of Congress Catalog Card No. 88-071506, CTFA, Inc.

The Cosmetics Trap: When the Truth Is Only Skin Deep, City of New York Department of Consumers Affairs, 1992

Drug and Cosmetic Industry Magazine, Advanstar Communications, Inc., Duluth, Minnesota

Rodale's Illustrated Encyclopedia of Herbs, Kowalchick and Hylton, ed., Rodale Press, Inc., Emmaus, Pennsylvania, 1987

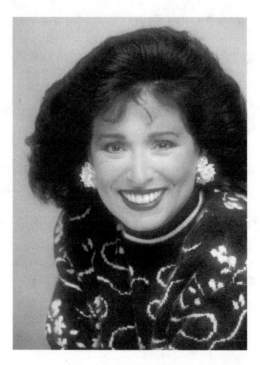

Paula Begoun is the recognized authority when it comes to candid and reliable information about all aspects of the cosmetics industry. Because of her reputation as the *Ralph Nader of Rouge* Ms. Begoun is a sought after guest on both television and radio talk shows. Even the fashion magazines, who can't always print what she has to say, call her for the inside scoop they can't get anywhere else. Besides having a science background in college, Paula also spent 10 years as a professional makeup artist, 2 years selling makeup at a department store (where she got fired for sparking too much controversy), and 4 years as an owner of a small chain of makeup stores. She also was a feature reporter on KIRO-TV and radio for 4 years in her home town of Seattle, Washington.

Paula Begoun is available as a guest speaker. Her informative, fun presentations are a great addition to any event where women are in attendance. For more information, call Beginning Press at (206) 723-6300.